S0-ABC-720

T73
e053
2008

Polk State Lakeland

CULTURAL COMPETENCE IN HEALTH EDUCATION AND HEALTH PROMOTION

Polk State College
Lakeland Library

CULTURAL COMPETENCE IN HEALTH EDUCATION AND HEALTH PROMOTION

Editors

MIGUEL A. PÉREZ
RAFFY R. LUQUIS

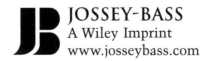 JOSSEY-BASS
A Wiley Imprint
www.josseybass.com

Copyright © 2008 by American Association of Health Education/American Alliance for Health, Physical Education, Recreation, and Dance (AAHE/AAHPERD). All rights reserved.

Published by Jossey-Bass
A Wiley Imprint
989 Market Street, San Francisco, CA 94103-1741—www.josseybass.com

No part of this publication may be reproduced, stored in a retrieval system, or transmitted in any form or by any means, electronic, mechanical, photocopying, recording, scanning, or otherwise, except as permitted under Section 107 or 108 of the 1976 United States Copyright Act, without either the prior written permission of the publisher, or authorization through payment of the appropriate per-copy fee to the Copyright Clearance Center, Inc., 222 Rosewood Drive, Danvers, MA 01923, 978-750-8400, fax 978-646-8600, or on the Web at www.copyright.com. Requests to the publisher for permission should be addressed to the Permissions Department, John Wiley & Sons, Inc., 111 River Street, Hoboken, NJ 07030, 201-748-6011, fax 201-748-6008, or online at www.wiley.com/go/permissions.

Readers should be aware that Internet Web sites offered as citations and/or sources for further information may have changed or disappeared between the time this was written and when it is read.

Limit of Liability/Disclaimer of Warranty: While the publisher and author have used their best efforts in preparing this book, they make no representations or warranties with respect to the accuracy or completeness of the contents of this book and specifically disclaim any implied warranties of merchantability or fitness for a particular purpose. No warranty may be created or extended by sales representatives or written sales materials. The advice and strategies contained herein may not be suitable for your situation. You should consult with a professional where appropriate. Neither the publisher nor author shall be liable for any loss of profit or any other commercial damages, including but not limited to special, incidental, consequential, or other damages.

Jossey-Bass books and products are available through most bookstores. To contact Jossey-Bass directly call our Customer Care Department within the U.S. at 800-956-7739, outside the U.S. at 317-572-3986, or fax 317-572-4002.

Jossey-Bass also publishes its books in a variety of electronic formats. Some content that appears in print may not be available in electronic books.

Library of Congress Cataloging-in-Publication Data

Cultural competence in health education and health promotion/Miguel A.
    Perez and Raffy R. Luquis, editors.
        p.   cm.
    Includes bibliographical references and index.
    ISBN 978-0-7879-8636-0 (pbk.)
        1. Transcultural medical care—United States.   2. Minorities—Medical care—United
    States.   3. Health education—United States.   4. Health promotion—United States.   I. Perez,
    Miguel A., 1969- II. Luquis, Raffy R., 1966-
    [DNLM: 1. Health Education.   2. Cultural Competency.   3. Cultural Diversity.   4. Health
Promotion.   WA 18 C968 2008]
    RA418.5.T73C853   2008
    362.1089—dc22

                                                                                    2008014871

Printed in the United States of America
FIRST EDITION

PB Printing   10 9 8 7 6 5 4 3 2 1

CONTENTS

CHAPTER EIGHT: COMMUNICATION AND CULTURAL COMPETENCE 147

Matthew Adeyanju

CHAPTER NINE: TOWARD A CULTURALLY COMPETENT HEALTH EDUCATION WORKFORCE 163

Eva I. Doyle

CHAPTER TEN: STRATEGIES, PRACTICES, AND MODELS FOR DELIVERING CULTURALLY COMPETENT HEALTH EDUCATION PROGRAMS 183

Miguel A. Pérez

CHAPTER ELEVEN: AGING AND HEALTH EDUCATION: PARTNERS FOR LEARNING 201

Carolina Aguilera, William H. Dailey Jr., and Miguel A. Pérez

FOREWORD

Cultural competency has been one of the essential skill sets for effective health education and promotion in locations where diverse populations exist. The dramatic demographic change that has taken place in the United States during the past two decades, however, means that undreamed of diversity now exists in small cities and towns across the country due to workforce recruitment from other countries, refugee resettlement, and a variety of other factors. It is now essential that all current and future health education specialists have knowledge and skills in cultural competency.

For more than fifteen years the American Association for Health Education (AAHE) has been working actively to advance cultural competency among health education and promotion professionals, and during the mid-1990s AAHE promulgated training in cultural competency through a series of AAHE-developed workshops funded by a grant from the U.S. Department of Education and conducted across the nation. Two written texts emerged from that work, and the authors of this book have reinforced a number of the guidelines and principles for cultural competency established at that time. However, the authors of this book have also greatly expanded upon that very early work. *Cultural Competence in Health Education and Health Promotion* fulfills current and future needs in cultural competency for both professional preparation and implementation by practitioners.

The authors of this book present a thorough exploration of up-to-date research about the impact of culture on health disparities, communication, wellness, belief systems, educational strategies, and a plethora of other factors essential to having a complete understanding of cultural competency. As Swartz and Tisdell point out in Chapter Five, delivering health education and promotion programs appropriately within a cultural framework requires taking into account the importance of not only health behaviors but also attitudes toward health and healing and the impact of leadership, religion, and spiritual beliefs within the culture.

The officers and staff of the American Association for Health Education (AAHE) wish to extend sincere appreciation to Dr. Miguel A. Pérez and Dr. Raffy R. Luquis for their excellent vision in conceptualizing and developing the content focus and organization of this important new resource for health education and promotion professionals. Their leadership and expertise coalesced to fill a need for the profession as well as for our organization.

We also wish to extend our sincere gratitude to all of the authors who contributed their expertise to *Cultural Competence in Health Education and Health Promotion*: Matthew Adeyanju, Carolina Aguilera, Kate Brindle, William H. Dailey Jr., Eva I. Doyle, Emogene Johnson Vaughn, Suzanne Kotkin-Jaszi, Nayamin Martinez-Cossio, Helda Pinzon-Pérez, Ann L. Swartz, Elizabeth J. Tisdell, and Kay Woodiel.

The Swahili word *harambe* means a coming together—not just physically but a coming together of spirit, of mind, and on a common ground. This is what these authors have accomplished in support of cultural competency for the American Association for Health Education. We believe *harambe* is also what the authors wish for all health education and promotion professionals and their clients or students.

The officers and staff of AAHE also wish to take this opportunity to recognize *Cultural Competence in Health Education and Health Promotion* as the launch of the American Association for Health Education/American Alliance for Health, Physical Education, Recreation, and Dance joint publishing venture with Wiley/Jossey-Bass. The anticipated outcome of this joint venture over a period of years is a series of books under our own imprint—AAHE Press. We are delighted to acknowledge the outstanding quality provided by Wiley/Jossey-Bass in health education, health promotion, and public health publications, and we look forward to a partnership that will set the standard for many years.

Becky J. Smith
Executive Director, AAHE

Katherine M. Wilbur
President, AAHE

March 2008

THE EDITORS

MIGUEL A. PÉREZ is a health educator who specializes in international health and applied research, adolescent health, and cultural competence. In 2001, he received a Fulbright award to teach at the Universidad El Bosque in Bogota, Colombia. In 2005, he was a Fulbright Senior Specialist Scholar in public/global health at the Nelson Mandela Metropolitan University in South Africa. In 2006, he was a Fulbright Senior Specialist Scholar in public/global health at the Universidad del Norte in Barranquilla, Colombia. He received his PhD degree in 1994 and his MS degree in 1993 in health education from the Pennsylvania State University, and his BS degree in research in mental health from California State University, Dominguez Hills.

RAFFY R. LUQUIS is a faculty member in the School of Behavioral Sciences and Education at the Pennsylvania State University, Harrisburg. He earned his PhD degree in health science at the University of Arkansas in 1996 and his MS degree in health education in 1991 and BS degree in science in 1988 at Penn State. His primary teaching and research interests are in community health education and health promotion, multicultural health, and sexuality.

THE CONTRIBUTORS

MATTHEW ADEYANJU is a professor and the director of the School of Health Sciences at the Ohio University, Athens, Ohio. Prior to joining Ohio University, Adeyanju was an associate professor and the graduate program coordinator for health education and health promotion at the University of Kansas. Before earning his PhD degree from the University of Illinois in 1985, Adeyanju served the World Health Organization in his native home in Nigeria, where he was also a public health educator.

CAROLINA AGUILERA obtained her MPH degree, with an emphasis in health promotion, in 2006 and her BS degree in health science, with an emphasis in community health, in 2001 from California State University, Fresno. Her current research interest is the effects of diabetes among Latino populations throughout the Central Valley region in California.

KATE BRINDLE has been at Eastern Michigan University since 2003, where she is program coordinator of the Lesbian, Gay, Bisexual and Transgender Resource Center. She holds an MLS degree in women's studies from Eastern Michigan University and a BFA degree from New York University. While a graduate student at EMU, she was recognized as a Woman of Excellence and was awarded the Margaret L. Rossiter Outstanding Graduate Paper Award. She is a recipient of the Stonewall Scholarship and has been recognized as an Outstanding Role Model and Mentor by the LGBT Resource Center. She has also been a nominee for the Gerri Collins Medal for Exemplary Service and the Best New Employee Gold Medallion Award.

WILLIAM H. DAILEY JR. is a lecturer in gerontology in the Health Science Department at California State University, Fresno, and also teaches periodically at Fresno City College in the Social Sciences Department. He works alongside Merlin, his guide dog of ten years, who is considered an "elder" dog. Dailey earned his MPA degree from California State University, Fresno, and is currently studying for his doctorate at Fielding Graduate University, focusing on educational leadership and change in dealing with disabilities related to aging. His doctoral dissertation will address practitioners' limitations, perceptions, and interactions as they work collaboratively to meet the needs of an increasing older population. Dailey was a delegate to the White House Conference on Aging held in December of 2005 in Washington, D.C., and he continues to collaborate with the California delegation to advocate for key aging issues. His research interests include the role of grandparents in raising their grandchildren, aging and disability issues facing elders, and also alternative housing and transportation issues.

EVA I. DOYLE is an associate professor and the director of health education in the Department of Health, Human Performance, and Recreation at Baylor University. She is a certified health education specialist (CHES) with a PhD degree in health education from the University of Maryland and an MS degree from Baylor University. She specializes in assessing health needs and providing cross-cultural health education in medically underserved communities. She regularly involves students in community-based health promotion projects in international and local settings.

EMOGENE JOHNSON VAUGHN is a professor in the Department of Health, Physical Education and Exercise Science at Norfolk State University, Norfolk, Virginia. Her teaching interests are in the areas of personal health and online instruction. Her other responsibilities have included serving as a wellness coordinator and coordinating the health education service course. Among her ongoing interests is the evaluation of teen pregnancy prevention programs with the Virginia Department of Health. She received her PhD degree from the University of Maryland.

SUZANNE KOTKIN-JASZI is an associate professor of health science in the College of Health and Human Services, California State University, Fresno, where she also serves as undergraduate adviser for the health administration option of the health science major and as the adviser for graduate study in the health policy and administration option in the Master of Public Health Program. She is a Health Policy Research Fellow at the Central Valley Health Policy Institute, and she was formerly director of the New Mexico Health Policy Commission, where she conducted research on Medicaid reform, the uninsured, health professional shortages, prescription drug coverage, pain management, and other critical health policy issues. She has taught and written about the financing, delivery, and organization of community health services; health policy; welfare reform and privatization; health law and legislation; and the integration of chronic care management into primary health care settings. She holds a DPH degree from the University of California, Berkeley.

NAYAMIN MARTINEZ-COSSIO has been working with Centro Binacional para el Desarrollo Indigena Oaxaqueño (CBDIO), Inc., since 2001 as the coordinator of Proyecto de Salud (Indigenous Health Project), a role that has involved her in partnerships with such health promotion initiatives as the Children's Health Initiative, the Multicultural Community Alliance, the HIV Surveillance Project, and the Fresno region Binational Health Task Force. Martinez earned her BA degree in international relations from Universidad Iberoamericana in Mexico City, and her MA degree in sociology from Instituto de Investigaciones Dr. José Maria Luis Mora, also in Mexico City. Her undergraduate and graduate theses addressed the sociopolitical dynamics of Mexican migration to the United States. She is currently studying for an MPH degree at California State University, Fresno, gaining skills and knowledge to apply to the development of community projects targeting indigenous migrants in California. She has also designed and implemented two health promotion programs (Comenzando Bien and

Na Vali Daatun) to provide prenatal education and assistance in accessing health and social services to pregnant, indigenous women.

HELDA PINZON-PÉREZ, a native of Colombia, South America, is a faculty member in the Department of Health Science at California State University, Fresno. Her research interests center on multicultural issues in health care, international health, and holistic health. She teaches multiple courses related to cultural competence and is a member of the Multicultural Involvement Committee of the American Association for Health Education. She received her RN degree from the Pontificia Universidad Javeriana in Bogota, Colombia, and her PhD degree from the Pennsylvania State University.

ANN L. SWARTZ is an instructor of nursing at the Pennsylvania State University, Harrisburg. She is a family nurse practitioner and psychiatric clinical nurse specialist. She has received an MSN degree with a family nurse practitioner certificate from Widener University, an MSN degree from the Catholic University of America, and a BSN degree from the University of Virginia. She is currently pursuing her EdD degree at the Pennsylvania State University.

ELIZABETH J. TISDELL is an associate professor of adult education at the Pennsylvania State University, Harrisburg. She researches and writes about culturally responsive education and spirituality in higher education. She earned her EdD degree at the University of Georgia, MA degree at Fordham University, and BA degree at the University of Maine, Orono.

KAY WOODIEL has been at Eastern Michigan University since 1998, where she serves as associate professor of health education. Since 2005, she has served as director of the Department of Diversity and Community Involvement, which includes the Center for Multicultural Affairs; the Lesbian, Gay, Bisexual and Transgender Resource Center (LGBTRC); the VISION (Volunteers in Service to our Neighborhoods) office; and the Women's Center. She has received two teaching awards at EMU: the LGBTRC has recognized her with its Role Model and Mentor Award and the Women's Center has recognized her as a Woman of Excellence. She has also received two faculty fellowships at EMU, one in diversity and the other in academic service learning. Woodiel received her PhD degree from the University of Arkansas.

ACKNOWLEDGMENTS

We would like to thank each of the chapter contributors for his or her work in this book, the American Association for Health Education for its continuous support of the content of this book, and especially the staff at Jossey-Bass for their careful review and assistance in the development of this book. Finally, we want to thank our respective families for their support and understanding; without them we would not have been able to spend the many hours on writing and editing that this book required.

M. A. P.
R. R. L.

CULTURAL COMPETENCE IN HEALTH EDUCATION AND HEALTH PROMOTION

CHAPTER

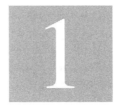

CHANGING U.S. DEMOGRAPHICS

Challenges and Opportunities for Health Educators

MIGUEL A. PÉREZ

RAFFY R. LUQUIS

LEARNING OBJECTIVES

After completing this chapter, you will be able to

- Explain the demographic changes and population trends in the United States.
- Describe characteristics of the major racial and ethnic groups in the United States.
- Discuss challenges and opportunities for health educators.

INTRODUCTION

On January 25, 2000, the U.S. surgeon general released *Healthy People 2010,* a document designed to provide a road map for improving the health status of all Americans. *Healthy People 2010* has two primary goals: increasing the quality of and extending the number of years of healthy life for individuals and eliminating health disparities among Americans (U.S. Department of Health and Human Services, 2000). In order to accomplish the second goal, we need to explore and embrace the shifting demographics of the U.S. population, the policies that have contributed to these changes, and the challenges and opportunities these demographics and policies represent for health educators.

The purpose of this chapter is to describe the *demographic shifts* that are affecting the U.S. population and to explore their impact on preparing a culturally competent health education workforce. These demographic shifts include the overall growth in population and the increase in the proportion of Hispanics, or Latinos, in that population; the increase in the number of foreign-born residents and related changes in immigration policy; the increase in the number of residents who do not speak English at home; the increase in the overall number of elderly and in the number of minority elderly; the increase in the number of women in the workforce; the population trends among lesbian, gay, bisexual, and transgender individuals; and the trends among people with disabilities. This chapter will also provide a brief description of relevant cultural characteristics for each of the major ethnic groups in the United States. These descriptions are essential background for the discussions of the challenges and responsibilities of health educators that follow in the remaining chapters of this book.

DEMOGRAPHIC SHIFTS

Population Growth

According to the U.S. Census Bureau the U.S. population passed the 300 million mark in 2006. This demographic shift[1] is not surprising given the trend of population increases observed between 2000 (282,216,952) and 2007 (301,621,157) (see Table 1.1). Exponential population growth is expected to continue for the next few decades, with an expected population increase from 296,507,061 residents in 2005 to 419,854,000 in 2050. Moreover, the Census Bureau projects that as the population increases, the majority of the population will be concentrated in urban areas, continuing a trend started in the late nineteenth century (see Figure 1.1).

Race and Ethnicity

A report by the Agency for Healthcare Research and Quality states that members of underrepresented groups are expected to make up more than 40 percent of the U.S. population by 2035 and 47 percent by 2050 (Brach & Fraser, 2000). The shifts in the ethnic and racial distribution and the age distribution of the U.S. population denote an urgent need for health educators to develop programs that are culturally appropriate

TABLE 1.1. **Estimates of U.S. Population, 2000–2007.**

July 1, 2007	301,621,157
July 1, 2006	298,754,819
July 1, 2005	295,895,897
July 1, 2004	293,191,511
July 1, 2003	290,447,644
July 1, 2002	287,888,021
July 1, 2001	285,112,030
July 1, 2000	282,194,308
April 1, 2000 (Estimates Base)	281,424,602
April 1, 2000 (Census 2000)	281,421,906

Source: U.S. Census Bureau, 2007f.

(Luquis & Pérez, 2005, 2006; Luquis, Pérez, & Young, 2006; Marín et al., 1995; Pérez, Gonzalez, & Pinzon-Pérez, 2006).

The 2000 Census marked a shift in how ethnic and racial data are collected. The Census Bureau introduced a larger pool of options, which allowed individuals, among other things, to select more than one ethnic or racial background. Although controversial, this measure allows the identification of individuals of mixed descent.[2]

Data from the American Community Survey conducted by the U.S. Census Bureau (2006) show that the U.S. population reached one of its most diverse stages in terms of race and ethnicity in 2005 (see Table 1.2). These data also show the richness in diversity found within the Hispanic population (see Table 1.3), which has become the fastest growing ethnic group in the United States.

Foreign-Born and Immigrant

In 2005, the foreign-born population numbered 35,689,467, or 12 percent of the U.S. population. The foreign-born population includes any resident who was not a U.S. citizen at birth. It includes legal permanent residents (immigrants), temporary migrants

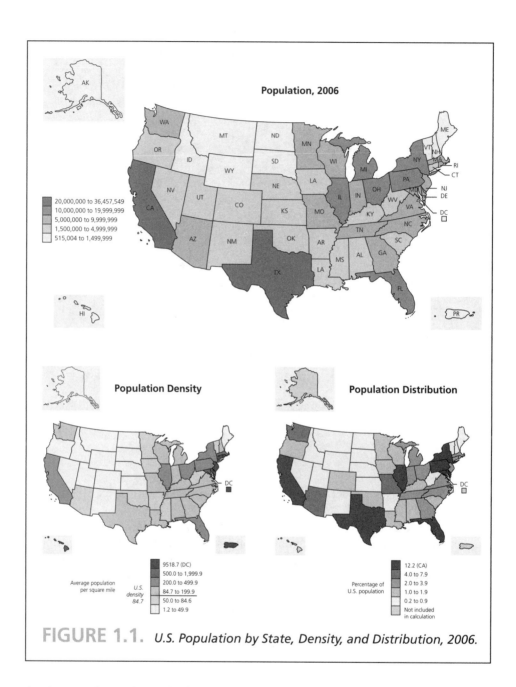

FIGURE 1.1. *U.S. Population by State, Density, and Distribution, 2006.*

(such as students), humanitarian migrants (refugees), naturalized U.S. citizens, and persons illegally present in the United States (U.S. Census Bureau, 2006).

The impact of the foreign-born population on the diversification of the U.S. population merits a little discussion of U.S. immigration policy, which not only affects the number of foreign-born nationals admitted to the United States but has also at times

TABLE 1.2. **U.S. Population Estimate by Race and Ethnicity, 2005.**

	Estimate	Percentage
Total population	288,378,137	100
White	192,615,561	66
African American	34,364,572	12
American Indian/Alaska Native	2,046,735	1
Asian	12,312,949	4
Native Hawaiian/Other Pacific Islander	355,513	<1
Hispanic	41,870,703	14
Other race	9,624,208	3

Source: U.S. Census Bureau, 2006.

TABLE 1.3. **Estimates of Hispanic Population by Country of Origin, 2005.**

	Estimate	Percentage
Total	41,870,703	100
Mexican	26,781,547	64
Puerto Rican	3,781,317	9
Cuban	1,461,574	3
Dominican (Dominican Republic)	1,118,265	3
Central American	3,084,580	7
South American	2,238,836	5
Other countries	3,404,584	8

Source: U.S. Census Bureau, 2006.

restricted the racial and ethnic composition of that immigration. U.S. immigration policy can be examined in terms of four distinct periods.

During the open-door era (1776 to 1882), the United States opened its doors without any restrictions to immigrants from all over the world (Yang, 1995). The era of selective exclusions (1882 to 1921) that followed was characterized by legislation such as the Chinese Exclusion Act of May 6, 1882, which contributed to the selectivity in the ethnic and racial composition of the U.S. population. This legislation was repealed in 1943, when China became an ally of the United States in the war with Japan (Briggs, 1984). Other laws that restricted immigration into the United States were the Immigration Act of August 3, 1882, which established a head tax of 50 cents and excluded individuals who could become a charge to the state; the Immigration Act of February 26, 1885, the first contract labor law, which prevented employers from importing "cheap foreign labor"; the Immigration Act of February 20, 1907, which severely restricted Japanese immigration; and the Immigration Act of February 5, 1917, which required individuals over 16 years of age to pass a literacy test before they could be considered for any type of employment (Briggs, 1984; Gomez-Quinones, 1981).

The next era severely limited the number of immigrants to the United States. On March 4, 1929, Congress passed a law that made it a felony for anyone to enter the country illegally. This law also provided severe sanctions against people who returned to the United States after being deported (Briggs, 1984; Gomez-Quinones, 1981). Thus the concept of the *illegal worker* was introduced.

President Lyndon B. Johnson signed into law the Immigration and Nationality Act Amendments of October 3, 1965, also known as the Hart-Cellar Act (Briggs, 1984), which attempted to eliminate national origin quotas yet strengthened numerical controls on immigration (Yang, 1995). The Immigration Reform and Control Act (IRCA) of November 6, 1986, contained the first major change in U.S. immigration policy since the 1960s (Lowell & Suro, 2002). One of the major IRCA provisions gave migrants who had lived in the United States since 1982 without proper documentation or who had been working in the United States in agriculture for at least six months the opportunity to legalize their migration status (Bean & Stevens, 2003). Sanctions were imposed on those employing individuals not authorized to work in the United States, in an effort to deter future illegal immigration.

Language

Nineteen percent of the people in the United States speak a language other than English at home (see Table 1.4). A closer look at this figure reveals that 9.5 percent of the native-born U.S. population report speaking a language other than English at home. Less surprisingly, 84.1 percent of the foreign-born population report speaking a language other than English at home. Similarly, 52 percent of the foreign-born population report speaking English "less than well," compared to 2 percent of native-born individuals (U.S. Census Bureau, 2006).

TABLE 1.4. **Language Spoken at Home and Ability to Speak English: Percentage of Population 5 Years of Age and Older.**

Category	Total	U.S. Native	Foreign Born
Language other than English	19.4%	9.5%	84.1%
Speak English "very well"	10.7%	7.5%	32.0%
Speak English less than "very well"	8.6%	2.0%	52.1%

Source: U.S. Census Bureau, 2006.

California has the largest percentage of residents who speak a language at home other than English (40.8 percent), followed by New Mexico (36.0 percent) and Texas (32.5 percent) (U.S. Census Bureau, 2006).

The Elderly

The number of elderly, those over the age of 65, is expected to more than double by the middle of this century, to 80 million. About one in eight Americans was elderly in 1994, but about one in five will be elderly in 2030 (U.S. Census Bureau, 1995). The oldest old (those 85 years old and older) form the fastest-growing segment of the elderly population; from 1960 to 1994, this group increased 274 percent, compared with an increase of 100 percent for persons 65 years of age and over, and an increase of 45 percent for the total population (U.S. Census Bureau, 2001). The elderly population is also expected to become more racially and ethnically diverse in the future. Hispanic elderly are expected to increase from less than 4 percent of the total population in 1990 to 16 percent by 2050. The proportion of elderly in each of the four major race groups (white, black, American Indian and Alaska Native, and Asian and Pacific Islander) and in the Hispanic-origin population is expected to increase substantially during the first half of the twenty-first century.

From 1990 to 2050, the proportion of elderly is projected to increase from 13 to 23 percent for whites, from 8 to 14 percent for blacks; from 6 to 13 percent for American Indians, Eskimos, and Aleuts; from 6 to 15 percent for Asians and Pacific Islanders; and from 5 to 14 percent for Hispanics (U.S. Census Bureau, 2001).

Gender

According to the 2005 American Community Survey the male to female ratio in 2005 in the United States was 96 males per 100 females. In 2005, of the 117 million women aged 16 and over in the United States, 69 million (almost 60 percent) were labor force participants, either working or looking for work.

Sexual Orientation

Although the U.S. Census Bureau asks respondents to identify their race and ethnicity, it does not contain a question about sexual orientation; hence it is difficult to estimate the prevalence of lesbian, gay, bisexual, and transgender (LGBT) individuals in the population. However, the Census does ask several questions about respondents' household composition by marital status and gender of partner (see Table 1.5). Twelve and 11 percent, respectively, of family households with an unmarried male or female householder and 8 and 6 percent, respectively, of nonfamily households with an unmarried male or female householder reported same-gender partners. Still, even in combination, these numbers represent less than 1 percent of the total households (U.S. Census Bureau, 2006).

Several studies have estimated that 5 to 10 percent of the U.S. population is lesbian, gay, bisexual, or transgender (National Coalition for LGBT Health & Boston Public Health Commission, 2002). Nonetheless, it is important to understand that the estimate that 10 percent of men are gay and 5 percent of women are lesbian is based on Kinsey Institute data, which may not accurately represent the percentage of LGBT individuals in the population (Gay and Lesbian Medical Association [GLMA] et al., 2001). Other studies have estimated the percentage of the gay and lesbian population to be from 1 to 10 percent. Thus the actual number of people who identify themselves as lesbian, gay, bisexual, or transgender is not known (GLMA et al., 2001).

The relative lack of research focusing on the size of this population and the fear that many LGBT people, especially youths, have concerning revealing their sexual identity make reliable data difficult to obtain (GLMA et al., 2001). Numbers may be underestimated, as many participants are fearful or reluctant to classify themselves as lesbian, gay, bisexual, or transgender when completing survey studies. A number of other factors that make estimates difficult are explored in Chapter Twelve. For example, many gay men and lesbians have participated in or continue to participate in sexual activities with member of the opposite sex and also choose not to identify as gay or bisexual. Others who have never participated in sexual activities at all may still identify as gay, lesbian, or bisexual.

People with Disabilities

In 2000, 49.7 million people aged 5 years old and older in the United States had some type of long-lasting, disabling condition. This number represented approximately 19 percent of the population, or one in every five persons (Waldrop & Stern, 2003). Moreover, the disability rate varied by race and ethnic group. Two groups, African Americans and American Indians/Alaska Natives, had the highest overall disability rate, 24 percent, whereas the rate for non-Hispanic whites was 18 percent. Approximately 21 and 19 percent, respectively, of Hispanics and of Native Hawaiians and Pacific Islanders reported having at least one disability in 2000. Asians had the lowest overall disability rate, 17 percent, of any racial and ethnic group (Waldrop & Stern, 2003).

By 2005, the overall estimated disability rate among people aged 5 and older had decreased to 15 percent of the population. Notwithstanding, disability continues to affect approximately 40 million people in the United States. In addition, the disability

TABLE 1.5. **Unmarried-Partner Households and Household Type by Sex of Partner, 2005.**

	Estimate	Percentage
Total households	111,090,617	100
Family households	74,341,149	67
Unmarried-partner households	2,512,744	3
Male householder, no wife present	1,129,921	45
Male householder and male partner	126,156	12
Male householder and female partner	1,003,765	88
Female householder, no husband present	1,382,823	55
Female householder and female partner	150,640	11
Female householder and male partner	1,232,183	89
Other family households	71,828,405	97
Nonfamily households	36,749,468	33
Unmarried-partner households	3,453,362	10
Male householder and male partner	286,939	8
Male householder and female partner	1,656,669	48
Female householder and female partner	213,208	6
Female householder and male partner	1,296,546	38
Other nonfamily households	33,296,106	90

Note: Percentages based on subcategory denominators.

Source: U.S. Census Bureau, 2006.

percentage is higher among older people than among any other age group (see Table 1.6) (U.S. Census Bureau, 2006). Moreover, people with disabilities are likely to have received less education than people who do not have disabilities. People aged 18 to 34 with any disability are less likely to be enrolled in college or graduate school than are people in the same age group with no disability. Moreover, people aged 16 to 64 with any disability are less likely than people with no disability to be employed. Finally, compared to people with no disability, a higher percentage of people with any disability aged 5 and older have incomes below the poverty level (21 percent compared to 11 percent) (U.S. Census Bureau, 2006).

TABLE 1.6. **Characteristics of the Population with a Disability, by Age: Estimates of Civilian Noninstitutionalized Population, 2005.**

Subject	Total
Population 5 years and over	**267,387,983**
With one type of disability	6.9%
With two or more types of disabilities	8.0%
Population 5 to 15 years	**44,586,147**
With any disability	6.5%
With a sensory disability	1.2%
With a physical disability	1.2%
With a mental disability	5.2%
With a self-care disability	0.9%
Population 16 to 64 years	**188,041,309**
With any disability	12.1%
With a sensory disability	2.8%
With a physical disability	7.2%

With a mental disability	4.5%
With a self-care disability	2.0%
With a go-outside-home disability	3.0%
With an employment disability	6.8%
Population 65 years and over	**34,760,527**
With any disability	40.5%
With a sensory disability	16.4%
With a physical disability	30.8%
With a mental disability	11.5%
With a self-care disability	9.7%
With a go-outside-home disability	16.6%
School Enrollment: Population 18 to 34 years	**64,647,330**
With any disability	4,505,696
Enrolled in college or graduate school	13.9%
Not enrolled and without a bachelor's degree or higher	73.2%
With a sensory disability	997,637
Enrolled in college or graduate school	14.0%
Not enrolled and without a bachelor's degree or higher	72.4%
With a physical disability	1,720,223
Enrolled in college or graduate school	11.7%

(continued)

(Table 1.6 continued)

Subject	Total
Not enrolled and without a bachelor's degree or higher	77.6%
With a mental disability	2,227,927
Enrolled in college or graduate school	13.4%
Not enrolled and without a bachelor's degree or higher	72.7%
No disability	60,141,634
Enrolled in college or graduate school	21.8%
Not enrolled and without a bachelor's degree or higher	56.0%
Poverty Status: Population 5 years and over	**266,588,142**
With any disability	39,646,722
Below poverty level	21.1%
With a sensory disability	11,551,860
Below poverty level	18.7%
With a physical disability	24,821,998
Below poverty level	20.9%
With a mental disability	14,638,611
Below poverty level	26.4%
No disability	226,941,420
Below poverty level	11.3%

Source: U.S. Census Bureau, 2006.

DEMOGRAPHICS OF RACIAL AND ETHNIC GROUPS

The following section provides a brief overview of the demographic characteristics of the major ethnic and racial groups in the United States. These descriptions will not, of course, apply to every individual who identifies as a member of a particular population group. Instead, they offer overarching generalizations about the characteristics shared by members of each group. As indicated earlier, significant differences exist within every racial and ethnic group.

African Americans

African Americans, or blacks, are defined as persons whose lineage includes ancestors who originated from any of the black racial groups in Africa. Contrary to popular belief, African Americans make up a diverse group that encompasses individuals of African descent, Caribbean descent, and South American descent.

African Americans are the second largest racial group in the United States, with approximately 39.7 million people, or 13 percent of the population, in July 2005 (Office of Minority Health [OMH], 2007). Over 50 percent of African Americans reside in the central cities of metropolitan areas, and the majority are concentrated in the southern states (McKinnon, 2003; U.S. Census Bureau, 2007c).

In comparison to the non-Hispanic white population, the African American population has a higher proportion of younger people, its members are less likely to be married, a large proportion of its households are maintained by women, and married couples in this group have larger families (McKinnon, 2003; U.S. Census Bureau, 2007c). In 2004, approximately 80 percent of African Americans aged 25 and older had completed high school and 17 percent had attained a bachelor's degree or higher level of education (U.S. Census Bureau, 2007c); yet these percentages are lower than the percentages obtained by their non-Hispanic white counterparts. Moreover, African Americans are less likely to be employed in management, professional, and related occupations (McKinnon, 2003; U.S. Census Bureau, 2007c), and their unemployment rate is twice that for non-Hispanic whites (OMH, 2007). Consequently, in 2005, the average African American family median income was less than the non-Hispanic white family median, and one-fourth of African American families were living at the poverty level (OMH, 2007). Finally, the life expectancy for African Americans is six years shorter than the life expectancy for the rest of the population (McKinnon, 2003; U.S. Census Bureau, 2007c). According to the Office of Minority Health (2007), in 2003 the death rate for African Americans was higher than the rate for non-Hispanic whites for heart disease, stroke, cancer, asthma, influenza and pneumonia, diabetes, HIV/AIDS, and homicide.

Hispanics

Hispanics are the fastest-growing population group in the United States. This group includes all those of Cuban, Mexican, Puerto Rican, South or Central American, or other Spanish culture or origin, regardless of race. In 2006, the U.S. Census Bureau estimated that this population represents more than 14 percent of the total U.S. population (OMH, 2007), almost a 40 percent increase since 1990. Moreover, it is estimated that by 2010 Hispanics will be the largest minority group and that by 2050 they will account for 24 percent of the total population (U.S. Census Bureau, 2004). Although Hispanics share many cultural characteristics, the many groups that make up the Hispanic population are also in many ways culturally and socially variant. For example, although a majority of Hispanics speak Spanish and follow the Roman Catholic faith, they speak their common language in many different dialects and practice their common religion with many spiritual variations (Marín & Marín, 1991).

In 2004, among Hispanic subgroups, Mexicans ranked as the largest, at 66 percent of the Hispanic population, followed by Central and South Americans, Puerto Ricans, and Cubans (OMH, 2007; Ramirez & de la Cruz, 2003; U.S. Census Bureau, 2007d). Hispanics are more likely than non-Hispanic whites to live in the U.S. West and South and to reside in central cities within metropolitan areas (OMH, 2007; Ramirez & de la Cruz, 2003; U.S. Census Bureau, 2007d). Hispanics are also younger on average than non-Hispanic whites, with approximately one in three Hispanics being under the age of 18, and with a median age of 26.9 years. The average age for the non-Hispanic white population was 40.1 years in 2004 (U.S. Census Bureau, 2007d). In 2004, nearly three-quarters of Hispanics were U.S. citizens, with three in five Hispanics having been born in the United States (Ramirez & de la Cruz, 2003; U.S. Census Bureau, 2007d). Although three-quarters of Hispanics spoke a language other than English (that is, Spanish) at home, almost two in five spoke English very well (U.S. Census Bureau, 2007d).

In 2004, Hispanic households were more likely to be family households than were non-Hispanic white households. These families also tended to be larger, with five or more people in the household (Ramirez & de la Cruz, 2003; U.S. Census Bureau, 2007d). Although half of Hispanics aged 15 and older were married, one in five households was maintained by a woman with no husband present (U.S. Census Bureau, 2007d). Moreover, approximately 60 percent of Hispanics aged 25 and older had graduated from high school and 13 percent had attained a bachelor's degree or higher level of education. However, this educational level varied among Hispanic subgroups. Hispanics from South America, Cuba, and Puerto Rico were more likely to have graduated from high school and to have completed a bachelor's degree or more education than were Hispanics from Mexico or Central America (U.S. Census Bureau, 2007d).

Hispanics were much more likely than non-Hispanic whites to be unemployed or to work in service, construction, and production jobs. Hispanics were also more likely to have a lower median income level and to live in poverty than non-Hispanic whites were (Ramirez & de la Cruz, 2003; U.S. Census Bureau, 2007d). In 2004, about 22 percent of Hispanics, in comparison to 9 percent of non-Hispanic whites, were living at the poverty level (U.S. Census Bureau, 2007d). Moreover, Hispanics had the highest uninsured rates of any racial or ethnic group in the United States. Still, the uninsured rate varied by Hispanic subgroup, with the Mexican and Central and South American subgroups having higher percentages of people without health insurance than the Puerto Rican and Cuban subgroups do (OMH, 2007).

Hispanic health is influenced by factors such as the language barrier, lack of access to preventive care, and lack of health insurance. The leading causes of illness and death among Hispanics are heart disease, cancer, unintentional injuries (accidents), stroke, and diabetes. In addition, Hispanics are significantly affected by asthma, chronic obstructive pulmonary disease, HIV/AIDS, obesity, suicide, and liver disease (OMH, 2007).

Asians

The Asian population in the United States is not homogeneous, as it includes many groups that differ in language and culture (U.S. Census Bureau, 2007b). *Asian* refers to people who have their origins in the Far East, in Southeast Asia, or on the Indian subcontinent, including people from Cambodia, China, the Philippines, India, Japan, Korea, Malaysia, Pakistan, and Vietnam (Reeves & Bennett, 2003). According to the 2005 Census Bureau population estimate, there were over 14 million Asians living in the United States in that year (OMH, 2007), with Chinese, Asian Indians, and Filipinos accounting for about 60 percent of this population (U.S. Census Bureau, 2007b). Moreover, in 2004, approximately 50 percent of the Asian population resided in three states: California, New York, and Texas (U.S. Census Bureau, 2007b).

The Asian population is younger on average than the non-Hispanic white population. In 2004, Asians had a median age of 34.8, about five years younger than non-Hispanic whites (U.S. Census Bureau, 2007b). Moreover, Asians were more likely than non-Hispanic whites to be married (62 percent) and to live in family households (74 percent), with a higher percentage of households maintained by married couples (60 percent). Although more than two-thirds of Asians were U.S. citizens, either through birth or naturalization, approximately 68 percent of Asians were foreign born (U.S. Census Bureau, 2007b). Most important, about 50 percent of foreign-born Asians arrived in the United States after 1990, and about 77 percent of all Asians in the United States spoke a language other than English at home. Moreover, the proportion of those 5 years of age and older who spoke a language other than English at home varied among Asians: 88 percent of Vietnamese, 83 percent of Chinese, 66 percent of Filipinos, and 47 percent of Japanese (U.S. Census Bureau, 2007b).

When it comes to education, approximately 85 percent of Asians 25 years old and older had at least a high school diploma and 48 percent had attained a bachelor's degree or higher level of education (U.S. Census Bureau, 2007b). Among specific Asian subgroups, Asian Indians, Filipinos, Japanese, and Koreans had the highest percentages of persons 25 years old and older with a bachelor's degree or higher. Moreover, Asians were more likely to be employed in management, professional, and related occupations than were non-Hispanic whites, 45 versus 38 percent respectively. Among Asian subgroups, higher percentages of Asian Indians (61 percent), Chinese (52 percent), and Japanese (48 percent) are employed in management, professional, and related occupations compared to other Asian subgroups (U.S. Census Bureau, 2007b). Finally, in 2005, the median income for Asian households was almost $15,000 higher than the national median income for all households (OMH, 2007). Among Asian subgroups,

Asian Indian and Filipino households had the highest median incomes (U.S. Census Bureau, 2007b). Still, about 12 percent of Asians lived below poverty level, compared to 9 percent of non-Hispanic whites (U.S. Census Bureau, 2007b).

In 2003, a high percentage of Asians had private health insurance coverage, but that also varied by subgroup. For example, 84 percent of Chinese had private insurance coverage, followed by 81 percent of Filipinos, and 76 percent of Vietnamese (OMH, 2007). It is also significant to note that Asian women have the highest life expectancy of any racial and ethnic group in the United States, and Chinese women have the longest life expectancy among all the Asian subgroups. Still, Asians contend with several factors affecting their health, including infrequent medical visits and language and cultural barriers (OMH, 2007). Finally, Asians are at higher risk than others for cancer, heart disease, stroke, unintentional injuries, diabetes, pulmonary disease, hepatitis B, smoking-related illnesses, tuberculosis, and liver diseases.

Pacific Islanders

Pacific Islanders are people who are natives of Hawaii and other Pacific islands, including people of Polynesian, Micronesian, and Melanesian backgrounds (U.S. Census Bureau, 2007e). Pacific Islanders differ in language and culture across many subgroups. According to the 2005 U.S. Census Bureau estimate, close to 1 million Pacific Islanders, or less than 1 percent of the U.S. population, were residing in the United States in that year. Over 50 percent of the Pacific Islander population resided in two states: California and Hawaii (OMH, 2007; U.S. Census Bureau, 2007e). In 2004, the median age for this group was 11 years less than the median age of non-Hispanic whites. Almost three-fourths of the population was under the age of 44, with nearly 30 percent under the age of 18 (U.S. Census Bureau, 2007e). In addition, approximately 53 percent of Pacific Islanders aged 15 years and older were married, compared to 57 percent of the non-Hispanic white population. The majority of Pacific Islander households were family households (78 percent), with over 50 percent maintained by married couples. Interestingly, approximately 10 percent of Pacific Islander grandparents were living with their coresident grandchildren, with 35 percent of grandparents responsible for grandchildren's care (U.S. Census Bureau, 2007e). Almost 86 percent of the Pacific Islanders were U.S. citizens by birth (78.7 percent) or by naturalization (6.8 percent), and 89 percent of them spoke only English at home or spoke English very well.

When it came to education, a high percentage of Pacific Islanders had graduated from high school (86 percent) and 16 percent had attained a bachelor's degree or higher level of education (OMH, 2007; U.S. Census Bureau, 2007e). In 2004, approximately one-third of Pacific Islanders were employed in sales or office occupations and almost one-fourth were employed in management, professional, and related occupations. The median household income for Pacific Islanders of $47,400 was similar to that for non-Hispanic whites. Still, 18 percent of Pacific Islanders were living under the poverty level compared to 9 percent of non-Hispanic whites (U.S. Census Bureau, 2007e).

Data on the health status of this population show that Pacific Islanders have higher rates of smoking, alcohol consumption, and obesity than other racial and ethnic groups do (OMH, 2007). Some leading causes of morbidity and mortality among Pacific Islanders are cancer, heart disease, unintentional injuries (accidents), stroke, diabetes, hepatitis B, and tuberculosis (OMH, 2007).

American Indians and Alaska Natives

In 2004, the U.S. Census Bureau estimated over 4 million people to be American Indians or Alaska Natives, entirely or in combination, representing slightly more than 1 percent of the U.S. population (U.S. Census Bureau, 2007a). In 2005, 4.5 million people were classified as American Indian or Alaska Native (OMH, 2007). This group is made up of individuals who have their origins in any of the original peoples of North, Central, and South America and who maintain tribal affiliation or community attachment (OMH, 2007; U.S. Census Bureau, 2007a). In 2004, American Indians and Alaska Natives other than those living in Alaska were most likely to live in one of four states: Arizona, California, Oklahoma, or New Mexico. Alaska had the highest proportion of any state of single-race American Indians and Alaska Natives in its population (U.S. Census Bureau, 2007a). Among American Indians, Cherokee, with 15 percent of the population, was the largest tribal grouping, followed by Navajo (11 percent). Among Alaska Natives, the Eskimo and Tlingit-Haida groups were the two largest tribal subgroups (U.S. Census Bureau, 2007a).

American Indians and Alaska Natives were younger than non-Hispanic whites in 2004, with a median age of 31.9 years. American Indians and Alaska Natives aged 15 and older were less likely to be married than non-Hispanic whites (42 and 57 percent, respectively). Approximately 68 percent of American Indian and Alaska Native households were family households, with a large percentage (21 percent) maintained by a female with no husband (U.S. Census Bureau, 2007a). Although only 7 percent of American Indian and Alaska Native grandparents lived in the same household as their grandchildren, a large percentage of them (58 percent) were responsible for the care of the grandchildren. Finally, approximately 75 percent of American Indians and Alaska Natives aged 5 and older spoke only English at home (U.S. Census Bureau, 2007a).

Information on educational attainment showed that approximately three-quarters of American Indians and Alaska Natives aged 25 and over had at least a high school diploma and 14 percent had attained a bachelor's degree or higher level of education (OMH, 2007; U.S. Census Bureau, 2007a). American Indians and Alaska Natives aged 16 and older were employed in a variety of occupations, including 25 percent in management, professional, and related occupations; 23 percent in sales and office occupations; and 22 percent in service occupations (U.S. Census Bureau, 2007a).

Still, the median household income of $31,600 for these two groups was $17,000 less than the median household income for non-Hispanic white households. Twenty-five percent of American Indian and Alaska Native households lived below the poverty level (U.S. Census Bureau, 2007a), and 30 percent had no health insurance coverage (OMH, 2007).

Presently, there are 561 federally recognized American Indian and Alaska Native tribes, and more than 100 state-recognized tribes (OMH, 2007). Federally recognized tribes receive health and educational assistance from the Indian Health Service (IHS), a governmental agency. This agency operates a comprehensive health service delivery system for 1.8 million American Indians and Alaska Natives, who reside mainly in reservations and rural communities. The IHS funds thirty-four urban Indian health organizations that provide services including medical and dental services; community services; alcohol and drug abuse prevention, education, and treatment services; mental health services; nutrition education; and counseling (OMH, 2007). Nonetheless, American Indians and Alaska Natives frequently are faced with issues such as cultural barriers, geographical isolation, inadequate sewage disposal, and low incomes that prevent them from receiving quality medical care.

American Indians and Alaska Natives are disproportionately affected by heart disease, cancer, unintentional injuries (accidents), diabetes, stroke, mental health issues, suicide, obesity, substance abuse, sudden infant death syndrome (SIDS), teenage pregnancy, and liver disease (OMH, 2007).

CONCLUSION

It is clear that members of underrepresented groups still face a number of barriers to obtaining optimal health. Health educators must work in conjunction with health care professionals not only to improve the health status of these groups but also to attempt to decrease the adverse health consequences for this population of the kinds of socioeconomic factors discussed in this chapter and also of events like the Tuskegee syphilis experiment (see Chapter Eight). Health educators must be cognizant of the differences existing between and among ethnic and racial groups in the United States. The following chapters discuss many ways of reaching out to these diverse populations.

POINTS TO REMEMBER

Demographic shifts in the U.S. population involving race, ethnicity, age, and sexual orientation make it imperative for health educators to learn how to deliver quality and culturally appropriate health education and prevention programs. An accurate understanding of the needs of different ethnic and cultural groups will go a long way toward achieving the goal of reaching diverse groups with prevention programs.

CASE STUDY

Almost all health promotion planning models require the collection of demographic data for the populations to be served. Using U.S. Census Bureau data, create a demographic profile for the county in which you currently reside. Be sure to collect the following information:

1. Total population

2. Age distribution

3. Sex distribution

4. Ethnic and racial composition

5. Educational level

6. Socioeconomic characteristics

    a. Family incomes

    b. Occupational categories

    c. Estimated level of unemployment

    d. Poverty ratios

7. Health characteristics

    a. Vital statistics (numbers and rates of births and deaths)

    b. Incidence and prevalence of diseases (morbidity)

    c. Leading causes of death (mortality)

8. Any other data you consider important for understanding the population in your county.

KEY TERMS

Demographic shift	Ethnicity	Race

NOTES

1. The term *demographic shift* refers to statistical changes in the socioeconomic characteristics of a population or consumer group. Typical characteristics examined are age, income, gender, occupation, education, family size, and similar descriptive variables (Lopez, 1999).

2. Note that more than one term may be used to refer to a particular population group. For instance, although some people prefer the term *African American,* others prefer the term *black.* Similarly, although some prefer the terms *Latino* and *Latina,* others prefer the term *Hispanic* and yet others prefer to list the name of their country first (for example, *Salvadoran American*). This chapter uses the terms used by the U.S. Census Bureau, including *Hispanic,* both *African*

American and *black,* and also *white, Alaska Native, American Indian, Asian, Native Hawaiian, and Pacific Islander.*

REFERENCES

Bean, F. D., & Stevens, G. (2003). *America's newcomers and the dynamics of diversity.* New York: Russell Sage Foundation.

Brach, C., & Fraser, I. (2000). Can cultural competency reduce racial and ethnic disparities? A review and conceptual model. *Medical Care Research and Review, 57*(Suppl. 1), 181–217.

Briggs, V. M. (1984). *Immigration policy and the American labor force.* Baltimore: Johns Hopkins University Press.

Chinese Exclusion Act of May 6, 1882, § 126, 22 Stat. 58 (1882).

Gay and Lesbian Medical Association et al. (2001). *Healthy people 2010 companion document for lesbian, gay, bisexual, and transgender (LGBT) health.* Retrieved October 24, 2007, from http://www.gayhealth.com/binary-data/GH_TEXT_BLOCK/attachment/1911.pdf.

Gomez-Quinones, J. (1981). Mexican immigration to the United States and the internationalization of labor, 1848–1980: An overview. In A. Rios-Bustamante (Ed.), *Mexican immigrant workers in the U.S.* (pp. 13–34). Los Angeles: University of California-Los Angeles, Chicano Studies Research Center Publications.

Lopez, E. (1999). *Major demographic shifts occurring in California.* Sacramento: California Research Bureau.

Lowell, L. B., & Suro, R. (2002). *How many undocumented: The numbers behind the U.S.-Mexico migration talks.* Washington, DC: Pew Hispanic Center.

Luquis, R. R., & Pérez, M. A. (2005). Health educators and cultural competence: Implications for the profession. *American Journal of Health Studies, 20*(3), 156–163.

Luquis, R. R., & Pérez, M. A. (2006). Cultural competency among school health educators. *Journal of Cultural Diversity, 13*(4), 217–222.

Luquis, R. R., Pérez, M. A., & Young, K. (2006). Cultural competence development in health education professional preparation programs. *American Journal of Health Education, 37*(4), 233–241.

Marín, G., Burhansstipanov, L., Connell, C. M., Gielen, A. C., Helitzer-Allen, D., Lorig, K., et al. (1995). A research agenda for health education among underserved populations. *Health Education Quarterly, 22*(3), 346–364.

Marín, G., & Marín, B. V. (1991). *Research with Hispanic populations.* Thousand Oaks, CA: Sage.

McKinnon, J. (2003). *The black population in the United States: March 2002* (Current Population Reports, Series P20-541). Washington, DC: U.S. Census Bureau.

National Coalition for LGBT Health & Boston Public Health Commission. (2002, June 28). *Double jeopardy: How racism and homophobia impact the health of black and Latino lesbian, gay, bisexual, and transgender (LGBT) communities.* Retrieved September 21, 2006, from http://www.lgbthealth.net/downloads/research/BPHCLGBTLatinoBlackHealthDispar.doc.

Office of Minority Health. (2007). *Minority population profile.* Retrieved September 17, 2007, from http://www.omhrc.gov/templates/browse.aspx?lvl=1&lvlID=5.

Pérez, M. A., Gonzalez, A., & Pinzon-Pérez, H. (2006). Cultural competence in health care systems: A case study. *California Journal of Health Promotion, 4*(1), 102–108.

Ramirez, R., & de la Cruz, G. P. (2003). *The Hispanic population in the United States: March 2002* (Current Population Reports, Series P20-545). Washington, DC: U.S. Census Bureau.

Reeves, T., & Bennett, C. (2003). *The Asian and Pacific Islander population in the United States: March 2002* (Current Population Reports, Series P20-540). Washington, DC: U.S. Census Bureau.

U. S. Census Bureau. (1995). *Sixty-five plus in the United States* (Statistical Brief). Retrieved September 22, 2007, from http://www.census.gov/population/socdemo/statbriefs/agebrief.html.

U.S. Census Bureau. (2001). *The elderly population.* Retrieved February 6, 2008, from http://www.census.gov/population/www/pop-profile/elderpop.html.

U.S. Census Bureau. (2004). *U.S. interim projections by age, sex, race, and Hispanic origin.* Retrieved February 9, 2008, from http://www.census.gov/ipc/www/usinterimproj.

U.S. Census Bureau. (2006). 2005 *American Community Survey.* Retrieved March 1, 2007, from http://factfinder.census.gov/servlet/ADPTable?_bm=y&-geo_id=01000US&-ds_name=ACS_2005_EST_G00_&-_lang=en&-_caller=geoselect&-format=.

U.S. Census Bureau. (2007a). *The American community—American Indians and Alaska Natives: 2004.* Retrieved September 22, 2007, from http://www.census.gov/prod/2007pubs/acs-07.pdf.

U.S. Census Bureau. (2007b). *The American community—Asians: 2004.* Retrieved September 22, 2007, from http://www.census.gov/prod/2007pubs/acs-05.pdf.

U.S. Census Bureau. (2007c). *The American community—Blacks: 2004.* Retrieved September 22, 2007, from http://www.census.gov/prod/2007pubs/acs-04.pdf.

U.S. Census Bureau. (2007d). *The American community—Hispanics: 2004.* Retrieved September 22, 2007, from http://www.census.gov/prod/2007pubs/acs-03.pdf.

U.S. Census Bureau. (2007e). *The American community—Pacific Islanders: 2004.* Retrieved September 22, 2007, from http://www.census.gov/prod/2007pubs/acs-06.pdf.

U.S. Census Bureau. (2007f). *Annual estimates of the population for the United States, regions, states, and Puerto Rico: April 1, 2000, to July 1, 2007* (NST-EST2007-01). Retrieved February 9, 2008, from http://www.census.gov/popest/states/NST-ann-est.html.

U.S. Department of Health and Human Services. (2000). *Healthy people 2010.* Washington, DC: Government Printing Office.

Waldrop, J., & Stern, S. M. (2003). *Disability status: 2000* (Census 2000 Brief C2KBR-17). Washington, DC: U.S. Census Bureau.

Yang, P. Q. (1995). *Post-1965 immigration to the United States: Structural determinants.* Westport, CT: Praeger.

CHAPTER

2

DISPARITIES IN HEALTH AMONG RACIAL AND ETHNIC GROUPS

Implications for Health Education

SUZANNE KOTKIN-JASZI

LEARNING OBJECTIVES

After completing this chapter, you will be able to

- Understand and explain the concept of health disparities.

- Understand and explain health and health care problems that disproportion-ately affect the major racial and ethnic groups.

- Provide an overview of morbidity and mortality patterns that affect each racial and ethnic group and the epidemiology of health and illness in each group.

- Describe the implications for health educators of these epidemiological pat-terns and health care access issues.

- List specific strategies that health educators can implement in their practices for overcoming access barriers for each of the groups.

INTRODUCTION

Carter-Pokras and Baquet (2002) suggest that "a health disparity should be viewed as a chain of events signified by a difference in: (1) environment, (2) access to, utilization of, and quality of care, (3) health status, or (4) a particular health outcome that deserves scrutiny" (p. 427). The National Institutes of Health (NIH), in its Strategic Research Plan to Reduce and Ultimately Eliminate Health Disparities (NIH, 2000), defines *health disparities* as the "differences in the incidence, prevalence, mortality and burden of diseases and other adverse health conditions that exist among several population groups in the United States" (p. 4). Research on health disparities related to socioeconomic status (SES) is also encompassed in this definition. The Institute of Medicine (IOM), in a landmark report titled *Unequal Treatment: Confronting Racial and Ethnic Disparities in Health Care,* documented and provided, for the very first time, evidence that the playing field is not equal—that ethnic and racial minorities receive lower quality health care than white people do, even when insurance status, income, age, and severity of conditions are comparable (Smedley, Strith, & Nelson, Committee on Understanding and Eliminating Racial and Ethnic Disparities in Health Care, Institute of Medicine, 2002). The IOM has taken a leadership role in advancing research efforts and polices to narrow these disparities and has partnered with private and public agencies to improve the way that care is delivered to people of color, to develop more effective communication strategies and tools to help the provider community more effectively interact with a broad range of patients, and to promote cultural competence in training health care professionals and in treatment.

The reasons why we observe these disparities are not clearly understood and may be due to such factors as individual choices, differences in disease processes, or systemic barriers to care, or to any combination of these factors. The IOM has produced a number of reports examining health care disparities and acknowledges that there are many possible reasons for the observed disparities in health and health care, including: language and cultural factors; distrust of the medical system among minority patients; a lack of minority physicians in clinical practice, who may be more culturally sensitized to the needs of minority patients; time limitations imposed by the pressures of clinical practice; and conscious or unconscious biases, prejudices, or negative racial and ethnic stereotypes that affect the ways in which health care providers deliver care to different populations (National Academy of Sciences, 2005, p. 4). It is most easy to identify a disparity in treatment for a particular condition when there is a clear clinical standard for quality health care for that condition and there is proof that this standard has not been met. Even when variations in individuals' disease state, severity of illness, and preferences are taken into account, there is a professional consensus that this standard of care has been breached (National Academy of Sciences, 2005). In a brief report targeted to health care administrators and managers, the IOM summarized the conclusions of its report *Unequal Treatment* by restating that "the sources of these disparities are complex, are rooted in historic and contemporary inequities, and involve many participants at several levels, including health systems, their administrative and bureaucratic processes, utilization managers, health care professionals and patients (National Academy of Sciences, 2002, p. 1).

A number of demographic changes in the United States over the past twenty years make it imperative that practicing health education and promotion professionals learn more about disparities for particular population groups, specifically low-income people and racial and ethnic groups. These demographic changes (discussed in detail in Chapter One), include an increase in the number of individuals belonging to minority racial and ethnic populations, an increase in the number of foreign-born residents, and an increase in the number of residents who do not speak English as their primary language at home. To compound these concerns, minorities and non-English speakers have greater difficulty in accessing needed health care services. Minorities are disproportionately more likely than the general population to be uninsured and are overrepresented among those in publicly funded insurance programs such as Medicaid.

The purpose of this chapter is to describe how these demographic shifts underscore the need to teach health care professionals and students studying to become health professionals concepts about health disparities, to describe these disparities in various ethnic and racial groups, and to train health care professionals, including health educators and managers, how to better meet the objective of providing high-quality care for all their patients. The term *demographic shift* is used to describe the totality of these changes and the beginning of the shift in the ethnicity of the U.S. population from a majority of non-Hispanic whites to a majority made up of other ethnicities. This chapter concludes with a discussion of how to address health care disparities in four major ethnic groups: African Americans, American Indians and Alaska Natives, Asians and Pacific Islanders, and Hispanics. (This chapter uses the terms *Hispanic* and *Latino* and also *African American* and *black* interchangeably.) Finally, a brief case study is presented that provides a hands-on opportunity for learners in a classroom or small-group setting to practice critical thinking skills concerning ways to overcome disparities in access to health promotion services for Mexican immigrant women.

HEALTH DISPARITIES BY CONDITION AND TREATMENT

There are numerous health disparities among racial and ethnic and low-income groups in the United States, and although the specific reasons why these disparities exist are not well understood, there is a consensus that in general they are largely due to complicated interrelationships among socioeconomic status, race, ethnicity, and culture. The following discussion highlights a number of the major disparities.

Cancer Screening and Management

Cancer is the second leading cause of death in the Unites States, causing more than 500,000 deaths each year (Centers for Disease Control and Prevention [CDC], 2006a). That is, one out every four deaths is due to cancer. There are many examples of important disparities in cancer screening and management. Health educators are in a unique position to begin to address these disparities. Much of the risk for developing cancer can be addressed by lifestyle modifications, including changes in diet and nutrition, exercise, and tobacco use. Tobacco use is estimated to be responsible for at least one-third of all cancer deaths (National Cancer Institute, 2007), and diet, weight control, and exercise can reduce cancer incidence by 30 to 40 percent (Dwyer, 2001; Antman et al., 2002; Freeman, 1989). Health educators are trained in theories of behavioral change, have excellent skills in communication, and are trusted members of the community. They need to help and support their clients in making lifestyle changes that will reduce cancer risk.

In addition to promoting lifestyle changes, health educators need to offer additional support to low-income and minority communities to bring their cancer-screening rates to a level of parity with rates for non-Hispanic whites. An important program for health educators to know about is the National Breast and Cervical Cancer Early Detection Program (CDC, 2007f) that provides low-income, uninsured women with access to screening services to detect breast cancer and cervical cancer at their earliest stages. Since 1991, this program has screened more than 2.9 million women, provided more than 6.9 million screening examinations, and diagnosed more than 29,000 breast cancers, 94,000 pre-cancerous lesions, and 1,800 cervical cancers.

Additional age-appropriate cancer-screening guidelines are important for health educators to communicate to their clients. A general cancer-related checkup is recommended every three years for all people aged 20 to 39 years and annually for people over 40. This checkup should include examination for cancers of the thyroid, testicles, ovaries, lymph nodes, skin, and oral cavity and "health counseling about tobacco, sun exposure, diet and nutrition, risk factors, sexual practices and environmental and occupational exposures" (American Cancer Society, 2007). Health educators are the ideal health care workers to provide this health counseling to patients because they are trained in discussing sensitive topics that may engender fear or be extremely personal. There is not much that is more anxiety provoking for a patient than talking with someone he or she does not know very well about his or her cancer risks, especially if the discussion is going to probe areas such as dietary choices, physical activity levels, weight control measures, and sexual practices. Specific screening tests recommended are a colonoscopy for all patients over 50 years old or, alternatively, a fecal blood test every year and a flexible sigmoidoscopy every five years. Mammograms are recommended for women over 40, combined with regular breast self-exams each month and a clinical exam by a health care professional, close to and preferably before the mammogram. Pap smears are recommended for all women over the age of 18, and if this test is normal for three years in a row, then the woman's health care provider will tell her how often to get this test. Digital rectal exams to screen for prostate cancer in men and rectal cancer in both genders are also recommended, along with prostate specific antigen tests for men starting at age 50, but some men who are at higher risk, including African American men and those with a first-degree relative diagnosed at a relatively young age, should consider earlier screening for prostate cancer. All men should be taught to practice regular testicular self-examinations.

To summarize the vast research on health care disparities and cancer, that research strongly suggests that African Americans and Hispanics are much more likely than non-Hispanic whites to receive a lower quality of health care for cancer, including lack of access to clinical trials, even when data are corrected for factors affecting access, such as insurance status (CDC, 2007b).

Diabetes

Diabetes was the sixth leading cause of death in the year 2000. More than 17 million people in the United States have diabetes, and each year over 200,000 people die from the complications associated with diabetes (CDC, 2007c). Minorities are much more likely to be diagnosed with diabetes than are non-Hispanic whites of a similar age. African Americans and American Indians also have higher rates of diabetes-related complications, including kidney disease and amputations. The Healthy People 2010 midcourse review, examining data available as of January 1, 2005, suggested that some progress has been made toward meeting the two overarching goals to increase quality and years of healthy life and reduce health disparities. However, when the data were disaggregated, the disparities among racial and ethnic populations were largely unchanged from the baseline assessments (CDC, 2006b). The most promising strategies to reverse these alarming statistics focus on early screening and treatment. Once diagnosed, individuals with diabetes need specialized self-management programs and improved tracking to ameliorate their risks for major complications. The federally qualified health centers (FQHCs) that serve low-income, largely minority, and often undocumented populations have taken part in a health care collaboratives study conducted with 9,558 patients in forty-four health centers nationwide. This study used nationally validated quality measures before and after each intervention, focusing on measures related to diabetes, asthma, and hypertension. The researchers found a 21 percent improvement in foot examinations for persons with diabetes and a 16 percent increase in the level of screening for glycated hemoglobin, a measure of diabetes. These efforts in improving chronic disease management involved focusing on tracking health screening efforts, communicating the results to the patients, and making sure that patients followed up on testing and examination results, along with making self-management efforts such as improving diet and nutrition, increasing physical activity, and tracking their efforts through patient logs (Agency for Healthcare Research and Quality [AHRQ], 2007).

Coronary Heart Disease

Overall, minority and low-income populations have a disproportionate share of morbidity and mortality from heart disease. Two goals of the Healthy People 2010 initiative address this disproportionate burden of cardiovascular disease in the African American community: one is to reduce deaths from heart disease among African Americans by 30 percent and the other is to reduce deaths from strokes among African Americans by 47 percent (CDC, 2006c).

There are many epidemiological disparities among African Americans that are related to this group's disproportionate share of heart disease. Numerous studies of African Americans consistently document differences in their access to care for heart disease and stroke. Study findings consistently suggest that African Americans are unfailingly less likely to receive diagnostic angioplasty and catheterization, pharmacological therapy, and invasive surgical treatment for heart disease and stroke than are non-Hispanic whites with similar disease characteristics (Mayberry, Mili, & Olifi, 2002).

The most promising preventive strategies target risk factors for cardiovascular disease (CVD) morbidity, mortality, and disability. These prevention programs target the conditions research has suggested are associated with CVD: having high blood pressure, having high cholesterol, smoking tobacco, being overweight, and being physically inactive. Again, for the two major cardiovascular disease killers, heart disease and stroke, health educators are in an excellent position to improve patient outcomes. They can convey critical health care information in a way that is culturally relevant and sensitive. The health educator can communicate during routine office visits that patients need to be screened for risk factors associated with CVD, and once risk factors are identified, he or she can provide individual and group classes that target smoking cessation, the importance of taking medications for hypertension, proper nutrition and exercise, stress reduction, and other heart-healthy behavioral modifications. Increasingly, these health education efforts are being conducted in schools and in the workplace and are also being supported by community-based groups, churches, and community partners such as the American Heart Association and other voluntary health agencies.

HIV and AIDS

HIV is now the fifth leading cause of death for people in the United States aged 25 to 44 and the leading cause of death for African American men aged 35 to 44 (CDC, 2007d). Racial, ethnic, and sexual minorities have been disproportionately affected by the HIV/AIDS epidemic in the United States. The disparities in pediatric HIV infection are most dramatic. Although non-Hispanic black children compose approximately 15 percent of the total child population, they represent almost 60 percent of all pediatric AIDS cases (Child Health USA, 2006). Two factors driving the increasing rate of new infections in minority communities are the growth of HIV infections in women transmitted through heterosexual contact and the spread of infection through injection drug use.

The goal of Healthy People 2010 is to eliminate these disparities by implementing strategies that focus on high-risk populations' knowing their HIV status and receiving appropriate counseling and treatment, on providing early access to health care and anti-retroviral drugs for at least 75 percent of people with HIV/AIDS, and on educating health care providers to target women and children on the Medicaid program with prevention and treatment strategies.

Health educators often have the linguistic and cultural competence to ensure that HIV/AIDS educational materials are provided to the community in languages other than English, in forms that populations with low levels of health literacy can understand

and act on, and in words that people actually use when talking about sexual and injection practices. Patients need to be counseled on prevention strategies, including harm reduction, in nonjudgmental ways. Patients need to be taught the benefits of knowing whether they are HIV positive or negative (their serostatus) and their right to receive effective drug therapies. It is also crucial that communities partner with health care professionals to reduce the impact of the HIV/AIDS epidemic on minority communities.

Adult and Child Immunization Rates

Although recent efforts have narrowed the gap in immunization rates between minority and non-Hispanic white populations, this nation is still below the goal set in Healthy People 2010 to achieve and maintain childhood immunizations at 90 percent and to increase influenza and pneumococcal immunizations to 60 percent among all older adults (65 years of age and older) (Niederhauser & Stark, 2005; Zimmerman, 2007). Also, although disparities in childhood vaccination coverage have decreased, largely due to the Childhood Immunization Initiative (CDC, 2007a), some disparities still exist.

The U.S. Department of Health and Human Services has developed a plan, the National Immunization Program (NIP), to improve adult and child immunization rates. This plan includes public and provider awareness campaigns, enhanced delivery of immunization services, and more assessment of the barriers to immunization. NIP has developed special programs for specific groups of people, including adults, infants and toddlers, pre-teens and adolescents, college students and young adults, parents, pregnant women, seniors, and racial and ethnic minorities. The program is community based and works with universities, clergy, health care professionals, churches, and senior centers to encourage vaccination (CDC, 2007g). Physicians and health educators must take leadership roles to help children and adults be vaccinated.

Vaccines for Children (VFC) is a program that funds free vaccines for low-income children and is administered through NIP. States and eligible U.S. projects enroll doctors, who then identify low-income children eligible for services (CDC, 2007h). Adult vaccination rates are lower than they need to be because of lack of information: adults may not know which immunizations are needed, and health care providers, including health educators, may not recommend vaccines to their adult clients. Many adults are also afraid of adverse reactions to vaccines and do not understand the threat of influenza and pneumococcal disease to older adults. Health educators have a vital role to work with their adult clients to educate them concerning the need to be vaccinated against influenza and pneumococcal disease.

Infant Mortality

The infant mortality rate (IMR) is an international measure used within and between nations to compare the health and well-being of populations. The IMR is often used as an overall measure of a country's health care status because it is sensitive to many of the underlying determinants of health status, including literacy, economic factors such as overall income, and the relative position of women in a society—their educational level, literacy, socioeconomic status, right to make their own reproductive health decisions, and overall access to primary care for themselves and their families. The United States ranked twenty-seventh among industrialized nations in 2000, with an IMR of 6.9 deaths per 1,000 live births (Child Health USA, 2004b). Another report by Child Health USA also found higher death rates for U.S. infants among minorities and disadvantaged groups. Only 17 percent of all U.S. births were to African American families, but 33 percent of all low birth weight babies were African American (Child Health USA, 2004a). Other data for African Americans reflect this disparity in infant mortality rates. What is interesting is that the African American infant mortality rate has been consistently reported to be double the white rate since the United States began to collect race-specific data. Some researchers have suggested that this disparity is occurring because, over the years, African Americans have experienced consistent deprivation as compared to whites (LaVeist, 2002). However, this apparently persistent 2:1 ratio shows more variation when the relative rate is aggregated over the years 1981 to 1985 for all U.S. cities that are at least 10 percent African American. LaVeist found that the degree of black to white relative disadvantage varied substantially across cities, from .56 to 5.02, and in eight cities found a higher rate of infant mortality for whites than for blacks. He suggests that these differences in disparity can be attributed to differences in racial residential segregation, poverty, and black political empowerment (LaVeist, 2002).

One of the goals of Healthy People 2010 is to eliminate the disparities among the racial and ethnic groups that have IMRs above the national average, including the American Indian, Alaska Native, and Puerto Rican populations. The strategy will consist of modifying the underlying determinants of birth outcomes including maternal substance abuse, poor nutrition and lack of prenatal care, smoking, and chronic illness. This plan to reduce infant mortality will require a partnership between health care professionals and minority communities to encourage and support healthy behaviors.

HEALTH DISPARITIES BY ETHNIC GROUP

Asians and Pacific Islanders

Asian women have the highest life expectancy (85.8 years) of any ethnic group in the United States (Office on Women's Health, 2006). This life expectancy for women does vary among Asian subgroups: Filipino women (81.5 years), Japanese women (84.5 years), and Chinese women (86.1 years). However, Asians in the United States also contend with numerous factors that threaten their health. Some negative factors are infrequent medical visits due to the fear of deportation, language and cultural barriers, and the lack of health insurance. Asians are most at risk for the following health conditions: cancer, heart disease, stroke, unintentional injuries (accidents), and diabetes. Asians also have a high prevalence of the following conditions and risk factors: chronic obstructive pulmonary disease, hepatitis B, HIV/AIDS, smoking, tuberculosis, and liver disease (Office of Minority Health and Health Disparities [OMHD], 2006). In 2004, Asians were 5.6 times more likely than the total U.S. population to have tuberculosis.

Tuberculosis was 13 times more common among such Asian subgroups as Cambodians, Chinese, Laotians, Koreans, Indians, Vietnamese, and Filipinos than it was among the total U.S. population. In 2001, Asians and Pacific Islanders aged 40 and older were 2.5 times more likely to have hepatitis B (14.2 per 100,000) than were non-Hispanic whites. Of the 12.5 million Americans living with chronic hepatitis B infection, approximately half are Asians. In 2002, the hepatitis B–related death rate among Asians was six times higher than the rate among whites (OMHD, 2006). In 2002, the AIDS rate among Asians and Pacific Islanders was 4.0 cases per 100,000 people. During 2003, 497 new AIDS cases were reported among this population, an increase of 9.9 percent over 2002, and 34.7 percent over the 1999 level (OMHD, 2006).

In terms of preventive services, Asians have the lowest utilization rate of any group for aspirin use, as well as for breast, cervical, and colorectal cancer screening. The report *Preventive Care: A National Profile on Use, Disparities and Health Benefits,* found that Asian men aged 40 and older and Asian women aged 50 and older are 40 percent less likely than their non-Hispanic white counterparts to use aspirin as part of a heart healthy regimen. When it comes to cancer screening, Asian adults aged 50 and older are 40 percent less likely than whites to be current on screening for colorectal cancer, Asian women aged 18 to 54 are 25 percent less likely than white women to have been screened for cervical cancer, and Asian women aged 40 and over are 21 percent less likely than white women to have been screened for breast cancer in the past two years (Partnership for Prevention, 2007).

Native Americans and Alaska Natives

American Indians and Alaska Natives are a heterogeneous population, with approximately 560 federally recognized tribes living in both the rural and urban areas of thirty-five states (U.S. Census Bureau, 2007). The 2004 American Community Survey estimated the number of American Indians and Alaska Natives to be about 4 million, or 1.4 percent of the U.S. households. The number of individuals who reported American Indian and Alaska Native as their only race was about 2.2 million, or 0.8 percent of the population. About another 1.9 million reported their race as American Indian and Alaska Native and one or more other races, including about 1.4 million people who reported their race as American Indian and Alaska Native and white. The American Indian and Alaska Native alone-or-in-combination population included about 561,000 Hispanics, and the American Indian and Alaska Native alone population included about 299,000 Hispanics (U.S. Census Bureau, 2007).

What is common to all tribal groups, both rural and urban, is a high rate of poverty; American Indians and Alaska Natives have the highest poverty rates of any racial or ethnic group. From 2001 to 2004, the three-year-average poverty rate for American Indians and Alaska Natives was 25.3 percent. The three-year-average poverty rate for Native Hawaiians and other Pacific Islanders was 12.2 percent. (The Census Bureau uses three-year-average medians for these groups because of their relatively small populations.) Although each tribal group has a unique history, culture, and economic outlook, there are some common trends in American Indian and Alaska Native health disparities (U.S. Census Bureau, 2006).

The American Indian and Alaska Native population has long experienced lower overall health status when compared with other populations, as evidenced by the statistics provided in this chapter. The reasons for this persistent and pervasive disparity are not entirely clear but are related to inadequate education, higher poverty rates, discrimination, and cultural differences.

On the health status measures of life expectancy at birth and the infant mortality rate, American Indian and Alaska Native populations are also disproportionately affected when compared with other U.S. populations. American Indian and Alaska Native people born today have a life expectancy 2.4 years less than the expectancy for all other races. Similarly, American Indian and Alaska Native infants die at a rate of 8.5 per every 1,000 live births, as compared to 5.8 per 1,000 for all U.S. races (2000 to 2002 rates) (Indian Health Service, 2007).

American Indians and Alaska Natives also die at higher rates than other U.S. racial and ethnic groups, from a variety of causes including tuberculosis (600 percent higher), alcoholism (510 percent higher), motor vehicle crashes (229 percent higher), diabetes (189 percent higher), homicide (61 percent higher), and suicide (62 percent higher), according to the Indian Health Service (2007).

It is important to note that American Indians and Alaska Natives frequently contend with issues that prevent them from receiving quality medical care. The American Indian and Alaska Native population is different in several key ways from the U.S. all-races population, and these differences affect that population's access to quality health care services at costs similar to costs for other U.S. populations. The American Indian and Alaska Native population is younger, due to having a higher mortality rate than other Americans do, and approximately 55 percent of this population receives health services from the Indian Health Service. The population is also predominantly rural, and a rural, younger population would suggest that personal health services could be provided at a lower cost than expected. The vast differences in health status between American Indian and Alaska Native people and non-Hispanic whites, reflecting American Indians' and Alaska Natives' disproportionate incidence of acute and chronic medical conditions, will require a continued commitment to funding ways to bring the health status of American Indians and Alaska Natives into parity with the health status measures for all Americans (Indian Health Service, 2007).

Hispanics

Although health disparities are narrowing for most U.S. minorities when their health is compared with that of non-Hispanics whites, Latinos may well be falling further behind, according to a study published by the Agency for Healthcare Research and Quality (2006). According to this report, which tracked disparities related to quality of health care and access using data from 2002 and 2003 that examined disparities in forty-six health care measures along with six categories of access to care, 59 percent of disparity measures were widening for Latinos, and 41 percent were decreasing. Treatment for diabetes, mental illness, and tuberculosis and also dental and preventive care were areas where the disparities for Latinos were widening (Henry J. Kaiser Family Foundation, 2006). AHRQ also reported that in five out of the six categories that measured access to care, disparities increased for Latinos even though they narrowed for other ethnic and racial groups, including blacks, Asians, and American Indians. Questioned as to the reason for the widening gap for Latinos, the director of AHRQ stated that perhaps a language barrier was contributing to the problem and also suggested that illegal immigration might play a role (Henry J. Kaiser Family Foundation, 2006).

A key report quantifying disparities in the use of preventive care services also reported that racial and ethnic minorities continue to receive less preventive care than non-Hispanic whites. The report highlighted three areas in which Hispanics use fewer preventive services: compared to similar non-Hispanic whites, Hispanic smokers are 55 percent less likely to get assistance from a health care professional when trying to quit smoking, Hispanic adults over the age of 50 are 39 percent less likely to be current on screening for colorectal cancer, and Hispanic adults over 65 are 55 percent less likely to be vaccinated against pneumococcal disease (Partnership for Prevention, 2007).

Ramsey, Wear, Labarante, and Nichman (1997) found no significant difference for bypass surgery and marginal differences for angioplasty between Mexican Americans and non-Hispanic whites in Corpus Christi, Texas. Other studies of Hispanics found different results. In a study conducted at a Veterans Administration hospital, Mickelson, Blum, and Geraci found Hispanics to be 71 percent less likely than whites to receive thrombolytic therapy (Mayberry et al., 2002).

The health profile of the Hispanic population in general and Mexican Americans in particular has seriously questioned the dominant paradigm that focuses on SES and access to medical care as the key explanatory factors for racial differences in health. In fact, first-generation Mexican Americans are often low in SES and have low utilization rates for health care services, insurance coverage, and preventive services but also have rates of infant mortality, overall mortality, and chronics illness that are lower than rates for African Americans and comparable to rates for non-Hispanic whites. This phenomenon is referred to as the *Hispanic paradox.* That acculturation may play a role is suggested by the fact that foreign-born Hispanics have a better health profile than their counterparts in the United States do. Rates of infant mortality, low birth weight, cancer, high blood pressure, adolescent pregnancy, and psychiatric disorders increase with length of stay in the United States (Vega & Amaro, 1994). Hispanic health status is nevertheless often shaped by factors such as language and cultural barriers, lack of access to preventive care, and the lack of health insurance. This is especially true in relation to length of time in the United States. As Mexican American and other Hispanic immigrants assimilate, they take on the diets, lifestyles, and health patterns of their adopted country. Their patterns of disease, mortality, morbidity, and chronic illness begin to look more like those of other Americans, and they quickly lose the health advantages described in the Hispanic paradox. The Centers for Disease Control and Prevention has cited heart disease, cancer, unintentional injuries (accidents), stroke, and diabetes as leading causes of illness and death among Hispanics.

Some other health conditions and risk factors that significantly affect Hispanics are asthma, chronic obstructive pulmonary disease, HIV/AIDS, obesity, suicide, and liver disease. Mexican American adults in the United States are considerably more obese than non-Hispanic whites, but the prevalence of obesity (defined as a body mass index, or BMI, greater than 30) has risen for all U.S. adults in the decade from 1999 to 2000 (American Obesity Association, 2007). There are also disparities among Hispanic subgroups. For instance, although the rate of low birth weight infants is lower for the total Hispanic population than it is for non-Hispanic whites, Puerto Ricans have a low birth weight rate that is 50 percent higher than the rate for non-Hispanic whites. Puerto Ricans also suffer disproportionately from asthma, HIV/AIDS, and infant mortality. Mexican Americans suffer disproportionately from diabetes. In a study to assess the health status of Mexican American, mainland Puerto Rican, and Cuban American children by examining the prevalence of poor pregnancy outcomes and chronic medical conditions, the health status of Cuban American children was similar to that of non-Hispanic white children and the Hispanic subgroup at greatest risk of poor health was Puerto Rican children (Mendoza et al., 1991).

African Americans

In the 2000 census, 36.4 million people identified themselves as black or African American, and 35.4 million of these individuals identified themselves as non-Hispanic. African Americans bear a disproportionate burden of disease, injury, death, and suffering. Although the top three causes of death and seven of the leading causes of death are the same for non-Hispanic and Hispanic whites, the risk factors and morbidity and mortality rates are greater among blacks than among whites and three of the leading causes of deaths for non-Hispanic blacks are not among the leading causes of deaths for non-Hispanic whites (CDC, 2005). Homicide is the sixth leading cause of death for non-Hispanic blacks, followed by HIV disease (seventh), and septicemia (ninth). African American men have the highest death rate of all racial and ethnic groups, male or female, as well as the lowest life expectancy. They are also negatively affected by high rates of incarceration, high unemployment, low college graduation rates, and problems with access to health care and quality of care (Henry J. Kaiser Family Foundation, 2007).

Cancer mortality rates are 35 percent higher in blacks than in whites (AHRQ, 2002). Although cancer is the second leading cause of death for both non-Hispanic blacks and non-Hispanic whites, the age-adjusted incidence per 100,000 population for 2000 is much higher for black women for colorectal cancer (57.2 versus 46.9) and for pancreatic and stomach cancer combined (21.2 versus 13.5). For black men the age-adjusted incidence was much higher for prostate (281.2 versus 169.4), lung/bronchus (109.2 versus 76.6), colorectal (72.0 versus 62.7), and stomach (18. 7 versus 9.9) cancers (National Center for Health Statistics, 2004, table 53).

What is striking is that even though African Americans have higher screening rates for breast and colorectal cancer than Asians and Hispanics do, increasing cancer screening in the African American population would have a bigger impact on African Americans' health because they have a higher mortality for these conditions. The Partnership for Prevention reports that if the 42 percent of African Americans aged 50 and older who are current with recommended screening could be increased to 90 percent, an additional 1,100 lives could be saved annually (Partnership for Prevention, 2007).

In 2002, non-Hispanic blacks who died from HIV disease had approximately eleven times as many age-adjusted years of life lost before age 75 per 100,000 population as non-Hispanic whites did (CDC, 2005). Blacks also had more years of potential life lost than non-Hispanic whites did for suicide (nine times as many), stroke (three times as many), and diabetes (three times as many).

The exact mechanism underlying these findings is not well understood but a growing body of literature suggests that they are not due just to difference in socioeconomic status, which accounts for many of the observed racial disparities in health, but rather to a complex interaction of race and SES. Racism, expressed as both individual and institutional discrimination, can adversely affect health status by restricting socioeconomic opportunity and mobility. Living in poor neighborhoods, experiencing discrimination, and accepting the social stigma of inferiority can have negative impacts on health (Williams, 1999). Blacks who challenged unfair treatment or reported that they had not experienced racial discrimination actually had systolic blood pressure 9 to 10 mg Hg lower than their African American neighbors, family, friends, and coworkers did in a study by Krieger and Sidney (1996). These results suggest that there may be a link between discrimination and health and that more research is needed to fully understand these differences.

Finally, in the area of substance abuse and mental health treatment, African Americans have a huge unmet need for services, as reported by numerous health services researchers (Hu, Snowden, Jerrell, & Nguyen, 1991; Wells, Klap, Koike, & Sherbourne, 2001; Fiscella, Franks, Doescher, & Saver, 2002; Chow, Jaffee, & Snowden, 2003).

HEALTH DISPARITIES AND HEALTH EDUCATION

This chapter has presented facts on health disparities among Americans that may seem on the surface to be insurmountable. For students in health education programs, it may feel as though the disparities in health care access and outcomes for the populations discussed in this chapter are almost impossible to address. It does seem that as we begin the twenty-first century in the United States, we are at a critical crossroads in the history of health education practice. For many Americans it is truly the best of times as technological advances in biology, genetics, and medicine mean that they can live long and prosperous lives with little or no morbidity and disability until their 80s. At the same time it is apparent that the racial and ethnic minority groups discussed in this chapter are living shorter lives, lives compromised by more morbidity and disability than other Americans face. The root causes of many of the disparities in health care status and access are inequalities in income and education, racial discrimination, lack of cultural understanding, and inability to modify health education programs to better target racial and ethnic minority groups. All health educators need to be aware of the statistics presented in this chapter and to understand the underlying determinants, insofar as they are currently known. In particular, theoretical models need to be developed and tested that can explain how variables interact to contribute to these observed disparities in health status.

Health educators have an important and pivotal role to play in addressing these pervasive health disparities. Health educators interact with the patient on a personal level and are in a unique position to try to overcome the correct perception of many ethnic minorities that the shadow of racism still looms large in the U.S. health care system and in the nation's medical and public health institutions. Health educators need to lead the charge to address the disparities identified in this chapter. The next generation of health educators and health promotion specialists needs opportunities to practice and internalize critical skills in culturally competent health education practice that recognizes and works with the inherent strengths of ethnic minority communities and patients in a new model of patient-centered care, characterized by more equitable decision making and power sharing between providers and patients.

In response to this challenge, the Society for Public Health Education (SOPHE) released special issues of its journals, *Health Promotion Practice* and *Health Education & Behavior,* focused on themes explored in SOPHE's inaugural summit, held in the summer of 2005, *Health Disparities and Social Inequities: Framing a Transdisciplinary Agenda in Health Education.* The special issue of *Health Education & Behavior* also presented ten new priorities for health education and social science research into racial and ethnic health disparities (SOPHE, 2006). During this summit, eighty health education leaders, including researchers, academics, practitioners, and students, came together to ask fundamental questions about health care disparities and to formulate a health education research agenda to address them, especially as our society becomes more diverse and the issues of multiculturalism more complex (Gambescia et al., 2006).

Although health educators, through the Society for Public Health Education, their professional association, have recognized this problem, held a summit, and dedicated special issues of their journals to further scholarship on disparities, it is alarming that the members of the general U.S. public have not recognized the impact of health care disparities on their neighbors and communities. Most Americans recognize that problems exist for many Americans in getting quality health care, but when asked about disparities for racial and ethnic minorities in specific aspects of health care, the majority of the population does not think that racial and ethnic minorities have worse problems with obtaining health care than non-Hispanic whites do. Whites in particular largely do not believe that problems of access or quality are any worse for African Americans or Hispanics than for whites. The most recent poll, which was conducted by the Harvard School of Public Health, the Robert Wood Johnson Foundation, and ICR (2005) and which examined a nationally representative sample of 1,111 adults 18 years of age and over in September 2005, found that only 32 percent of Americans think the problem of getting quality health care is worse for minorities than for whites. Another striking finding from this report is that 23 percent of African Americans reported they had received poor quality care because of their race or ethnicity, as compared to only 1 percent of whites. Twenty-one percent of Hispanics also reported that they received poor quality medical treatment that was due to their having an accent and to their lack of ability with English.

CONCLUSION

It is obvious from this brief review of the statistics on health disparities that although some disparities are diminishing, the overall picture is mixed. For every minority group, measures can be identified on which that group received worse care than the reference group (non-Hispanic whites) did and on which the difference was getting worse rather than better. For the racial and ethnic minority groups reported on in AHRQ's 2006 *National Healthcare Disparities Report,* the disparities found for blacks, Asians, and Hispanics crossed all the domains of quality that could be tracked and included preventive services, treatment of acute illness, management of chronic disease and disability, timeliness, and patient centeredness. For the American Indian and Alaska Native populations, the disparities reported were concentrated in the treatment of chronic illness and also in the management of chronic disease and disability. The other alarming findings presented in this report were the measures of disparities in access to care for Hispanics and the poor. For Hispanics, both not having health insurance and lacking a usual source of care (a medical home) were getting worse, whereas for the poor, not having a usual source of care and experiencing delays in getting care were getting worse. The *National Healthcare Disparities Report* is the biggest annual examination of disparities in health care access in the United States, and AHRQ has now added new information sources to track the nation's progress toward the elimination of disparities. AHRQ has also developed partnerships with health plans, states, coalitions of business leaders, and community partners to address these persistent disparities.

This pervasive disconnect between the facts on health care disparities and popular beliefs suggests yet another critical role for health care professionals, especially those involved in health education and promotion. They have a critical role to play in championing and advocating a partnership between health care professionals and the federal government to address these troubling disparities. The poll discussed earlier suggests overwhelming public support for the medical profession (66 percent of the total respondents) and for the federal government (65 percent) to do more to ensure racial and ethnic equality in health care (Harvard School of Public Health, Robert Wood Johnson Foundation, & ICR, 2005).

The Partnership for Prevention has concluded that an additional 100,000 lives could be saved annually just by increasing the currently low utilization rates of five cost-effective prevention services. It is racial and ethnic minorities who are getting even less preventive care than the U.S. population in general (Partnership for Prevention, 2007, p. 3). Health educators have to take a leadership role to transform the U.S. health care system from one that focuses on providing acute care to the few to one that emphasizes preventive care for all Americans.

POINTS TO REMEMBER

- Health care disparities are persistent and pervasive. This chapter has focused on disparities due to race and ethnicity; however, disparities are also associated with disability status, geography, sexual orientation, and gender.

- Knowing key health disparities by race and ethnicity is critical for health educators if they are to take a leadership role in collaborating with key partners in the community to address these disparities.

- Health educators need to create their own research agenda, one that focuses on how to create an infrastructure to support health care disparities research; how to increase the dialogue with the community, researchers, and policymakers; how to measure progress in addressing health care disparities; and how to advocate for more funding for health disparities research.

- As Gambescia and his colleagues (2006) state, "the issues of race, ethnicity and culture will become more complex as we develop into a rich, multiethnic nation" (p. 537).

CASE STUDY

Alicia Garcia is a 25-year-old migrant farmworker born in Zacatecas, Mexico. You hear from her neighbor who is your patient that she is two months pregnant with her third child but has not seen a health care provider, not even a lay midwife (*partera*). Her neighbor tells you that Alicia does not think it is important to take time off from work to make an appointment to see a health care provider. You are the health educator and your responsibility is to encourage farmworker women to enter prenatal care by the first trimester. Please discuss with the other students, in small groups, some strategies you could use to encourage Alicia to enter prenatal care within the next month and then to continue to follow the protocols for a health pregnancy and delivery.

1. How would you approach Alicia about the need for early prenatal care?

2. What inherent strengths of Latino culture can you identify that might help you convince Alicia of the need to take care of her unborn child?

3. What do you think are some of the barriers faced by Alicia in seeking prenatal care?

4. What are some of the strategies that might help her to overcome these barriers?

5. What resources and agencies in the community can you identify that could partner with health educators to help Alicia have a successful pregnancy, labor, and delivery?

6. How would you assess Alicia's and her family's need for continuing support and counseling?

7. What are the steps of your action plan for Alicia?

KEY TERMS

Demographic shift   Health disparity

Cultural competence   Hispanic paradox

REFERENCES

Agency for Healthcare Research and Quality. (2002). *Disparities in health care: AHRQ focus on quality.* Retrieved October 10, 2007, from http://www.ahrq.gov/news/focus/disparhc.htm.

Agency for Healthcare Research and Quality. (2006). *National healthcare disparities report.* Retrieved September 20, 2007, from http//www.ahrq.gov/qual/nhdr06/highlights/nhdr06high.htm.

Agency for Healthcare Research and Quality. (2007, February 28). *Chronic disease management quality improvement efforts yield better care delivery.* Retrieved October 29, 2007, from http://www.arghr.gov/news/press/pre2007/cdmqipr.htm.

American Cancer Society. (2007). *Screening guidelines.* Retrieved September 17, 2007, from www.overlakehospital.org/services/cancerservices/detection/acscreenings.aspx.

American Obesity Association. (2007). *Obesity in minority populations* (AOA Fact Sheet). Retrieved October 9, 2007, from http://obesity1.tempdomainname.com/subs/fastfacts/Obesity_Minority_Pop.shtml.

Antman, K., Abraido-Lanza, A. F., Blum, D., Browfield, E., Cicatelli, B., Debor, M. D., et al. (2002). Reducing disparities in breast cancer survival: Columbia University and Avon breast cancer research and care network symposium. *Breast Cancer Research and Treatment, 75*(3), 269–280.

Carter-Pokras, O., & Baquet, C. (2002). What is a health disparity? *Public Health Reports, 117*(5), 426–434.

Centers for Disease Control and Prevention. (2005). Health disparities experienced by black or African Americans. *Morbidity and Mortality Weekly Report, 54*(1), 1–3.

Centers for Disease Control and Prevention. (2006a). *Healthy people 2010: Midcourse review* (Focus Area 3: Cancer). Retrieved September 21, 2007, from http://www.healthypeople.gov/data/midcourse/html/focusareas/FA03TOC.htm.

Centers for Disease Control and Prevention. (2006b). *Healthy people 2010: Midcourse review* (Focus Area 5: Diabetes). Retrieved September 19, 2007, from http://www.healthypeople.gov/data/midcourse/pdf.fa05.pdf.

Centers for Disease Control and Prevention. (2006c). *Healthy people 2010: Midcourse review* (Focus Area 12: Heart disease and stroke). Retrieved September 12, 2007, from http://www.healthypeople.gov/data/midcourse/html/tables/dt/DT-12a.htm.

Centers for Disease Control and Prevention. (2007a). *The childhood immunization initiative* (HHS Fact Sheet). Retrieved February 15, 2007, from http://www.hhs.gov/news/press/2000pres/200000706a.html.

Centers for Disease Control and Prevention. (2007b). *Eliminate disparities in cancer screening and management* (Factsheet). Retrieved February 15, 2007, from http://www.cdc.gov/omhd/AMH/factsheets/cancer.htm.

Centers for Disease Control and Prevention. (2007c). *Eliminate disparities in diabetes* (Factsheet). Retrieved February 12, 2007, from http://www.cdc.gov/omhd/AMH/factsheets/diabetes.htm.

Centers for Disease Control and Prevention. (2007d). *Eliminate disparities in HIV and AIDS* (Factsheet). Retrieved February 15, 2007, from http://www.cdc.gov/omhd/AMH/factsheets/hiv.htm.

Centers for Disease Control and Prevention. (2007e). *Eliminate disparities in infant mortality* (Factsheet). Retrieved February 15, 2007, from http://www.cdc.gov/omhd/AMH/factsheets/infant.htm.

Centers for Disease Control and Prevention. (2007f). *National breast and cervical cancer early detection program*. Retrieved September 21, 2007, from http://www.cdc.gov/cancer/NBCCEDP.

Centers for Disease Control and Prevention. (2007g). *Vaccines and immunizations*. Retrieved October 29, 2007, from http://www.cdc.gov/vaccines/spec-grps/default.htm.

Centers for Disease Control and Prevention. (2007h). *Vaccines for Children program*. Retrieved October 16, 2007, from http://www.cdc.gov/vaccines/programs/vfc/default.htm.

Child Health USA. (2004a). *Infant mortality*. Retrieved November 16, 2007, from http://mchb.hrsa.gov/mchirc/chusa_04/pages/0406im.htm.

Child Health USA. (2004b). *International infant mortality rates*. Retrieved September 17, 2007, from http://mchb.hrsa.gov/mchirc/chusa_04/pages/0405iimr.htm.

Child Health USA. (2006). *Pediatric AIDS*. Retrieved November 16, 2007, from http://www.mchb.hrsa.gov/chusa_06/healthstat/children/0310pa.htm.

Chow, J. C., Jaffee, K., & Snowden, L. (2003). Racial/ethnic disparities in the use of mental health services in poverty areas. *American Journal of Public Health, 93*(5), 792–797.

Dwyer, J. T. (2001, July 16). *Nutritional guidelines and education of the public*. Paper presented at the 11th annual research conference on diet, nutrition and cancer of the American Institute for Cancer Research, Washington, DC.

Fiscella, K., Franks, P., Doescher, M. P., & Saver, B. (2002). Disparities in health care by race, ethnicity, and language among the insured: Findings from a national sample. *Medical Care, 40*(1), 52–59.

Freeman, H. P. (1989). Cancer in the socioeconomically disadvantaged. *CA: A Cancer Journal for Clinicians, 39*(1), 266–288. Retrieved November 16, 2007, from http://caonline.amcancer.org.

Gambescia, S. F., Woodhouse, L. D., Auld, E. M., Green B. L., Quinn, S. C., & Airhihenbuwa, C. O. (2006). *Framing a transdisciplinary research agenda in health education to address health disparities and social inequities: A road map for SOPHE action*. Retrieved October 29, 2007, from http://www.heb.sagepub.com/cgi/content/abstract/33/4/531.

Harvard School of Public Health, Robert Wood Johnson Foundation, & ICR. (2005). *Americans' views of disparities in health care: A poll*. Retrieved October 29, 2007, from http://www.rwjf.org/file/research/Disparties_Survey_Report.pdf.

Henry J. Kaiser Family Foundation. (2006). *Disparities in health care growing for Latinos, gap closes for other minorities*. Retrieved September 20, 2007, from http://www.kaisernetwork.org/Daily_reports/rep_index.cfm?DR_ID=34967.

Henry J. Kaiser Family Foundation. (2007). *The health status of African American men in the United States*. Retrieved October 10, 2007, from http://www.kff.org/minorityhealth/7630.cfm.

Hu, T. W., Snowden, L. K., Jerrell, J. M., & Nguyen, T. D. (1991). Ethnic populations in public mental health: Services choice and level of use. *American Journal of Public Health, 81*(11), 1429–1434.

Indian Health Service. (2007). *Facts on Indian health disparities*. Retrieved February 15, 2007, from http://www.ihs.gov/Files/DispartiesFacts_Jan2007.doc.

Krieger, N., & Sidney, S. (1996). Racial discrimination and blood pressure: The CARDIA study of young black and white adults. *American Journal of Public Health, 86*(10), 1370–1378.

LaVeist, T. A. (2002). *Segregation, poverty, and empowerment: The health consequences for African Americans*. In T. A. LaVeist (Ed.), *Race, ethnicity, and health: A public health reader* (pp. 76–96). San Francisco: Jossey-Bass.

Mayberry, R. M., Mili, F., & Olifi, E. (2002). *Racial and ethnic differences in access to medical care*. In T. A. LaVeist (Ed.), *Race, ethnicity, and health. A public health reader* (pp. 163–197). San Francisco: Jossey-Bass.

Mendoza, F. S., Ventura, S. J., Valdez, R. B., Castillo, R. O., Saldivar, L. E., Baisden, K., et al. (1991). Selected measures of health status for Mexican-American, mainland Puerto Rican, and Cuban-American children. *Journal of the American Medical Association, 265*(2), 227–232.

National Academy of Sciences. (2002). *Unequal treatment: What health care system administrators need to know about racial and ethnic disparities in health care*. Retrieved February 15, 2007, from http://www.iom.edu/Object.File/Master/14/973/DisparitiesAdm.8pg.pdf.

National Academy of Sciences. (2005). *Addressing racial and ethnic health care disparities.* Retrieved February 15, 2007, from http://www.iom.edu/?id=33252.

National Cancer Institute. (2007). *Research topics: Tobacco control monograph series.* Retrieved November 15, 2007, from http://cancercontrol.cancer.gov/tcrb/monographs.

National Center for Health Statistics. (2004). *Health, United States, 2004: With chartbook on trends in the health of Americans.* Retrieved November 15, 2007, from http://www.cdc.gov/nchs/data/hus/hus04.pdf.

National Institutes of Health. (2000). *NIH strategic research plan to reduce and ultimately eliminate health disparities.* Retrieved September 13, 2007, from http://www.nih.gov/about/hd/strategicplan.pdf.

Niederhauser, V. P., & Stark, M. (2005). *Narrowing the gap in childhood immunization disparities.* Retrieved October 15, 2007, from http://www.pediatricnursing.net/ce/2007/article10380388.pdf.

Office of Minority Health and Health Disparities. (2006, May). *Highlights in minority health and health disparities.* Retrieved October 29, 2007, from http://www.cdc.gov/omhd/Highlights/2006/HMay06AAPI.htm.

Office on Women's Health. (2006, November). *Minority women's health: Asian American/Pacific Islanders and Native Hawaiians.* Retrieved October 16, 2007, from http://www.4women.gov/minority/asianamerican.

Partnership for Prevention. (2007). *Preventive care: A national profile on use, disparities, and health benefits.* Retrieved October 15, 2007, from http://www.prevent.org/content/view/129/72.

Ramsey, D. J., Wear, M. L., Labarante, D. R., & Nichman, M. Z. (1997). Sex and ethnic differences in the use of myocardial revascularization procedures in Mexican American and non-Hispanic whites. *Journal of Clinical Epidemiology, 50*(5), 603–609.

Smedley, B. P., Strith, A. Y., & Nelson, A. R., Committee on Understanding and Eliminating Racial and Ethnic Disparities in Health Care, Institute of Medicine (Eds.). (2002). *Unequal treatment: Confronting racial and ethnic disparities in health care.* Washington, DC: National Academies Press.

Society for Public Health Education. (2006). *SOPHE journals to examine new research and practice solutions to eliminate health disparities* (Press Release). Washington, DC: Author.

U.S. Census Bureau. (2006). *Income climbs, poverty stabilizes, uninsured rate increases.* Retrieved October 16, 2007, from http://www.census.gov.

U.S. Census Bureau. (2007). *The American community—American Indians and Alaska Natives: 2004.* Retrieved October 16, 2007, from http://www.census.gov/prod/2007pubs/acs-07.pdf.

U.S. Department of Health and Human Services. (2006, December). *Healthy people 2010: Midcourse review.* Washington, DC: Government Printing Office.

U.S. Department of Health and Human Services. (2007). *Data/statistics.* Retrieved October 16, 2007, from http://www.omhrc.gov/templates/browse.aspx?lvlID=53.

Vega, W. A., & Amaro, H. (1994). Latino outlook: Good health, uncertain prognosis. *Annual Review of Public Health, 15,* 39–67.

Wells, K., Klap, R., Koike, A., & Sherbourne, C. (2001). Ethnic disparities in unmet need for alcoholism, drug abuse, and mental health care. *American Journal of Psychiatry, 158*(12), 2027–2032.

Williams, D. R. (1999). Race, socioeconomic status, and health: The added effects of racism and discrimination. *Annals of the New York Academy of Science, 89*(1), 173–188.

Zimmerman, R. K. (2007). Impact of the 2004 influenza vaccine shortage on patients from inner city health centers. *Journal of Urban Health, 84*(3), 389–399.

CHAPTER

3

CULTURAL COMPETENCE AND HEALTH EDUCATION

EMOGENE JOHNSON VAUGHN

LEARNING OBJECTIVES

After completing this chapter, you will be able to

- Understand the broader meaning of the term *cultural competence.*
- Recognize principles and practices used in the application of cultural competence.
- Recognize the importance of training and of acquiring skills in cultural competence.

INTRODUCTION

In this chapter, the multiple dimensions of *cultural competence* will be covered, including models, frameworks, and constructs that exemplify the principles and practices used in a variety of health education settings and the training and related skills needed by the health educator.

Although the ongoing Healthy People initiative continues to emphasize and promote the adoption of healthy behaviors for all Americans, the successes of this initiative are dimming as old problems like obesity and lack of physical activity exacerbate poor health and as challenges continue to abound, as measured by the initiative's longstanding goals. First, gaps in life expectancies and years of quality health still exist disproportionately; second, access to and availability of health care and services are still limited for minorities and are being made worse by inflationary health care costs and a lack of affordable health insurance; and third, health disparities among Americans remain a major concern.

For at least two decades, according to Braithwaite and Taylor (1992), too little focus has been given to cultural competence as a strategy for effective health education or as a strategy to close the prevailing health gaps and disparities. In 1999, with the launching of the Reach 2010 project (American Association for Health Education [AAHE], 2007), greater and growing interest has been directed toward culturally appropriate and community-driven strategies to address selected diseases and health problems disproportionately affecting specific racial and ethnic groups. The future quality of the health and wellness of all cultural groups depends not only on the quality of U.S. health education in relation to the diversity of the population but also on how well prepared the new generation of health professionals is for working with that diverse population. Professional organizations like the American Association for Health Education are responding to this challenge. The AAHE has published *Cultural Awareness and Sensitivity: Guidelines for Health Educators* (1994), and a position statement on cultural competence (2006). Also, in a joint venture with the Health Resources and Services Administration (HRSA), AAHE published a supplemental issue of its journal (the *American Journal of Health Education*) that highlighted cultural competence as a strategy for "eliminating health disparities for vulnerable populations" (see, for example, Montes, Johnston, Airhihenbuwa, & Gotsch, 1998). Whereas the demographics of health professionals remain rather constant and homogeneous, the demographics of their minority clients are growing more and more varied. Consequently, the demand for cultural skills in the health professional is becoming more challenging to meet. In the interim, health education programs continue to have too little regard for culture-specific content, for the cultural qualifications of the messenger, and for how the message should be delivered. That is, the process of *translating* programs has been underused and overlooked as a strategic action plan. Many community health promotion programs have failed due to lack of financial support, an inability to reach target populations, especially those of high risk, and of equal concern, an inability to design content that is meaningful in light of the health beliefs, practices, and behaviors of the community to be served. The future realization of healthy lifestyles among specific target populations traditionally underserved, or yet to be served, and underrepresented may depend on this country's ability to effect changes in currently unhealthy lifestyles and on its efforts to prepare health professionals for working with racially and culturally diverse individuals and groups. When we ignore multicultural differences, then a void exists in the health education process.

Health gaps and disparities continue to widen because goals and behavioral outcomes may be set that are not shared by those of a different race or culture (Sue, 2001).

With the establishment of the National Center for Cultural Competence, the Centers for Minority Health Initiatives and Cultural Competency, and other national and state resources (Johnston, Denboba, & Honberg, 1998), a more concerted effort is being directed toward making improvements in the skills, practices, attitudes, policies, and environments of health professionals working in culturally diverse settings (Ahmann, 2002). Today's concern is that those providing the product, service, or education actually look, talk, and act like those receiving the product, service, or education. This "look like me" approach is very convincing in visual media advertising. So this approach may be just as effective in health education and the related areas of health services and health promotion. Whether the product is an intervention or training program, a prescription drug, a call-in to a radio talk show host, a seminar with a nutritionist, a set of pictures in a magazine, or the text message in a health pamphlet, there is a need for a common *translator.* People who share similar cultural patterns, values, experiences, and problems are more likely to feel comfortable with and understand each other, and this enables translation (Levy, 1985). This "look like me" approach becomes a greater challenge as the U.S. population becomes more and more racially and culturally diverse. Thus the need for cultural competence becomes greater too.

The goal should be to increase health educators' skill, knowledge, and comfort levels when interacting with people of color and people from diverse backgrounds. Within this goal the aim is to provide *multicultural training* and experiences that challenge, stretch, and expand the health professional's world and local view in any health setting. Higher cultural competence is perceived when programs or services are culturally responsive, cultural differences are acknowledged and reframed, and images of color and racial blindness are projected (Atkinson, Thompson, & Grant, 1993). Addressing the cultural competence of health professionals, individually and collectively, and particularly those who are health educators, has now gained attention as another strategy to increase America's adoption of healthy behaviors.

Because health and social practices are usually the manifestations of cultural beliefs and individual life experiences (Braithwaite & Taylor, 1992), understanding and developing cultural competence should be of growing concern to health educators and other health professionals. Luquis and Pérez (2003) and Pérez, Gonzalez, and Pinzon-Pérez (2006, p. 102) urge health educators to "assume their inherent responsibility" and to be proactive in forging a partnership and collaboration with federal agencies in establishing "discipline-specific" guidelines and interventions for cultural competence in the field of health education. In the academic arenas of counseling, psychology, education, business, and advertising, the consensus is that through being able to act as translators, the culturally competent are more likely to be the key to success in getting people to adopt healthy behaviors and in creating supportive environmental conditions, thereby reducing the health gaps and disparities in this country. "Cultural competence may mean the difference between a successful and an unsuccessful program" (Davis & Rankin, 2006, p. 250).

DEFINING CULTURAL COMPETENCE

Full consensus on a definition for *cultural competence* does not exist. The meaning of the term may vary with a user's perspective. Luquis and Pérez (2003) explore several professional organizations' definitions of this term. Their identification of key terms within their sample of definitions helps to show both the commonalities and contrasts in the meaning and usage of this term.

An example from a professional organization is that the 2000 Joint Committee on Health Education and Promotion Terminology of the AAHE (Joint Committee on Health Education and Promotion Terminology, 2002) has added this term to its updated terminology list and has defined cultural competence as "the ability of an individual to understand and respect values, attitudes, beliefs, and mores that differ across cultures, and to consider and respond appropriately to these differences in planning, implementing, and evaluating health education and promotion programs and interventions" (p. 5).

More commonly, the term is defined from a racial or culture-specific perspective. Defining cultural competence from this perspective involves a simplistic view. That is, an individual with cultural competence is the person who looks, talks, and acts like health education program clients (students, patients, and other participants) and who shares, understands, and respects their culture, history, values, preferences, and social status and their community. This person is a translator and is seen as "one of us," invited and welcomed, and received and valued by the participant, the group, and the community.

In contrast, cultural competence may be defined from the more universal vantage point of an institution or system. From this perspective a culturally competent health service delivery institution or system is one that "acknowledges and incorporates— at all levels—the importance of culture, assessment of cross-cultural relations, vigilance toward the dynamics that result from cultural differences, expansion of cultural knowledge, and adaptation of services to meet culturally unique needs" (Betancourt, Green, Carillo, & Ananeh-Firempong, 2003, p. 294). In this organizational context, *cultural competence is the ability to serve multicultural populations.* This perspective implies that cultural competence can be defined as a set of values, behaviors, attitudes, practices, and policies within an organization or program or among staff that enables people to work effectively with diverse groups. From a practical view, greater consensus and commonality are found when cultural competence is expansively and collectively viewed from a multidimensional perspective that includes knowledge of the health beliefs, values, preferences, practices, and skills involved and also general knowledge of the race, ethnic group, individuals, communities, systems, and organizations involved.

Multiple Dimensions of Cultural Competence

The dimensions of cultural competence may vary across multidimensional models. However, some of the more complex models actually combine the simplistic view of cultural competence with a more universal and system perspective. Even from a simplistic view, the dimensions of cultural competence are more than a list of descriptors; rather, they represent the interaction and integration of an individual's or group's health beliefs, values, preferences, and practices with knowledge of the race and ethnic group. Likewise, from a universal perspective, the dimensions of cultural competence are more than a list of elements of the health service system. From this expansive perspective they represent an organizational, structural, and clinical framework that entails an understanding of the importance of social and cultural influences on clients' health beliefs and behaviors and the integration and interaction of these factors with those who provide the product, service, or health education. Dumas, Rollock, Prinz, Hops, and Blechman (1999) argue that all such dimensions are legitimate aspects of cultural competence, but also advocate the reorganization of the dimensions into a unified concept that provides a useful sense of direction for practice, education and training, and research. A look at selected models, frameworks, and constructs provides a structural view of how the many dimensions can be reorganized.

Models, Frameworks, and Constructs

Although models, frameworks, and constructs provide guidance and direction in explaining complex and abstract ideas, understanding cultural competence is a challenge magnified by that competence's own diversity. Cultural competence draws from the knowledge base of many disciplines in an attempt to establish a theoretical orientation for translating the many sociodemographic variables of a given group. Addressing the ways the term *multiculturalism* obscures the reality that race and culture present many different aspects, Helms and Richardson (1997) suggest a philosophical theoretical construct that is responsive to the dynamics of diverse demographic groups. They also acknowledge that a philosophical approach allows a focus on the strengths, competencies, and skills of a demographic group, rather than an emphasis on group deficiencies and a group's need for remediation based on a standard of the majority group.

The multiple dimensions of cultural competence (MDCC) model proposed by Sue (2001) is both comprehensive and inclusive. This three-dimensional model addresses the attributes of competence from a race- and culture-specific dimension; focuses on culture at individual, professional, organizational, and societal levels; and builds on knowledge, awareness of attitudes and beliefs, and skills as the components of cultural competence. The model is expansive because each of its elements involves a confluence of these three major dimensions.

The MDCC model's three-dimensional concept can be helpful to health professionals in defining cultural competence. There are three points of interest here. First, the model moves the definition of cultural competence beyond mere racial identification and allows a comfortable dialogue in order to address cultural competence with multicultural understanding and sensitivity. This comprehensive and inclusive approach is one of the model's strengths. Further, the MDCC model allows analysis to focus on the individual (a single or micro unit of measure) or on other units all the way up to the full society (a composite or macro unit of measure). In this way the model allows inclusive recognition of the uniqueness of the individual, the shared values and beliefs of the group, and universal societal attributes. The model also takes multiple forces (gender, religion, socioeconomic class, and so forth) in addition to race into account when considering cultural competence in relation to the individual, group, or society.

Second, the MDCC model uses three groups of components to clarify the meaning of cultural competence. The culturally competent health professional, organization, or system is expected to hold a set of beliefs, a knowledge base, and a set of skills that add to the successful responsiveness of the individual, group, organization, or system. Inherent to this successful responsiveness is a hint of social justice in that the culturally competent individual or health professional, group, organization, or system should provide equal access and opportunity, be inclusive, and remove individual and systemic barriers. With these three groups of components of cultural competence outlined, the term *cultural competence* can be defined more clearly as "the ability to engage in actions or to create conditions that maximize the optimal development of client and client systems" (Sue, 2001, p. 802).

Third, the MDCC model is useful to the health professional because it advocates a top-down approach to acquiring cultural competence. In simple terms, the model recognizes that organizations and systems must be reconditioned to become culturally competent before their frontline workers, such as health educators, can be similarly reconditioned. Cultural competence is seen as the thread that links society to the organization, the organization to the professionals, and the professionals to the individuals and groups they serve. Without this top-down reconditioning, a clash is imminent between the professionals who are using cultural knowledge and skills and the culturally incompetent organization that employs them. With the MDCC model, Sue advises organizational leaders to proceed through the social reconditioning process in a concerted fashion, driving cultural competence downward through the organizational, professional, and individual levels.

Another model of potential interest to the health educator defines cultural competence within a framework that links communication to health outcomes (Betancourt et al., 2003). Betancourt's framework establishes three points of intervention—organizational, structural, and clinical—to represent the many dimensions of cultural competence at multiple levels useful to the health educator. The complexity of cultural competence is highlighted within each intervention point and in relation to sociocultural barriers that affect health education and the adoption of healthy behaviors.

For an organization, the first question raised by this framework is the following: *Does the diversity of the leadership and the workforce representing the health needs of individuals, groups, and communities reflect the racial and ethnic composition of the general population?* (Betancourt et al., 2003). Further, are the policies, procedures, and delivery systems suited to serve the intended population? Lastly, do the persons providing health education serve as role models, and as teachers, do they "look like me"? The sociocultural barriers that make it necessary to ask these questions also point to a need for health education that arises from diversity in leadership and in the workforce and that is supported by policies, procedures, and delivery systems that provide services from which the targeted population can receive benefits. It is expected that the organization can ensure that services are available and accessible, that they are provided by a diverse health education team, and that the targeted population uses the services and finds satisfaction in the quality of the service and a racial concordance with the providers (Betancourt et al., 2003, p. 296). Thus, using Betancourt's framework, cultural competence at the organizational level is measured by the outcomes of a communication process used by the health professional.

Some of the same sociocultural barriers found at the organizational level may be present in the structural interventions of this framework. Betancourt addresses sociocultural barriers in such areas as oral and written language, comprehension and compliance, and access to health education providers. Cultural competence in using structural interventions may require an interpreter during appointments to read materials aloud and to verify instructional communications between provider and client. Awareness and adoption of healthy behaviors—the ultimate goals in the health education process—are more likely to result when the target population understands the health education process, the messenger, and the message.

Clinical or community barriers in Betancourt's cultural competence framework are found in the interaction between the provider and the participant or family. Effective interventions at the clinical or community level depend on the health educator's creation and capture of opportunities to understand, accept, appreciate, explore, and integrate the sociocultural differences that exist between the provider and the receiver. Without such opportunities the health educator–participant relationship may fail to be mutually productive. A lack of trust and differences in spiritual values and in health beliefs, practices, and attitudes are linked to participant dissatisfaction with the health education process, programs, and providers; failures in compliance; and poor communications, all of which are deterrents to the adoption of healthy behaviors.

In summary, organizationally, structurally, and clinically, cultural competence entails a framework that allows an understanding of the importance of social and cultural influences on an individual's health beliefs and behaviors and that allows a consideration of these personal factors at any point of intervention. Succinctly, Betancourt's framework defines organizational cultural competence as the ability to ensure that the leadership and workforce of a system is diverse and representative of its target population. Structural cultural competence is the ability of a system to provide full access to quality services and programs for everyone in the target population. Cultural competence in relation to the community is the ability of providers to communicate with clients to acquire and integrate knowledge of their sociocultural factors and to use that knowledge to encourage awareness and adoption of healthy behaviors. In essence Betancourt's concept provides direction for the implementation of programs, and it offers an expanded view of cultural competence that is useful to the health professional in the effective delivery of health education information, programs, and services to a multicultural population.

For the health educator the challenge is to identify the model, framework, or construct that best identifies the characteristics most important to the health education process.

These characteristics vary among individuals and groups, and the process must be adaptable. The health education process is not "one size fits all." Therefore cultural competence is an evolving ability to identify which competencies work best for what aspects of diversity and an ability to integrate client demographics in order to understand the client; to identify problems, issues, and concerns; and to bring forth the resources useful to the mutually agreed upon solution that best suits the client. (Additional models, frameworks, and constructs are discussed in Chapter Six.)

RELATED AND DISCIPLINE-SPECIFIC CULTURAL COMPETENCE PRINCIPLES

The 2000 Joint Committee on Health Education and Promotion Terminology (2002) defines *health education* as "any combination of planned learning experiences based on sound theories that provide individuals, groups, and communities the opportunity to acquire information and the skills needed to make quality health decisions" (p. 6). From this vantage point the field of health education may be explained by, first, what it covers (content and scope). As a content area, health education is an umbrella structure; its knowledge base and scope run the gamut of health determinants, from lifestyles to environment, heredity, media, health care, and culture. Because health and health education are multidisciplinary, their scope is broad and far reaching.

Second, taking a traditional approach and drawing from a concept of health as a process or function, Green, Kreuter, Deeds, and Partridge (1980) describe health education as "any designed combination of methods to facilitate voluntary adaptations of behavior conducive to health" (p. xiv). As a process this design involves planning, influencing, motivating, and supporting individuals, families, groups, and communities to adopt healthy lifestyles. Thus the skills and competencies of the health educator must include a broad knowledge base and a wide skill set. Further complicating the qualifications of professionals is their need for cultural competence in a variety of settings and often in a culture other than their own.

The following discussions present some helpful principles that can guide the individual health educator and the profession in developing personal and discipline-specific cultural competence.

Principles for Personal Cultural Competence

Sue (2001) offers four principles to achieve personal cultural competence that can be readily applied to health education. First, cultural competence comes from the kind of firsthand knowledge and varied experiences that teach health educators about the beliefs, behaviors, values, preferences, and so forth of one or more races or ethnic groups. The caveat here is not to rely on the media and the opinions of others, which are often fraught with misinformation, misunderstandings, stereotypes, discrimination, prejudices, and biases. Rather, cultural competence should evolve from a variety of personal experiences. The second principle is to learn about other cultures by interacting with a wide sample, one that includes variety in age and gender and also the rich and the poor, educated and uneducated, strong and weak, and healthy and sick. Following this principle guides health educators to a balanced view of the culture under study. The third principle is for health educators to add to their factual knowledge base real-life experiences shared with the cultural group. The fourth principle is for health educators to address, through informal and formal assessments, their own biases and the biases of persons around them. This last principle is especially difficult to follow for it requires health educators to accept responsibility for moving out of their comfort zones.

These four principles make it obvious that developing cultural competence requires personal growth. It may be uncomfortable, even painful, to undertake the close, critical, and honest inspection needed to evaluate one's own sense of decency, morality, fairness, and justice. Thus, personal growth is the outcome of one's willingness to challenge one's own social conditioning and cultural incompetence.

Principles for Discipline-Specific Cultural Competence

The field of health education and the professional organizations associated with this field are also guided by set of principles that are helpful in making the health professional culturally competent. Several discipline-specific principles are briefly explored here. Perhaps paramount among the many principles in this field is that the adoption of healthy behaviors is voluntary (Green et al., 1980). The impact of lifestyle exceeds all other health determinants. Healthy and unhealthy behaviors are decided upon primarily by the individual. Coercion is not the desired means of changing behavior, nor is it effective in getting people to adopt what should be *voluntary* healthy behaviors. In addition to motivating the adoption of health-promoting behaviors, culturally competent health educators show sensitivity and responsiveness in identifying and supporting healthy behaviors that are culturally related.

A second principle that the profession follows is that health and social practices are usually the manifestations of cultural beliefs and individual life experiences (Braithwaite & Taylor, 1992). Implicit in this principle is that behavioral change can occur only within the context of a person's culture and life experiences. For some minority groups, pedagogically tying past history into current sociopolitical issues is essential in motivating behavioral change (Marbley, Bonner, McKisick, Henfield, & Watts, 2007). For example, all cultures do not agree that today's obesity problem is escalating. Whereas in one cultural group the height-weight charts may be the rule to follow, in another culture a little extra weight may mean "eating fine."

A third principle that the health education profession follows is tied to the medical model that is built on the premise that the causes and cures of diseases are scientifically founded. Conversely, certain cultural groups may be guided by beliefs passed down through generations that support the existence of a higher being or spirit that will grant them good health. A group with cultural practices that reflect harmony with the environment may find its practices challenged by the use of medicines prescribed by the medical profession. Thus cultural awareness and sensitivity become essential in accepting, establishing, and promoting compliance to medical treatment.

A growing concern over the lack of multicultural representation in leadership roles and in the workforce in the field of health education relates to the fourth principle, which is that compliance with and adoption of healthy behaviors are strongly linked to the cultural orientation of the messenger. Clients' "look like me," "talk like me," and "act like me" perceptions are critical to the influence that the health educator has on them. The absence of language barriers, of differences in health beliefs, and of problems with accessing health care produces a trusting relationship that promotes comprehension, compliance, and hope for a mutually acceptable health resolution.

Inherent in the personal and discipline-specific health education principles described here are the basic principles of participation, empowerment, and cultural sensitivity, which must also be addressed if health education programs are to be successful in any setting. These and the many other principles that relate to the field of health education help us to further define cultural competence in health education and to adopt codes of ethics, standards, and practices that are multiculturally sensitive to the persons in the profession and to those who are served by the profession (Deeds, Cleary, & Neiger, 1996).

CULTURALLY COMPETENT PRACTICES IN DIVERSE SETTINGS

Cultural beliefs and experiences, when properly understood, can be used to promote the success of health education programs in any cultural setting (Braithwaite & Taylor, 1992, 2001). The health educator is trained to work appropriately in a variety of settings—including the community, schools, churches, industry, hospitals, and businesses—and with individuals, families, and groups. Each of these settings is culture bound and may require the health educator to possess cultural competence that is unique, sensitive, and linguistically appropriate to the setting of the target culture (Braithwaite & Taylor, 1992).

The Community

In the community, the health educator interacts with key formal and lay leaders and large groups of people sharing an interest in a health problem or issue. The cultural competence needed here must address the global health beliefs, practices, and preferences of this group. Programs, services, and resources must match what the community deems to be important and must be provided at a time that fits the conditions of this targeted population.

Schools

In the school setting, factors such as age, language styles, peer influence, crowded curriculum schedules, part-time jobs and extra class activities, full-time working parents, and technological devices may be external forces competing with the recruitment of students to participate in the adoption of healthy behaviors. Teenagers see themselves as invincible; thus they care little about choosing the nutrient density of milk over the extra calories in sweet drinks. Social-networking platforms, such as Facebook, MySpace, e-mail, chat rooms, and podcasting, supersede the desire to "shoot some hoops" for the nonathletic youth. The cultural competence of the health educator in the school setting requires creativity to influence this age group to adopt health-enhancing behaviors. Ideas involving hip-hop dancing and changing fashions in clothes and hairstyles may be typical of the kinds of approaches the health educator can use to motivate youths and teens to exercise and to become more nutrition and weight conscious. Cultural competence in the school setting implies knowledge of the specific needs and interests of this target population. Marbley et al. (2007) suggest that cultural competence also requires a culture-specific pedagogy that bridges the gap between the cultural past of the group and the daily issues of the present in the hope of directing participants' future aspirations.

Churches and Other Faith-Based Organizations

Health educators often rely on theoretical frameworks like health belief models to explain health behaviors. Health beliefs that advocate that the power to achieve lies within the inner self of the individual may be in direct contrast to the teachings of a client's church or the beliefs of his or her faith. The cultural competence of the health educator working or volunteering in a church or faith-based organization requires knowledge of religion, spiritual beliefs, and practices and their impact on the attitudes, beliefs, and behaviors of the churchgoer. Oftentimes there is a conflict between what the health educator views as scientifically factual and what the congregation or church leaders believe or preach as spiritually acceptable. For example, congregations may learn that to practice a faith "as small as a mustard seed" is sufficient to guide them through challenges of disease, death, and other misfortunes, secure in the belief that their faith will prevail. The spirituality of many cultures requires the culturally competent health educator to balance science with faith. Compliance with and adoption of healthy behaviors rest upon this balance. (See Chapter Five for a full discussion on the topic of religion and spirituality.)

Individual and Family Settings

The health educator working with individuals and families is often confronted with personal and family values that differ from the values among the majority population or those held by the educator. Encouraging individuals and families to adopt healthy behaviors voluntarily may be more successful when a partnership is established that acknowledges and respects these differences. Here cultural competence implies a flexible and collaborative effort by all parties involved. There may be an opportunity here (one not unique to this setting) for the individual or the family to recognize that reaching the goal of being a healthier person or a healthier family is a solution-seeking venture where one's culture may either hinder or help in the adoption of healthy behaviors. Consider a family where children who complete their schoolwork early are rewarded with unlimited television watching and thus they oversleep each morning and miss breakfast. Such a family lifestyle and values probably limit the academic success of the children. The culturally competent health educator will explore with the family a mutually agreeable solution that maximizes the children's success in school, provides a morning nutrition source, promotes limits on television watching and on selection of programs, and sets a reasonable bedtime hour. In this example, cultural competence is the ability to see the whole problem and to apply the appropriate skills to engage the whole family in its own solution.

ISSUES, CONCERNS, AND STRATEGIES IN MULTICULTURAL TRAINING

The need for cultural competence is apparent in a variety of health education settings, but what are the concerns and strategies when it comes to training people for that competence? The issues surrounding the ongoing lack of cultural competence and the strategies for achieving that competence appear to be global and individual, respectively. Globally, there appears to be a perception that cultural competence is important and needed; yet resources for achieving cultural competence are limited, as pointed out in a national survey by Redican, Stewart, Johnson, and Frazee (1994), conducted more than a decade ago. Of the college and university professional preparation programs in health education responding to the survey, slightly more than half offered training in cultural competence. This training, they reported, was provided by individual faculty or occurred during an internship experience. Redican et al. (1994) suggested that this finding indicated benign neglect toward providing these educational opportunities. Two other surveys have followed Redican et al.'s research. Doyle, Liu, and Ancona (1996) conducted a similar study, and their results suggested that the commitment by the professional preparation programs of colleges and universities to course-based cultural diversity was weak and that cultural competence training was particularly lacking.

More recently, Luquis, Pérez, and Young (2006) conducted a similar survey distributed to about 255 college and university professional preparation programs in health education. About 27 percent reported offering a course entirely directed toward cultural competence, 88 percent reported that cultural competence was addressed in core courses, and 82 percent reported that cultural competence training was offered through instructional activities. Oddly enough, 87 percent of the reporting programs referred students to other departments or programs for courses dealing with topics related to cultural competence. Almost as high a percentage (88 percent) of these programs indicated that they did not provide cultural competence training to the faculty. The benign neglect characterized by Redican et al. (1994) has seemingly continued to the present day.

On the individual level, numerous strategies exist through which the health educator can attempt, almost alone, to gain the experiences, skills, and resources that will lead to a higher level of personal cultural competence. Yet a review of the models of Sue (2001) and Betancourt et al. (2003) or of the basic principles for planning or practicing cultural competence shows that having support from within the work environment is consistently advocated. Working individually, the health educator is limited by what can be accomplished by one person, whereas support (opportunities for training and resources) given at the organizational level could make such training exponentially further reaching. However, organizational benign neglect persists, forcing the health educator to forge ahead as a lone ranger in acquiring the cultural competence that will be a critical component of his or her skill repertoire.

Further, the weak interest and efforts shown by professional preparation programs and the reality that certification or licensing agencies do not currently use cultural competence models or frameworks make it imperative for health educators to take the initiative for their own professional development. In alignment with the AAHE (2006) position statement on cultural competency, Stoy (2000) advocates an action plan for improving intercultural competence that the health educator can follow in an individual effort to expand his or her skill repertoire. Stoy emphasizes the need and provides examples of activities to do to acquire knowledge, increase awareness, and accept emotional challenges as a part of a personal commitment to improve cultural competence applicable in a variety of health education settings. More specifically, Stoy promotes the activities of exploring culture and reviewing the works of anthropologists to grasp a more meaningful view of culture and an understanding of culture theory. Stoy recognizes the important benefits that can be gained by health educators in becoming more aware of and knowledgeable about the cultural differences and commonalities that exist. Equally as important is health educators' need to expand personal opportunities to be a part of and to interact with individuals from cultures outside of the educators' own environment. Capitalizing on the opportunity just to talk to persons of cultures dissimilar to one's own, reading about the health issues and problems of other cultures, and participating in cross-cultural simulations are a few of the strategies for acquiring real or near-real experiences. Lastly, Stoy strongly encourages health educators to accept the emotional challenge that results from confronting what is learned about cultures and, just as important, the challenge that results from becoming aware of cultural ideas that need to be unlearned.

The Competencies Update Project and Professional Expectations

The work done by the National Commission for Health Education Credentialing, Society for Public Health Education, and American Association for Health Education (2006) helps to identify the responsibilities and competencies of a health educator. Further, these 7 responsibilities, 35 competencies, and 163 subcompetencies, which specify the scope of practice in the field of health education, can also be and should be used to conduct a personal assessment of one's progress toward reaching cultural competence in each of the 7 responsibility areas. The health educator, once a needs assessor and a program planner, must extend those roles to become a culturally competent needs assessor and program planner, one whose responsibility may be appropriately displayed in seeking sources of information that help to identify the cultural needs of the community to be served. This extension also includes determining the resources needed to get diverse youths to participate in community programs designed to help them develop culturally based life skills, such as saying no to drugs or abstaining from sexual activity. The culturally competent health educator can be instrumental in guiding youths toward learning via role playing and applying refusal skills in simulated and real-life situations that represent and fit the culture in question.

As advocate, communicator, and planner, the culturally competent health educator can be instrumental in seeking resources that relate to a minority culture, such as using brochures written in the group's language or translating a script for a role play into the desired language. Strategies for ensuring that a health education program is culturally and linguistically appropriate are offered by Davis and Rankin (2006) and include the identification of the intended audience, use of appropriate terminology, and use of native speakers to both translate and back translate.

In the role of culturally competent facilitator or evaluator, the health educator's role may be to bring groups of participants together to share in forums or focus groups to identify specific needs and concerns of a particular neighborhood. Here, the health educator may aim to create a tapestry effect by *weaving* in the views of all participants while highlighting the way each view adds to the color and texture of the tapestry while also strengthening its representation. Developing a sense of *bonding,* as described by Dordoni and Larson (2003), can result in a greater diversity of participation in a less threatening environment.

In the roles of implementer, administrator, and evaluator the health educator may work closely with someone with cultural and political ties to the community to address, in the most culturally appropriate manner, the strategies and resources for removing the cause of a neighborhood issue. Health educators can increase their level of cultural competence in this setting by using the facsimile case study approach suggested by Pinzon and Pérez for studying the Latino community (1997) and by using AAHE's 1994 guidelines for health educators to grasp a capsule view of the historical and ethnographic profiles of the major minority groups in the United States.

Lastly, in the role of resource person, the culturally competent health educator works well with persons responsible for decision making and implementation. Here the educator may actually study a health issue, such as the identification of factors that lead to poor communication due to language barriers. Or the health educator may seek training in the use of complementary, alternative, or holistic medicine and integrative healing to increase his or her cultural competence (Pinzon-Pérez, 2005) and to understand the resistance and reluctance of members of a minority group when they are asked to use modern medicine and technology.

In any role that they play, health educators are asked to assess the issue at hand from the perspective of the dissimilar culture represented. To do so is to recognize that every cultural transaction is likely to be racialized (Hassouneh-Phillips & Beckett, 2003), genderized, age prompted, or value laden. This is to say that race, gender, age, values, and beliefs, as cultural variables, add an extra layer of complexity to the principles of participation, empowerment, and cultural sensitivity that must be addressed if health education programs are to be successful in any setting (Braithwaite & Taylor, 2001, p. 130). (Further discussion can be found in Chapter Nine, which addresses cultural competence in the health education workforce.)

Stage Development in Cultural Competence Training

Recognizing that the development of cultural competence is an evolving process over time, Carney and Kahn (1984) developed a five-stage model to address the acquisition of the attitudes, sensitivity, knowledge, and skills needed to achieve cultural competence. The model is general but progressive; it is constructed around the concept that one's ability to reach the higher stages is influenced by the challenges and resources in one's work environment. Thus the development of cultural competence is a collaborative effort between the health educator and the work environment. If resources such as appropriate supervision and job-related experiences are available, the health educator is able to mature from stage one toward the higher stages of development.

In stage one, health educators have limited knowledge, stereotypical attitudes, and little to no counseling experience. Lacking accurate views of cultures dissimilar to their own, health educators may construct programs and materials that represent only their own culture. Thus health educators in stage one need training to build a knowledge base on culture theory; this base will include direct experiences gained from internships and volunteer experiences with the dissimilar culture of interest.

Progression from this initial stage involves equipping health educators with a knowledge of the dissimilar culture and its current lifestyle patterns that assists the educators in adapting their attitudes in order to build working relationships with individuals and groups within the culture. Health educators who progress to stage two become more aware of their own cultural views, but they are still challenged by stereotypical and ethnocentric views held by themselves or others. Training in stage two requires a more structured environment that permits a deeper knowledge of the culture and exposure to experiences that challenge the ability to communicate within the venues of the culture. Carney and Kahn (1984) suggest that these training needs can be met through supervision, role modeling, and critical incident experiences that help health educators to deal more critically in assessing their own attitudes, sensitivities, knowledge, and skills. Carney and Kahn also suggest that it is an educator's own critical assessment that really moves him or her to stage three of cultural competence development.

In stage three the health educator may experience a greater sense of personal inadequacy for working with culturally dissimilar groups. Carney and Kahn (1984) account for this effect by pointing out the educator's immaturity in this stage and his or her focus on self. This observation explains why health educators in this stage can find it a struggle to move away from doing things the old way to doing things in a new way to fit a cultural group to which they are still learning how to relate. The training goal of stage three is to assist health educators in appreciating and respecting the differences of others. Supervisory assistance may include experiences that allow health educators to walk in the shoes of the culturally different group, continuing academic study, participation in lectures and workshops, and ongoing self-examination of personal attitudes and sensitivity awareness. The training environment should be supportive in addressing the challenges of these kinds of experiences and should provide diversity and balance in the cultural groups represented by those providing the academic study, lectures, workshops, and self-examination experiences.

In stage four the progress toward cultural competence is measured by health educators' ability to validate the worldview of others while blending their own training and direct experiences to form a new *self-identity.* Training in stage four requires supervision that supports autonomous decisions. The goal at this stage is to assist health educators in making autonomous decisions about their newly altered and emerging personal and professional identities. The field experiences should match the level of cultural competence attained by a health educator. It is at the end of stage four and the beginning of stage five that health educators may seek to change policies and procedures that represent the old way of working with dissimilar cultural groups.

In the last stage, the thrust of a health educator's efforts is to seek action that represents a new way of addressing diversity and embracing the values of social equality and cultural pluralism. Carney and Kahn (1984) suggest that the training needs of stage five can be met by using mentors or professional coaches to guide health educators in exploring their effectiveness as change agents. The mentors or coaches provide a supportive environment, allowing health educators to process the experiences and encouraging them to continue their development of a cultural knowledge base, personal assessments, and skills in working with cultural groups.

Prerequisites to Cultural Competence

Three prerequisites aid in achieving cultural competence: cultural desire, cultural awareness, and cultural sensitivity. Prerequisite to addressing the concerns and needs of a culturally dissimilar client, classroom, small group, or large community audience in a culturally competent way is *cultural desire,* a term defined by Campinha-Bacote (1999) as a "want to" to engage in the process of becoming culturally aware, culturally knowledgeable, and culturally skillful. Further, seeking cultural encounters leads to awareness of and sensitivity to clients' racial, ethnic, or cultural backgrounds. As defined by Redican et al. (1994) *cultural awareness* is being conscious of cultural similarities and differences and *cultural sensitivity* is the knowledge that cultural differences as well as similarities exist. Possession of these three prerequisites allows the development of credibility and trust that promotes a working relationship that can achieve the outcomes and goals set by both the health educator and the dissimilar client, group, or audience. Following the basic principles (Sue, 2001) that should guide the development of cultural competence, and proceeding with respect and consideration, the health professional will find that trust, sensitivity, and credibility will minimize and make resolvable any unintentional errors that result from any lingering cultural incompetence.

In spite of the limited training opportunities that exist in cultural sensitivity and cultural competence (Doyle et al., 1996; Luquis, Pérez, & Young, 2006) and the attitude of benign neglect in college and university health education preparation programs (Redican et al., 1994), "health educators hold an inherent responsibility in assisting organizations to comply with standards and best practices supported by federal funds and in becoming leaders in the development and implementation of programs which are culturally competent" (Pérez et al., 2006, p. 102). Specific personal skills are needed to ensure client compliance and to exhibit the leadership expected of the health educator. Fueled by cultural desire, strengthened by cultural awareness, and reinforced by cultural sensitivity, health educators can develop the sensitivity, trust, and credibility that are pivotal for integrating cultural competence into the work of the profession and its members. This effort can also bring about the trust, sensitivity, and connectedness needed for the target population's participation in successful programs.

Sensitivity. When individuals value and respect their differences in personalities, attitudes, beliefs, behaviors, and environments, they are said to be *culturally sensitive.* These differences can be addressed in many training settings that will provide for political correctness. In workshops, seminars, and other learning adventures, sensitivity experiences are used to bring about a sense of connectedness between the health educator and the client in a working relationship. Often walking in another's shoes, open discussions, role playing and reverse role playing, and questions and responses are used as reflective practices in order to share information, reveal inadequacies, and examine myths and stereotypes. All these activities can bring about an honest exchange that helps health educators to become sensitive to differences and to appreciate diversity and sameness simultaneously. In minority settings the importance of health professionals' sensitivity often comes through when they are judged by how much they care rather than how much they know. The knowledge base of the health professional is valued only when it is obvious to the participant that that knowledge is relevant to the knowledge that the participant's cultural group already holds, needs, desires, or values.

Health educators, individually and collaboratively, can heighten their own and others' awareness of and sensitivity to the importance of cultural diversity and cultural competence in health care settings. The National Center for Cultural Competence (NCCC) offers a self-assessment checklist that can be used by individuals, agencies, or organizations. This thirty-item checklist identifies the frequency of specific behaviors and practices in relation to physical environment, use of materials and resources, communication styles, and values and attitudes. The NCCC also provides further guidance in the planning and implementation of culturally competent principles and practices in the workplace (Ahmann, 2002). Individual assessments promote cultural self-awareness, a vital first step toward cultural sensitivity (Ponterotto, Casas, Suzuki, & Alexander, 1995). This perspective is consistent with the underlying philosophy of many multicultural experiences for health educators, which emphasizes that counselors and educators must understand themselves before they can expect to help or educate others. Being comfortable with both one's own and others' cultural groups indicates an advanced developmental state of cultural awareness and competence.

Trust. Acquiring sensitivity to likenesses and differences between individuals, groups, and communities leads to connectedness and eventually to a sense of trust that transcends racial, age, gender, and economic differences. This transcending trust, according to Thomas and Quinn (1993), may neutralize racial discordance between the health professional and those who are being served when there is a high degree of community engagement and empowerment aimed at maximizing the use of available resources in a concordant environment. Trust or connectedness is evidenced by the use of kinship terms and by efforts to find familiar ways to assist and reinforce survival skills. Culturally competent health professionals recognize the role and recognition of elders in the family and in the community. The "grandmother" in one family may also be the community's "matriarch." Before a family or community can strategize with a health professional to keep kids off the street, in school, employed, or volunteering, that family or community must trust the health professional to know and understand the specific characteristics, needs, and interests of the community being served.

Credibility. A limited sample study conducted by Price and Sidani (2007) asked a group of 200 health clinic patients to identify their preferred characteristics in a clinic health educator. The results failed to show a preference toward race, age, or gender. Rather, a majority in this group believed that a health educator should be a healthy role model. Such a role model is one who does not smoke, has girth control, and practices those behaviors that lead to a higher quality of life. Having visual (looking the part), professional (having been trained and being knowledgeable), and practical (living the role) credibility is essential in influencing others to adopt what the health educator wants them to do.

By experiencing growth and progression toward cultural competence and by acquiring and expressing trust, sensitivity, and credibility, health educators are able to advance in attaining the professional capacities supported by AAHE. More specifically, health educators are expected to have the capacity to communicate respect, to personalize knowledge, to display empathy, to be nonjudgmental, to be flexible in different roles, to demonstrate reciprocal concern, and to tolerate ambiguity (AAHE, 1994, p. 11).

THE COUNSELING ROLE IN HEALTH EDUCATION

There is a strong counseling component in the professional role of the health educator. Thus training for cultural competence centers on the roles of the health educator as a multicultural counselor for dissimilar others. Atkinson et al. (1993) enumerate three factors to consider in selecting an appropriate counseling role. The first factor is identification of the locus of problem etiology. The second factor is acculturation. The third factor is the goals of counseling. An exploration of these three factors helps health educators to understand the different roles that they must play when counseling others from a different culture and when counseling others from a similar culture.

Etiology. The impact of the locus of problem etiology may differ with a group's culture. For some groups, if the problem is external then the resolution may be seen as beyond group members' control or as environmental. Atkinson uses the example of an American from an Asian group who may feel insecure about his new management role because, throughout his life, people have overlooked his interpersonal skills and rewarded his computational skills. Another example can be seen in the case of the health educator who is faced with gender issues when a female student refuses to seek a male-dominated career. The internal origin of gender issues appears in this individual who feels more comfortable in a caring and nurturing position, such as being a nurse or a teacher. The success of health educators in addressing cultural values and practices rests in part with their consideration of the etiology of the problem.

Acculturation. The interactions that come out of circumstances when two cultures meet are numerous and fluid. Sometimes the health educator recognizes that the minority culture looks and acts like the majority culture. At other times the majority culture may be totally immersed in the minority culture. For example, at a health fair for a minority group, a health educator may provide an infrastructure that displays American information about health problems while the health fair workers from the minority community bring their own food, music, dress, and folk medicine and their extended family members. The health fair may be a culmination of the impact that the health educator has had on the dissimilar cultural group and the impact of the dissimilar cultural group on the health educator and the work environment. Thus the health fair becomes a credible celebration of connectedness and of diversity.

Goals of counseling. As a counselor the health educator may facilitate decision making, prevent problems, or remediate problems. Although using the skills of assessment, planning, and identifying resources, the health educator's counseling role is guarded by the basic principles of the profession. For example, the goals of counseling, which determine the health educator's role, are set by the youth or student in a school setting. It is the student who decides the goal for a weight loss effort or a drug, self-image, or school attendance problem. Knowledge of the problem-solving process and the ability to identify antecedents surrounding the problem, and the resources available to remediate the problem, are valuable skills when the health educator determines the role to be played with clients of dissimilar cultures. How much counseling influence (to facilitate decision making, prevent problems, or remediate problems) the health educator has in this setting may readily be determined through knowledge of the student, the student's home life, the community the student represents, previous and current interactions and any rapport between the student and health educator, and a host of other variables that will affect expectations, readiness, and the goals of counseling.

Once consideration is given to these three factors (etiology, acculturation, and counseling goals), the roles of the health educator as a counselor become more extensive. This three-dimensional model constructed by Atkinson can support delineation of the health educator's roles as an adviser, advocate, facilitator, change agent, and consultant. Training for cultural competence should center on these roles.

Many academic and walk-in-my-shoes learning adventures and strategies can assist the health educator who has gained others' trust and has exhibited sensitivity and connectedness in providing advice, speaking for, making happen, altering environmental conditions, and serving as a resource for information. In essence, following a model or a framework, the health educator's progress toward cultural competence evolves through diverse activities encountered in training, experience, guidance, and self-evaluation (Jackson-Carrol, Graham, & Jackson, 1996).

The task of becoming culturally competent is enormous when one considers the desire, the commitment, and the training that are needed and the resources that are only marginally available. If health educators and the health education profession fail to recognize, support, and build cultural competence, a void will continue to exist in the health education process. Nevertheless, making personal efforts to become culturally competent and forging partnerships and collaborations with governmental agencies and other organizations at the professional level to encourage cultural competence are worthy strategies to extend the quality of life of all cultures, to reduce health disparities, and to make health care and services available, accessible, and afforded to all.

CONCLUSION

This chapter has examined diverse meanings of the term *cultural competence,* has addressed basic principles and practices to be considered in the application of cultural competence in different health care and health education settings, and has described the importance of cultural competence training and the acquisition of cultural competence skills. Cultural competence is recognized as a strategy that can be used to increase the effectiveness of health education programs and to reach the nation's health goals. Health education programs are more effective when they are designed and delivered with a specific culture in mind, using basic principles and practices appropriate for the intended audience.

POINTS TO REMEMBER

This chapter examined the need for cultural competence in health education as a strategy to meet the goals of the Healthy People initiative. Selected models, frameworks, and constructs have been used to exemplify and integrate related and basic principles, practices, and training needs for the health educator.

CASE STUDY

Chris graduated from a big Eastern university with a degree in health education over twenty years ago. He then spent twenty years working as program coordinator for college health education in a Midwestern university. Recently, Chris was hired as the program coordinator for the patient health education department in a large hospital in Nevada that serves a largely working-class and diverse population. Chris's new staff consists of three young, well-educated health educators—a Hispanic man, an African American woman, and a white man. These three individuals have a lot of enthusiasm but not much experience in the field of health education and health promotion. A review of a health status profile prepared by the hospital reveals that African American mortality rates from cardiovascular problems are three to four times higher than the rates for the rest of the population. The data also reveal that behavior modification could significantly decrease morbidity and mortality in this population group. Chris has read about successful efforts to reach African Americans through faith-based organizations and decides that given the hospital's lack of rapport with the members of this population group, this would be a good way to reach them. Discuss the following questions:

1. What three cultural competence factors are presented in this case study? Discuss these factors.

2. What additional information would be useful to Chris and his team as they embark on this new initiative?

3. What particular issues do they need to be concerned about as they implement this new initiative?

4. What are three steps that they could take to ensure that their health education endeavor is successful? Discuss these steps.

KEY TERMS

Cultural awareness

Cultural competence

Cultural diversity

Cultural sensitivity

Multicultural training

REFERENCES

Ahmann, E. (2002). Developing cultural competence in health care settings. *Pediatric Nursing, 28*(2), 133–137.

American Association for Health Education. (1994). *Cultural awareness and sensitivity: Guidelines for health educators.* Reston, VA: Author.

American Association for Health Education. (2006). *Cultural competency in health education.* Retrieved February 6, 2008, from http://www.aahperd.org/aahe/pdf_files/CulturalCompetencyInHealthEd.pdf.

American Association for Health Education. (2007). *Eliminating racial and ethnic health disparities* (Fact Sheet). Retrieved August 8, 2007, from http://www.aahperd.org/aahe.

Atkinson, D. R., Thompson, C. E., & Grant, S. K. (1993). Three-dimensional model for counseling racial/ethnic minorities. *The Counseling Psychologist, 21*(2), 257–277.

Betancourt, J. R., Green, A. R., Carillo, J. E., & Ananeh-Firempong, O. (2003). Defining cultural competence: A practical framework for addressing racial/ethnic disparities in health and health care. *Public Health Reports, 118,* 293–302.

Braithwaite, R. L., & Taylor, S. E. (Eds.). (1992). *Health issues in the black community.* San Francisco: Jossey-Bass.

Braithwaite, R. L., & Taylor, S. E. (Eds.). (2001). *Health issues in the black community* (2nd ed.). San Francisco: Jossey-Bass.

Campinha-Bacote, J. (1999). A model and instrument for addressing cultural competence in health care. *Journal of Nursing Education, 38*(5), 203–207.

Carney, C. G., & Kahn, K. B. (1984). Building competencies for effective cross-cultural counseling: A developmental view. *The Counseling Psychologist, 12*(1), 111–119.

Davis, P. C., & Rankin, L. L. (2006). Guidelines for making health education programs more culturally appropriate. *American Journal of Health Education, 37*(4), 250–254.

Deeds, S. G., Cleary, M. J., & Neiger, B. L. (Eds.). (1996). *The certified health education specialist: A self-study guide for professional competency* (2nd ed.). Allentown, PA: National Commission for Health Education Credentialing.

Dordoni, G., & Larson, K. L. (2003). The campus tapestry: A nonthreatening multicultural awareness program. *American Journal of Health Education, 34*(1), 60–63.

Doyle, E. I., Liu, Y., & Ancona, L. (1996). Cultural competence development in university health education courses. *Journal of Health Education, 27*(4), 206–213.

Dumas, J. E., Rollock, D., Prinz, R. J., Hops, H., & Blechman, E. A. (1999). Cultural sensitivity: Problems and solutions in applied and preventive intervention. *Applied and Preventive Psychology, 8,* 175–195.

Green, L., Kreuter, M., Deeds, S., & Partridge, K. (1980). *Health education planning: A diagnostic approach.* Mountain View, CA: Mayfield.

Hassouneh-Phillips, D., & Beckett, A. (2003). An education in racism. *Journal of Nursing Education, 42*(6), 258–265.

Helms, J. E., & Richardson, T. Q. (1997). How "multiculturalism" obscures race and culture as differential aspects of counseling competency. In D. B. Pope-Davis & H.L.K. Coleman (Eds.), *Multicultural counseling competencies: Assessment, education and training, & supervision* (pp. 60–79). Thousand Oaks, CA: Sage.

Jackson-Carrol, L. N., Graham, E., & Jackson, J. C. (1996). *Beyond medical interpretation: The role of interpreter cultural mediators in building bridges between ethnic communities and health institutions.* Seattle, WA: Community House Calls, Harborview Medical Center.

Johnston, L. L., Denboba, D. L., & Honberg, L. (1998). Reducing health disparities: Ideas for resource development and technical assistance. *Journal of Health Education, 29*(5), S54–S58.

Joint Committee on Health Education and Promotion Terminology. (2002). Report of the 2000 Joint Committee on Health Education and Promotion Terminology. *Journal of School Health, 72*(1), 3–7.

Levy, D. R. (1985). White doctors and black patients: Influence of race on the doctor-patient relationship. *Pediatrics, 75*(4), 639–643.

Luquis, R. R., & Pérez, M. A. (2003). Achieving cultural competence: The challenges for health educators. *American Journal of Health Education, 34*(3), 131–138.

Luquis, R. R., Pérez, M. A., & Young, K. (2006). Cultural competence development in health education professional preparation programs. *American Journal of Health Education, 37*(4), 233–241.

Marbley, A. F., Bonner, A., II, McKisick, S., Henfield, M. S., & Watts, L. M. (2007). Interfacing culture specific pedagogy with counseling: A proposed diversity training model. *Multicultural Education, 14*(3), 8–16.

Montes, J. H., Johnston, L. L, Airhihenbuwa, C. O., & Gotsch, A. R. (1998, September/October). Eliminating health disparities for vulnerable populations. *American Journal of Health Education, 29*(5, Suppl.), S1–S64.

National Commission for Health Education Credentialing, Society for Public Health Education, & American Association for Health Education. (2006). *A competency-based framework for health educators–2006.* Whitehall, PA: National Commission for Health Education Credentialing.

Pérez, M. A., Gonzalez, A., & Pinzon-Pérez, H. (2006). Cultural competence in health care systems: A case study. *California Journal of Health Promotion, 4*(1), 102–108.

Pinzon, H. L., & Pérez, M. A. (1997). Multicultural issues in health education programs for Hispanic-Latino populations in the United States. *Journal of Health Education, 28*(5), 314–316.

Pinzon-Pérez, H. (2005). Complementary and alternative medicine, holistic health, and integrative healing: Applications in health education. *American Journal of Health Education, 36*(3), 174–178.

Ponterotto, J. G., Casas, M. J., Suzuki, L. A., & Alexander, C. M. (1995). *Handbook of multicultural counseling.* Thousand Oaks, CA: Sage.

Price, S., & Sidani, J. E. (2007). Characteristics of health educators desired by inner-city health clinic patients: A case study. *American Journal of Health Education, 38,* 4–8.

Redican, K., Stewart, S. H., Johnson, L. E., & Frazee, A. (1994). Professional preparation in cultural awareness and sensitivity in health education: A national survey. *Journal of Health Education, 25,* 215–217.

Stoy, D. B. (2000). Developing intercultural competence: An action plan for health educators. *Journal of Health Education, 31*(1), 16–19.

Sue, D. W. (2001). Multidimensional facets of cultural competence. *The Counseling Psychologist, 29*(6), 790–821.

Thomas, S. B., & Quinn, S. C. (1993). An evaluation of HIV education messengers in a black low income housing complex. *Journal of Health Education, 24*(3), 135–140.

CHAPTER

4

COMPLEMENTARY AND ALTERNATIVE MEDICINE IN CULTURALLY COMPETENT HEALTH EDUCATION

HELDA PINZON-PÉREZ

LEARNING OBJECTIVES

After completing this chapter, you will be able to

- Recognize the similarities and differences among complementary healing, alternative medicine, and holistic health.
- Discuss the impact of complementary healing, alternative medicine, and holistic health on the practice of culturally competent health education.
- Identify the potential challenges and future applications of complementary healing, alternative medicine, and holistic health for health educators.

INTRODUCTION

With the emergence of such health-related fields as complementary and alternative medicine (CAM), a new body of knowledge is expanding the horizons of health educators' practice. Culturally competent health educators need to understand the value of scientific and cultural constructs related to alternative forms of healing.

Health educators are being called on to explore their role in educating the public at large about complementary and alternative medicine, holistic health, and integrative healing (Johnson & Johnson, 2004). This chapter provides an overview of the principles involved in the practice of complementary healing, alternative medicine, and holistic health, as well as a description of the use of these modalities in the United States and worldwide. It also includes an analysis of the applications and future challenges for health education posed by these emerging fields.

USE OF CAM

The use of CAM among adults in the United States has been documented by the 2002 National Health Interview Survey, conducted by the Centers for Disease Control and Prevention and the National Center for Health Statistics (Barnes, Powell-Griner, McFann, & Nahin, 2004). This study collected information from 31,044 adults, 18 years of age and older, through computer-assisted personal interviews. Selected results of this study are presented in Exhibit 4.1.

Pearson, Johnson, and Nahin (2006) mention that over 1.6 million Americans use CAM practices for insomnia or sleeping disorders. Of those, 65 percent use herbal products and 39 percent use mind-body therapies. Barnes et al. (2004) found that CAM has most commonly been used to treat low-back pain, neck-related problems, joint pain, and depression. Other uses mentioned by Barnes et al. include the treatment of sinusitis (1.2 percent), cholesterol problems (1.1 percent), asthma (1.1 percent), hypertension (1.0 percent), and menopause (0.8 percent).

The 2002 National Health Interview Survey revealed that 19 percent of U.S. adults used herbal medicine, functional foods such as garlic, and animal-based supplements such as glucosamine during the twelve months preceding the survey. Among the natural products most often used by respondents were echinacea (40.3 percent), ginseng (24.1 percent), Ginkgo biloba (21.1 percent), and garlic supplements (19.9 percent) (Barnes et al., 2004).

A review of the use of traditional, complementary, and alternative medicine among 123 member states of the World Health Organization (WHO) revealed that CAM and traditional medicine are widely used around the world. In Africa, over 80 percent of Ethiopians use traditional medicine. In the Americas, a 1999 study revealed that 70 percent of Canadians have used one or more natural health products. In the Eastern Mediterranean region, 70 percent of the Pakistani rural population have used CAM and traditional medicine. In Europe, one-eighth of the British population have tried complementary or alternative medicine, and 90 percent of these people are ready to use

EXHIBIT 4.1. Selected Results of the 2002 National Health Interview Survey: Complementary and Alternative Medicine Use Among Adults, United States, 2002.

USE OF COMPLEMENTARY AND ALTERNATIVE MEDICINE

- Seventy-five percent of adults age 18 and over have ever used CAM when prayer specifically for health reasons was included in the definition.

- Sixty-two percent of adults have used CAM during the past 12 months when prayer specifically for health reasons was included in the definition.

- The ten CAM therapies most commonly used within the past 12 months measured in terms of the percentage of U.S. adults were prayer specifically for one's own health (43.0%), prayer by others for one's own health (24.4%), natural products (18.9%), deep breathing exercises (11.6%), participation in prayer group for one's own health (9.6%), meditation (7.6%), chiropractic care (7.5%), yoga (5.1%), massage (5.0%), and diet-based therapies (3.5%).

- Of the ten CAM therapies most commonly used within the past 12 months, most were mind-body interventions. Forty-five percent of adults used some method of prayer for health reasons within the past 12 months.

- The two most widely used diet-based therapies by U.S. adults were the Atkins diet (1.7%) and the vegetarian diet (1.6%).

USE OF CAM BY SELECTED CHARACTERISTICS

- Women were more likely than men to use CAM. The largest sex differential is seen in the use of mind-body therapies including prayer specifically for health reasons.

- For all therapies combined, CAM use was more likely among older adults than younger adults.

- If prayer specifically for health reasons is excluded from the definition of CAM, all the CAM categories demonstrated inverse "U" relationships with age, with the youngest and oldest groups reporting the least use of CAM.

- Black adults (68.3%) were more likely to use mind-body therapies including prayer specifically for health reasons than white adults (50.1%) or Asian adults (48.1%).

- Asian adults were more likely (43.1%) to use CAM (excluding megavitamin therapy and prayer specifically for health reasons) than white adults (35.9%) or black adults (26.2%).

- White adults (12.0%) were more likely to use manipulative and body-based therapies than Asian adults (7.2%) or black adults (4.4%).

- Non-Hispanic adults were more likely than Hispanic adults to use mind-body therapies excluding prayer specifically for health reasons and less likely to use mind-body therapies including prayer specifically for health reasons.

- Except for the groups of therapies that included prayer specifically for health reasons, use of CAM increased as education level increased.

Source: Barnes et al., 2004.

it again. In Southeast Asia, 70 percent of rural Indonesians have used CAM practices. In the Western Pacific region, 95 percent of Chinese hospitals have units for traditional medicine (WHO, 2001).

According to WHO (2001), the most commonly cited reasons for the use of these healing practices in the world are that they are more affordable, more closely related to the patient's ideology, and less paternalistic than biomedicine. CAM and traditional medicine constitute important sources of medical care in various nations around the globe.

DEFINITIONS OF CONCEPTS IN NONTRADITIONAL HEALING

Health educators need to have a clear understanding of each of the terms used in non-traditional healing, including *complementary* and *alternative medicine, conventional medicine, integrative medicine* or *healing, holistic health,* and *folk* and *traditional medicine.* Understanding what each of these areas encompasses is important for health educators because they are among the educational agents whom consumers of nontraditional healing will consult for clarification.

Complementary medicine and alternative medicine have been defined as the medical and health care practices, systems, and products that are not included yet in the conventional medicine delivery system and are now in the process of being studied under rigorous scientific inquiry (National Center for Complementary and Alternative Medicine [NCCAM], 2007a). In contrast, the conventional medicine delivery system, also known as *allopathic care* or *biomedicine,* has been defined as the body of scientific knowledge practiced by doctors of medicine, doctors of osteopathic medicine, and allied health professionals such as psychologists, physical therapists, and registered nurses, among others (NCCAM, 2003). Health educators have been active educational agents in the field of conventional medicine; now they need to increase their presence in the areas of complementary and alternative medicine.

Complementary medicine and alternative medicine are terms with distinct meanings. *Complementary medicine* describes practices used simultaneously with conventional medicine (NCCAM, 2007a). An example of this is the use of aromatherapy following surgery to alleviate discomfort. In contrast, *alternative medicine* is used instead of conventional medicine, as in using a specific diet for the therapeutic treatment of cancer instead of using chemotherapy (NCCAM, 2007b). Health educators may find that health care professionals have less initial resistance to becoming involved in complementary medicine, because it acknowledges the value of conventional and traditional healing.

Traditional medicine and *folk medicine* are often associated with CAM. These approaches employ indigenous health traditions and cultural healing constructs involving the use of plants, animal remedies, mineral-based medicines, and spiritual means (WHO, 2001).

Traditional and folk medicine have gained recognition among health educators because of these educators' interest in culturally competent health care. Conducting further studies on these forms of medicine is important for the growth of the health education profession.

The National Center for Complementary and Alternative Medicine (NCCAM) also uses the term *integrative medicine,* which it defines as a combination of conventional medical practices and CAM therapies. Integrative medicine systems promote the equal importance and scientific value of mainstream and alternative healing mechanisms. An example of integrative medicine is the simultaneous use of massage therapy and conventional medications to alleviate low-back pain (NCCAM, 2007a). No current data exist on the number of practitioners and customers of integrative medicine. According to the American Association of Integrative Medicine (2006), additional research in this area is greatly needed. Health educators ought to contribute toward the understanding of this new field by becoming actively involved in research exploring the number of people using this modality, their reasons for such use, and their experiences with it.

These conceptual terms were clarified and differentiated in 2002 by the National Center for Complementary and Alternative Medicine. This differentiation is an attempt to provide a clear basis for the understanding of CAM and other modalities among health practitioners.

Pinzon-Pérez (2005) has advocated for a broader understanding of these concepts and the use of more inclusive terms such as holistic, complementary, alternative, and integrative *healing.* Currently, the focus on medical practices denoted in terms such as complementary, alternative, and integrative *medicine* narrows the scope of these practices and limits their applications to the field of medicine. There is a need to expand the focus of these terms to embrace *healing* and thus to make them more applicable in fields such as health education and allied health professions. Health education publications such as book chapters, journal articles, and conference proceedings on holistic and integrative healing are needed.

Patterson and Graf (2000) have described the relevance of integrating complementary and alternative medicine into the health education curriculum. Chng, Neill, and Fogle (2003) have advocated for conducting research on CAM and integrative medicine among college student populations and for exploring the application of these terms in the field of health education.

Holistic health describes practices oriented toward integration of the body, the mind, the spirit, and the environment. Holistic health should be an important domain in the field of health education because this discipline ought to view health in a comprehensive manner.

Integrative medicine or *healing* refers to a multidisciplinary process that has resulted in benefits such as improved clinical outcomes, reduction in hospital days, decreased hospitalizations, decreased pharmacological costs, and fewer outpatient surgeries (Sarnat & Winterstein, 2004). Integrative healing is comprehensive and multisectorial.

Health educators need to conduct further studies to expand the understanding of these conceptual definitions and their applications to health education. It is important that health educators create a body of knowledge unique to the domains and needs of the health education practice. Some recommendations for health educators in this regard are (1) conducting research on holistic health and integrative healing; (2) expanding the competencies and responsibilities of health educators to address newly emerging fields such as CAM, integrative healing, and holistic health; and (3) designing culturally appropriate strategies to educate individuals and communities on these new forms of healing.

MODALITIES OF CAM

The National Center for Complementary and Alternative Medicine divides CAM therapies into five major categories, as shown in Exhibit 4.2. These categories are based on mechanisms of action and modalities of treatment.

Barnes et al. (2004) used the definitions of CAM modalities presented in Exhibit 4.3 for the 2002 National Health Interview Survey on complementary and alternative medicine use among adults in the United States. Exhibit 4.4 displays a selection of recent NCCAM definitions of additional CAM modalities.

Exhibits 4.2, 4.3, and 4.4 provide important theoretical definitions for health educators that will enhance their ability to deliver health education about CAM effectively. The responsibilities and competencies delineated by the National Commission for Health Education Credentialing (NCHEC) (2002) are directly linked to health educators' knowledge of concepts and theories. Responsibilities such as acting as a resource person in health education and communicating health and health education needs, concerns, and resources related to CAM require the health educator to have a solid understanding of these operational and theoretical definitions.

The Competencies Update Project (CUP), undertaken between 1998 and 2004 by the American Association for Health Education (AAHE), the National Commission for Health Education Credentialing, and the Society for Public Health Education (SOPHE), delineated the role of the health educator as a three-tiered hierarchical model. This new framework defined the responsibilities and competencies of health educators based on their level of practice (NCHEC, 2007).

Entry-level health educators, defined as those with a bachelor's or master's degree and fewer than five years of experience, need to expand their body of knowledge on the types and modalities of CAM. Advanced 1 level health educators, those with a bachelor's or master's degree and five years or more of experience, ought to engage in the design, implementation, and evaluation of educational programs related to CAM. Advanced 2 level health educators, defined as those with a doctoral degree and five or more years of experience, ought to engage in research projects and scientific discovery related to CAM (NCHEC, 2007).

EXHIBIT 4.2. Categories of Complementary and Alternative Medicine as Defined by NCCAM.

WHOLE MEDICAL SYSTEMS

Whole medical systems are built upon complete systems of theory and practice. Often, these systems have evolved apart from and earlier than the conventional medical approach used in the United States. Examples of whole medical systems that have developed in Western cultures include homeopathic medicine and naturopathic medicine. Examples of systems that have developed in non-Western cultures include traditional Chinese medicine and Ayurveda.

MIND-BODY MEDICINE

Mind-body medicine uses a variety of techniques designed to enhance the mind's capacity to affect bodily function and symptoms. Some techniques that were considered CAM in the past have become mainstream (for example, patient support groups and cognitive-behavioral therapy). Other mind-body techniques are still considered CAM, including meditation, prayer, mental healing, and therapies that use creative outlets such as art, music, or dance.

BIOLOGICALLY BASED PRACTICES

Biologically based practices in CAM use substances found in nature, such as herbs, foods, and vitamins. Some examples include dietary supplements, herbal products, and the use of other so-called natural but as yet scientifically unproven therapies (for example, using shark cartilage to treat cancer).

MANIPULATIVE AND BODY-BASED PRACTICES

Manipulative and body-based practices in CAM are based on manipulation and/or movement of one or more parts of the body. Some examples include chiropractic or osteopathic manipulation, and massage.

ENERGY MEDICINE

Energy therapies involve the use of energy fields. They are of two types:

- Biofield therapies are intended to affect energy fields that purportedly surround and penetrate the human body. The existence of such fields has not yet been scientifically proven. Some forms of energy therapy manipulate biofields by applying pressure and/or manipulating the body by placing the hands in, or through, these fields. Examples include qi gong, Reiki, and Therapeutic Touch.

- Bioelectromagnetic-based therapies involve the unconventional use of electromagnetic fields, such as pulsed fields, magnetic fields, or alternating-current or direct-current fields.

Source: NCCAM, 2007a.

EXHIBIT 4.3. Selected Modalities of CAM as Defined for the 2002 National Health Interview Survey.

Ayurveda—This comprehensive system of medicine, developed in India over 5,000 years ago, places equal emphasis on body, mind, and spirit. The goal is to restore the natural harmony of the individual. An ayurvedic doctor identifies an individual's "constitution" or overall health profile by ascertaining the patient's metabolic body type (Vata, Pitta, or Kapha) through a series of personal history questions. Then the patient's "constitution" becomes the foundation for a specific treatment plan designed to guide the individual back into harmony with his or her environment. This plan may include dietary changes, exercise, yoga, meditation, massage, herbal tonics, and other remedies.

Biofeedback—This method teaches clients, through the use of simple electronic devices, how to consciously regulate normally unconscious bodily functions (e.g., breathing, heart rate, blood pressure) to improve overall health. Biofeedback has been used to reduce stress, eliminate headaches, recondition injured muscles, control asthmatic attacks, and relieve pain.

Chelation therapy—This therapy involves a series of intravenous injections of a binding (chelating) agent, such as the amino acid EDTA, to remove toxic metals and wastes from the bloodstream. Following injection, the binding agent travels through the bloodstream attaching itself to toxic metals and wastes, which are subsequently excreted through the patient's urine. Used initially to treat lead poisoning, chelation therapy is used by a growing number of practitioners to treat and reverse the process of arteriosclerosis (hardening of the arteries).

Energy healing therapy/Reiki—This method helps the body's ability to heal itself through the flow and focusing of healing energy (Reiki means universal healing energy). During treatment, this healing energy is channeled through the hands of a practitioner into the client's body to restore a normal energy balance and health. Energy healing therapy has been used to treat a wide variety of ailments and health problems and is often used in conjunction with other alternative and conventional medical treatments.

Folk medicine—These systems of healing (such as Curanderismo and Native American healing) have persisted since the beginning of culture and have flourished long before the development of conventional medicine. Folk healers usually participate in a training regimen of observation and imitation, with healing often considered a gift passed down through several generations of a family. Folk healers may employ a range of remedies including prayer, healing touch or laying on of hands, charms, herbal teas or tinctures, magic rituals, and others. Folk healers are found in all cultures and operate under a variety of names and labels.

Guided imagery—This method involves a series of relaxation techniques followed by the visualization of detailed images, usually calm and peaceful in nature. If used for treatment, the client may visualize his/her body as healthy, strong, and free of the specific problem or condition. Sessions, conducted in groups or one-on-one, are typically 20–30 minutes and may be practiced several times a week. Guided imagery has been advocated for a number of chronic conditions, including headaches, stress, high blood pressure, and anxiety.

Healing circles—These spiritual gatherings usually occur in informal settings, may involve invocations (calling upon a higher power or authority), and may use other healing approaches such as prayer, energy healing therapy/Reiki, and natural herbs.

High dose or megavitamin therapy—This therapy refers to the use of vitamins in excess of the Recommended Daily Allowances (RDA) established by the National Academy of Sciences, Food and Nutrition Board. Although these therapies have been used for the prevention and treatment of diseases and illnesses such as cancer, heart disease, schizophrenia, and the common cold, some high dose or megavitamin regimens can produce adverse or toxic effects.

Laying on of hands—This religious ceremony involves the placement of hands, by one or more persons (lay or clergy), on the body of the recipient. Usually including prayer, the ceremony may occur in a church or less formal setting and may be used for minor as well as more serious ailments and illnesses.

Macrobiotic diet—This low fat diet emphasizes whole grains and vegetables and restricts the intake of fluids. Consumption of fresh, unprocessed foods is especially important. Daily intakes break out as follows: 50–60% whole grains; 25–30% fresh vegetables; 5–10% beans, soy-based products, and sea vegetables; and 5–10% soups. Meat, poultry, dairy products, eggs, alcohol, coffee, caffeinated tea, sweets and sugar, and strong spices are to be avoided.

Meditation—Mental calmness and physical relaxation is achieved by suspending the stream of thoughts that normally occupy the mind. Generally performed once or twice a day for approximately 20 minutes at a time, meditation is used to reduce stress, alter hormone levels, and elevate one's mood. In addition, a person experienced in meditation can achieve a reduction in blood pressure, adrenaline levels, heart rate, and skin temperature.

Tai chi—This Chinese self-defense discipline and low-intensity, low-impact exercise regimen is used for health, relaxation, and self-exploration. Usually performed daily, tai chi exercises include a set of forms, with each form comprising a series of body positions connected into one continuous movement. A single form may include up to one hundred positions and may take as long as 20 minutes to complete. Some of the proposed benefits of tai chi include improved concentration, circulation, and posture, reduction of stress, and prevention of osteoporosis.

Source: Barnes et al., 2004.

EXHIBIT 4.4. Modalities of CAM as Defined by NCCAM.

Acupuncture is a method of healing developed in China at least 2,000 years ago. Today, acupuncture describes a family of procedures involving stimulation of anatomical points on the body by a variety of techniques. American practices of acupuncture incorporate medical traditions from China, Japan, Korea, and other countries. The acupuncture technique that has been most studied scientifically involves penetrating the skin with thin, solid, metallic needles that are manipulated by the hands or by electrical stimulation.

Aromatherapy involves the use of essential oils (extracts or essences) from flowers, herbs, and trees to promote health and well-being.

Ayurveda is a CAM alternative medical system that has been practiced primarily in the Indian subcontinent for 5,000 years. Ayurveda includes diet and herbal remedies and emphasizes the use of body, mind, and spirit in disease prevention and treatment.

Chiropractic is a CAM alternative medical system. It focuses on the relationship between bodily structure (primarily that of the spine) and function, and how that relationship affects the preservation and restoration of health. Chiropractors use manipulative therapy as an integral treatment tool.

Dietary supplements. Congress defined the term "dietary supplement" in the Dietary Supplement Health and Education Act (DSHEA) of 1994. A dietary supplement is a product (other than tobacco) taken by mouth that contains a "dietary ingredient" intended to supplement the diet. Dietary ingredients may include vitamins, minerals, herbs or other botanicals, amino acids, and substances such as enzymes, organ tissues, and metabolites. Dietary supplements come in many forms, including extracts, concentrates, tablets, capsules, gel caps, liquids, and powders. They have special requirements for labeling. Under DSHEA, dietary supplements are considered foods, not drugs.

Electromagnetic fields (EMFs, also called electric and magnetic fields) are invisible lines of force that surround all electrical devices. The Earth also produces EMFs; electric fields are produced when there is thunderstorm activity, and magnetic fields are believed to be produced by electric currents flowing at the Earth's core.

Homeopathic medicine is a CAM alternative medical system. In homeopathic medicine, there is a belief that "like cures like," meaning that small, highly diluted quantities of medicinal substances are given to cure symptoms, when the same substances given at higher or more concentrated doses would actually cause those symptoms.

Massage therapists manipulate muscle and connective tissue to enhance function of those tissues and promote relaxation and well-being.

Naturopathic medicine is a CAM alternative medical system. Naturopathic medicine proposes that there is a healing power in the body that establishes, maintains, and restores health. Practitioners work with the patient with a goal of supporting this power, through treatments such as nutrition and lifestyle counseling, dietary supplements, medicinal plants, exercise, homeopathy, and treatments from traditional Chinese medicine.

Osteopathic medicine is a form of conventional medicine that, in part, emphasizes diseases arising in the musculoskeletal system. There is an underlying belief that all of the body's systems work together, and disturbances in one system may affect function elsewhere in the body. Some osteopathic physicians practice osteopathic manipulation, a full-body system of hands-on techniques to alleviate pain, restore function, and promote health and well-being.

Qi gong is a component of traditional Chinese medicine that combines movement, meditation, and regulation of breathing to enhance the flow of qi (an ancient term given to what is believed to be vital energy) in the body, improve blood circulation, and enhance immune function.

Reiki is a Japanese word representing Universal Life Energy. Reiki is based on the belief that when spiritual energy is channeled through a Reiki practitioner, the patient's spirit is healed, which in turn heals the physical body.

Therapeutic Touch is derived from an ancient technique called laying on of hands. It is based on the premise that it is the healing force of the therapist that affects the patient's recovery; healing is promoted when the body's energies are in balance; and, by passing their hands over the patient, healers can identify energy imbalances.

Traditional Chinese medicine (TCM) is the current name for an ancient system of health care from China. TCM is based on a concept of balanced qi (pronounced "chee"), or vital energy, that is believed to flow throughout the body. Qi is proposed to regulate a person's spiritual, emotional, mental, and physical balance and to be influenced by the opposing forces of yin (negative energy) and yang (positive energy). Disease is proposed to result from the flow of qi being disrupted and yin and yang becoming imbalanced. Among the components of TCM are herbal and nutritional therapy, restorative physical exercises, meditation, acupuncture, and remedial massage.

Source: NCCAM, 2007b.

THE NATIONAL CENTER FOR COMPLEMENTARY AND ALTERNATIVE MEDICINE

The National Center for Complementary and Alternative Medicine (NCCAM), created in 1998, is the lead federal entity supporting scientific research initiatives in the areas of complementary and alternative medicine. Studies on the applications of holistic health and alternative medicine in realms of scientific discovery such as health education, medicine, social work, nursing, and others have been supported by NCCAM. (A precursor agency, the Office for Alternative Medicine, existed from 1992 to 1998.)

As one of the twenty-seven institutes and centers of the National Institutes of Health this agency promotes rigorous scientific inquiries on healing practices, educates complementary and alternative medicine researchers, and informs the public on the latest findings related to complementary and alternative medical practices. The primary focus areas of the NCCAM are presented in Exhibit 4.5.

Exhibit 4.5 presents information of particular relevance for health educators within the framework of the new responsibilities and competencies delineated by the Competencies Update Project. Responsibility VII states that health educators should communicate and advocate for health and health education (Gilmore, Olsen, Taub, & Connell, 2005). The NCCAM focus areas reveal a need for health educators

EXHIBIT 4.5. NCCAM Focus Areas.

ADVANCING SCIENTIFIC RESEARCH

As of August 2006, NCCAM had funded more than 1,200 research projects at scientific institutions across the United States and around the world.

TRAINING CAM RESEARCHERS

NCCAM supports training opportunities for new researchers and encourages experienced researchers to study CAM.

SHARING NEWS AND INFORMATION

NCCAM provides timely and accurate information about CAM research through a Web site, a national information clearinghouse, fact sheets, a distinguished lecture series, continuing medical education models, and publications.

SUPPORTING INTEGRATION OF PROVEN CAM THERAPIES

NCCAM's sponsored research programs help the public and health professionals understand which CAM therapies have been proven to be safe and effective.

Source: Adapted from NCCAM, 2006a.

to take an active and leading role in advocating for advancing scientific research on CAM, sharing news and information on emerging CAM practices, and supporting the integration of proven CAM therapies.

NCCAM provides funding for research centers intended to advance scientific knowledge on alternative and complementary medicine. The budget for NCCAM in 2006 was $ 122.7 million dollars, a significant increase from 1992, when the Office of Alternative Medicine (OAM) was first created. In 1992, the operating budget for the OAM was $2 million dollars (NCCAM, 2006a).

Twenty-six research centers are currently sponsored by NCCAM. They deal with such topics as acupuncture, antioxidants, botanicals, phytotherapy, botanical medicine, cancer, chiropractic, bioenergetics, touch therapy, Chinese herbal therapy, mind-body medicine, osteopathy, and traditional Chinese medicine. The 2006 funding research priorities of NCCAM include CAM approaches to anxiety and depression; secondary prevention and management of hypertension, atherosclerosis, and congestive heart failure; ethnomedicine; immune modulation and enhancement; inflammatory bowel syndrome and irritable bowel syndrome; insomnia; liver diseases; obesity and metabolic syndrome; infectious respiratory diseases; gender health; and health disparities (NCCAM, 2006b).

NCCAM also offers funding for training and educational programs at the undergraduate, graduate, and postdoctoral level. The focus of these training opportunities is the development of culturally competent research and delivery systems for complementary and alternative medicine.

The health education profession needs to extend its body of knowledge to new domains such as CAM. Health educators can find CAM research and training opportunities at the National Center for Complementary and Alternative Medicine.

APPLICATION TO HEALTH EDUCATION

Health educators have embraced the concepts promoted by holistic health and integrative healing (Chng et al., 2003). According to Pinzon-Pérez (2005), the practice of health education is based on a holistic understanding of human life and the multidimensional nature of health. Terms such as *holistic health* and *integrative medicine* or *healing* are traditional in the health education vocabulary and have become an integral part of the practice of this profession.

Health educators are defined by NCHEC (2002) as practitioners who have scientific training in the design, development, and evaluation of activities that help to improve the health of all people. The emerging fields of CAM, holistic health, and integrative healing pose new challenges for health educators in the areas of advocacy, needs assessment, program planning, and program evaluation. Multiple strategies for educating the public on CAM, in settings such as schools, communities, health care facilities, businesses, colleges, and government agencies, will need to be developed.

NCCAM has made a call to health professionals to educate the public on how to select a CAM provider. Responsibility VI of responsibilities and competencies of health educators says that these professionals should act as resource persons in health education (NCHEC, 2002). Health educators should be knowledgeable about CAM so they can educate others. An important goal in this educational process is to educate consumers on how to select CAM practitioners. Selecting the appropriate CAM provider will protect the consumer and increase the likelihood of success in treatment. The NCCAM guidelines for selecting a CAM practitioner may need to be transmitted by health educators to their clients. These guidelines are presented in Exhibit 4.6.

Currently, the body of knowledge on the application of CAM in the field of health education is limited. Patterson and Graf (2000), Chng et al. (2003), Johnson and Johnson (2004), Pinzon-Pérez (2005), and Synovitz, Gillan, Wood, Martin-Nordness, and Kelly (2006) have published valuable articles or presented papers at national conferences or on the importance of CAM in health education. Synovitz et al. (2006) have conducted research on college students' complementary and alternative medicine use in relation to health locus of control and spirituality level. Their findings indicated that internal locus of control was positively associated with use of CAM therapies and with spirituality level.

Pinzon-Pérez (2005) discusses the applications of the studies conducted by Patterson and Graf; Chng, Neill, and Fogle; and Johnson and Johnson and provides valuable insights on the applications and challenges for health education posed by these emerging fields (see Exhibit 4.7).

The nursing profession could serve as a valuable example to health educators on the importance of establishing formal education programs and standards of practice on CAM, traditional medicine, and holistic health. The American Holistic Nurses Association (AHNA), an organization founded in 1981, has served as a bridge between the biomedical perspective in nursing and the alternative and complementary healing paradigm (AHNA, 2004). This organization has developed philosophical principles that can be adopted by health educators interested in CAM, traditional medicine, and holistic health.

EXHIBIT 4.6. NCCAM Guidelines for Selecting a CAM Practitioner.

- If you are seeking a CAM practitioner, speak with your primary health care provider(s) or someone you believe to be knowledgeable about CAM regarding the therapy in which you are interested. Ask if he or she has a recommendation for the type of CAM practitioner you are seeking.

- Make a list of CAM practitioners and gather information about each one before making your first visit. Ask basic questions about their credentials and practice.

Where did they receive their training? What licenses or certifications do they have? How much will the treatment cost?

- Check with your insurer to see if the cost of therapy will be covered.

- After you select a practitioner, make a list of questions to ask at your first visit. You may want to bring a friend or family member who can help you ask questions and note answers.

- Come to the first visit prepared to answer questions about your health history, including injuries, surgeries, and major illnesses, as well as prescription medicines, vitamins, and other supplements you may take.

- Assess your first visit and decide if the practitioner is right for you. Did you feel comfortable with the practitioner? Could the practitioner answer your questions? Did he respond to you in a way that satisfied you? Does the treatment plan seem reasonable and acceptable to you?

- Ask what training or other qualifications the practitioner has. Ask about her education, additional training, licenses, and certifications. If you contacted a professional organization, see if the practitioner's qualifications meet the standards for training and licensing for that profession.

- Ask if it is possible to have a brief consultation in person or by phone with the practitioner. This will give you a chance to speak with the practitioner directly. This consultation may or may not involve a charge.

- Ask if there are diseases or health conditions in which the practitioner specializes and how frequently he treats patients with problems similar to yours.

- Ask if the practitioner believes the therapy can effectively address your complaint and if there is any scientific research supporting the treatment's use for your condition.

- Ask how many patients the practitioner typically sees in a day, and how much time she spends with each patient.

- Ask about charges and payment options. How much do treatments cost? If you have insurance, does the practitioner accept your insurance or participate in your insurer's network? Even with insurance, you may be responsible for a percentage of the cost.

- Ask about the hours appointments are offered. How long is the wait for an appointment? Consider whether this will be convenient for your schedule.

- Ask about office location. If you are concerned, ask about public transportation and parking. If you need a building with an elevator or a wheelchair ramp, ask about them.

- Ask what will be involved in the first visit or assessment.

- Observe how comfortable you feel during these first interactions.

Source: Adapted from NCCAM, 2004.

EXHIBIT 4.7. **CAM, Holistic Health, and Integrative Healing: Applications and Challenges for Health Education.**

■ The increasing pattern of use of CAM, holistic health and integrative healing practices has motivated health educators and other practitioners in the behavioral and medical fields to conduct and publish research in this area.

■ In the field of health education, professional development organizations such as AAHE, SOPHE and others have started to provide grants, under the umbrella of cultural competence, to find out the applications of CAM, holistic health and integrative healing in this field. Although this is a promising start, more funding is needed to motivate health education practitioners to conduct research in these areas.

■ CAM, holistic health and integrative healing are now being addressed in professional development agendas for health educators.

■ According to Johnson and Johnson (2004), health educators need to be aware of the current status of CAM use in the U.S., become familiar with different forms of CAM therapy, discuss commonly used CAM therapies with clients, assist clients in their selection of appropriate CAM therapies to promote health and prevent disease, encourage clients to communicate the use of CAM therapies to their health care providers, have continuing education opportunities in CAM from professional organizations, and offer CAM courses in professional health education preparation programs.

■ In health education . . . no national standards have been developed yet to unify the curriculum for the training of health educators on CAM, holistic health and integrative healing. Most efforts to teach health educators about these issues have been developed as part of curriculums that address cultural competence and cultural proficiency.

■ Patterson and Graf (2000) wrote a cornerstone article in defense of requiring complementary and alternative medicine training in the curriculum for health educators. These authors presented a well-founded rationale to support their premise that CAM should be taught as a separate course, or in the absence of enough resources, be integrated into existing health education courses.

■ Section 3 of Article VI of the Code of Ethics for the Health Education Profession: "Responsibility in Professional Preparation," indicates that health educators should be involved in professional preparation and professional development programs that provide them with materials that are accurate, up-to-date and timely.

■ It is essential that entry-level health educators become knowledgeable of the scientific and cultural basis of the various forms of CAM, holistic health practices, and integrative healing therapies. This knowledge will provide health educators with the professional skills to become accurate health resources.

- Academic training on CAM, holistic health and integrative healing should be included at the undergraduate and graduate levels.

- Creating standards related to CAM, holistic health and integrative healing for the professional preparation of health educators implies a revision of the requirements for Certified Health Education Specialists (CHES). Although CHES certification addresses issues related to cultural competence and proficiency, it needs to be extended to assess health educators' knowledge and scientific understanding of . . . basic forms of CAM, holistic health and integrative healing. . . . This indicates that health educators with CHES designation should be professionals with scientific and socio-cultural knowledge on alternative and complementary healing practices.

- An additional challenge for health educators is to generate knowledge on the applications of integrative healing to the practice of health education. . . . Theses, doctoral dissertations and professional research on this issue should be encouraged at all levels of professional preparation.

Source: Pinzon-Pérez, 2005. Reprinted with permission.

Some of the philosophical principles for holistic nurses that health educators and other health professionals could adhere to include the understanding that they (1) can have a professional practice that promotes wholeness; (2) can motivate individuals to become responsible health consumers; (3) should provide services to individuals, families, and communities in ways that integrate the body, the mind, and the spirit; and (4) should advocate for the understanding that illness is an opportunity for individuals to regain their wholeness (AHNA, 2004). According to AHNA, nurses should begin by developing lifestyles congruent with a philosophy of wholeness. Health educators too should consider embracing this concept and developing for themselves lifestyles oriented toward inner-self enhancement and holistic health, lifestyles that will ultimately enable them to provide a better quality of health education services.

A possible strategy for enhancing the understanding of CAM in health education would be to create ad hoc and standing committees in professional organizations, such as the American Association for Health Education and the Society for Public Health Education, to stimulate scientific inquiry and develop a specific body of knowledge on the integration of CAM into health education. As mentioned earlier, Patterson and Graf (2000) have made a call to health educators to incorporate CAM into the health education curriculum. Of particular relevance in the development of a specific body of knowledge on CAM for health education is the study of culturally competent health education programs in relation to complementary and alternative medicine, holistic health, and integrative healing.

Culturally competent health education programs should include constant dialogue and further research on how to incorporate training, publications, and professional development in CAM, traditional medicine, and holistic health into the delivery of health education services. Examples of culturally competent health education programs on CAM should be published and made known to the professional health education body. Funding for research and publications on this area ought to be a priority for professional health education organizations and individual members.

There is also a need to add classes at the undergraduate and graduate levels in which future health educators can learn about and discuss the implications of CAM for their professional practice. Synovitz et al. (2006) have supported this need, finding it relevant in light of the results of their study on college students' use of CAM therapies. There is also a need to consider the development of academic certificate programs and international research cooperative agreements on CAM.

Potential challenges in future applications of complementary healing, alternative medicine, and holistic health for the health education profession include (1) defining health educators' competencies and responsibilities associated with CAM practices, (2) enhancing the body of knowledge relating to CAM in health education professional practice, and (3) stimulating dialogues in the health education professional community on alternative, complementary, and holistic healing practices and on their use within a context of cultural respect and rigorous scientific inquiry.

CONCLUSION

Complementary and alternative medicine practices are amply used in the United States. The 2002 National Health Interview Survey documented that approximately 62 percent of the U.S. adult population has used CAM modalities, including prayer. The major modalities of CAM, as described by the National Center for Complementary and Alternative Medicine, are whole medical systems, mind-body medicine, biologically based practices, manipulative and body-based practices, and energy medicine. NCCAM is the lead federal entity supporting scientific research initiatives related to complementary and alternative medicine. The clarification of terms such as complementary and alternative medicine, conventional medicine, folk or traditional medicine, integrative medicine or healing, and holistic health is of special relevance for the health education practice.

POINTS TO REMEMBER

- Health educators face a new body of knowledge related to the emergence of fields such as complementary and alternative medicine. There are new challenges for health educators regarding their role in complementary and alternative healing practices.

- It is vital that health educators create a body of knowledge on CAM unique to the domain and needs of the health education practice. Further research in this area is needed.

■ Of particular relevance in the development of a specific body of knowledge on CAM for health education is the study of culturally competent health education programs related to complementary and alternative medicine, holistic health, and integrative healing.

CASE STUDY

A significant number of clients in a health care facility have reported using CAM and traditional healing practices. As a member of the health care team, you, the health educator, have been commissioned to provide culturally competent health education on CAM, traditional medicine, and holistic health to these clients.

1. What steps would you follow to assess the health education needs of this group?

2. What topics would you suggest including in the educational plan for this group?

3. What resources (Web sites, articles, organizations) would you use in designing the health education program for this group?

4. What elements would you take into account when designing a culturally competent health education program for this group?

KEY TERMS

Alternative medicine

Complementary medicine

Cultural competence

Cultural proficiency

Folk and traditional medicine

Holistic health

Integrative healing

REFERENCES

American Association of Integrative Medicine. (2006). *Member testimonials.* Retrieved April 30, 2007, from http://aaimedicine.com/about_testimonials.php.

American Holistic Nurses Association. (2004). *About AHNA.* Retrieved September 28, 2006, from http://www.ahna.org/about/about.html.

Barnes, P., Powell-Griner, E., McFann, K., & Nahin, R. (2004). *Complementary and alternative medicine use among adults: United States, 2002* (CDC advance data from Vital and Health Statistics, Report #343). Hyasttsville, MD: National Center for Health Statistics. Retrieved October 3, 2007, from nccam.nih.gov/news/camstats.htm.

Chng, C. L., Neill, K., & Fogle, P. (2003). Predictors of college students' use of complementary and alternative medicine. *American Journal of Health Education, 34*(5), 267–271.

Gilmore, G. D., Olsen, L. K., Taub, A., & Connell, D. (2005). Overview of the National Health Educator Competencies Update Project, 1998–2004. *American Journal of Health Education, 32*(6), 363–370.

Johnson, P., & Johnson, R. (2004). *Current status of complementary and alternative health practices in the U.S.: Implications for health education professionals.* Paper presented at the 2004 AAHPERD national convention, New Orleans.

National Center for Complementary and Alternative Medicine. (2003). *About chiropractic and its use in treating low back pain.* Retrieved September 30, 2006, from http://nccam.nih.gov/health/chiropractic.

National Center for Complementary and Alternative Medicine. (2004). *Selecting a CAM practitioner.* Retrieved September 27, 2006, from http://nccam.nih.gov/health/practitioner/index.htm.

National Center for Complementary and Alternative Medicine. (2006a). *NCCAM facts-at-a-glance.* Retrieved September 22, 2006, from http://nccam.nih.gov/about/ataglance.

National Center for Complementary and Alternative Medicine. (2006b). *Research funding priorities.* Retrieved September 22, 2006, from http://nccam.nih.gov/research/priorities/index.htm#5.

National Center for Complementary and Alternative Medicine. (2007b). *CAM basics.* Retrieved October 3, 2007, from http://nccam.nih.gov/health/whatiscam/pdf/D347.pdf.

National Center for Complementary and Alternative Medicine. (2007a). *What is CAM?* Retrieved February 9, 2008, from http://nccam.nih.gov/health/whatiscam.

National Commission for Health Education Credentialing. (2002). *What is a certified health education specialist (CHES)?* Retrieved April 30, 2007, from http://www.nchec.org.

National Commission for Health Education Credentialing. (2007). *Competencies Update Project.* Retrieved April 30, 2007, from http://www.nchec.org/aboutnchec/cup/cup.htm.

Patterson, S., & Graf, H. (2000). Integrating complementary and alternative medicine into the health education curriculum. *Journal of Health Education, 31,* 346–351.

Pearson, N. J., Johnson, L. L., & Nahin, R. L. (2006). Insomnia, trouble sleeping, and complementary and alternative medicine: Analysis of the 2002 National Health Interview Survey data. *Archives of Internal Medicine, 166,* 1775–1782.

Pinzon-Pérez, H. (2005). Complementary and alternative medicine, holistic health, and integrative healing: Applications in health education. *American Journal of Health Education, 36*(3), 174–178.

Sarnat, R. L., & Winterstein, J. (2004). Clinical and cost outcomes of an integrative medicine IPA. *Journal of Manipulative Physiological Therapies, 27*(5), 336–347.

Synovitz, L., Gillan, W., Wood, R., Martin-Nordness, M., & Kelly, J. (2006). An exploration of college students' complementary and alternative medicine use: Relationship to health locus of control and spirituality level. *American Journal of Health Education, 37*(2), 87–96.

World Health Organization. (2001). *Legal status of traditional medicine and complementary/alternative medicine: A worldwide review.* Retrieved September 27, 2006, from http://whqlibdoc.who.int/hq/2001/WHO_EDM_TRM_2001.2.pdf.

CHAPTER

5

A SPIRITUALLY GROUNDED AND CULTURALLY RESPONSIVE APPROACH TO HEALTH EDUCATION

ANN L. SWARTZ

ELIZABETH J. TISDELL

LEARNING OBJECTIVES

After completing this chapter, you will be able to

- Demonstrate a general familiarity with the state of research on spirituality related to health.

- Understand through case examples ways to develop spiritually grounded and culturally responsive education and clinical practice.

- Begin to formulate a personal model of such practice.

INTRODUCTION

Education for health happens in many contexts. It happens formally when it is presented by health educators in classes in schools, communities, and universities and by health care professionals in hospitals or health clinics. But it also happens less formally in families, in cultural communities, and in religious institutions and other settings, presented by those who educate to promote a holistic view that sees caring for the body, mind, soul, and spirit as an important way to promote health. The word *health* actually comes from the root term *hal,* which means "to be whole" (Sanford, 1977). Thus one could easily argue that education for health is about education for wholeness. Such a definition is in keeping with the World Health Organization's (1948) definition, which describes health as "a state of complete physical, mental and social wellbeing and not merely the absence of disease or infirmity." Further and more recently, the World Health Organization (WHO) (1998) noted that "quality of life" relates to how individuals perceive their lives in relation to their cultural context and value systems and is also related to their physical health, social relationships, spirituality, and salient environmental factors.

The purpose of this chapter is to discuss a spiritually grounded and culturally responsive approach to education for health, in light of both the literature and the authors' experience. Because the health education literature on spirituality is sparse, it is hoped that this chapter, through its sharing of experiences in health and education related practice, will inspire the reader to develop the concept of spirituality within health education. We, the authors of this chapter, are educators for health in the broad sense of that term. We recognize that health education is a defined field in which neither of us practices. One of us (Ann Swartz) is an educator for health in the expected sense in that she teaches practicing registered nurses (RNs) as they work to complete their bachelor of science degrees. The other (Elizabeth "Libby" Tisdell) is not a health care professional but teaches in a doctoral program in adult education with part-time adult students who themselves work as educators of adults in many contexts, including health education settings. One class she teaches is titled "Spirituality and Culture in the Health and Education Professions" and is based on her research into spirituality, culture, and health in adult education. Both of us attempt to be spiritually grounded, culturally responsive educators, working for the health of both individuals and society as a whole.

According to our shared perspective, body, mind, soul, and spirit are one in the individual who is inextricably linked to her or his context, the rest of society, the environment, and the sacred. Health is that which fosters the interconnection and expression of all these aspects of self. Because society is broad and individuals are unique, they must be allowed to define health for themselves. Sometimes that definition is related to the absence of disease, sometimes it is a more culturally determined construct. Often it is directly tied to spirit.

This chapter will outline the understanding we have arrived at of what it means to educate for health, and it will discuss how we carry this understanding into practice.

The chapter begins with a brief overview of society's perception of religion and health and then reviews spirituality and culture in the health education literature. Because we often teach by example, this chapter then provides a spiritually grounded and culturally responsive example of our approach, showing how we taught in a workshop at an immigrant women's health conference. Then it outlines the components of a spiritually grounded, culturally responsive approach to education for health (Tisdell, 2003). A basic assumption we make is that such an approach requires an understanding of health that is beyond the medical model and that educates the whole person and hence makes the person visible. At times in our teaching we speak in the first person about ourselves to make ourselves as educators visible, in the same way that we want to make our students or our patients visible. At other times we speak in the third person, when we are talking about theory and the professional literature, for example. This use of multiple voices is intentional and is meant partially to embody and make visible a holistic understanding of education for health. Even with a group, our work is individual and personal. This is part of what makes it spiritual. We have carried that practice and principle into this chapter.

DEFINING SPIRITUALITY

Spirituality is individually determined, often finding expression and meaning in life's most ordinary aspects. An individualistic approach to its definition allows the word to remain mysterious, making room for the analogy and symbolism used throughout history to reflect and inspire connection with divinity (McSherry, 2006).

WHO's definition of spirituality can only be inferred, but that organization does believe it is something that can be measured and has designed an instrument for that purpose. WHO conceives of spirituality as a subset of quality of life, related to religiousness and personal belief (Saxena, 2007). This definition influences the public health emphasis on religion and faith-based health programs when programs are seeking to operationalize spirituality. Faith-based programs in the United States do achieve positive effects by increasing knowledge of disease, improving screening and changing behavior, and reducing risk associated with disease symptoms. This is especially true among African Americans (DeHaven, Hunter, Wilder, Walton, & Berry, 2004). However, there is a possible downside to attempting to induce behavioral change through religion, as WHO is learning. WHO has been criticized because its regional offices have supported religion-based tobacco control activities, family planning, and HIV/AIDS/STD responses in some Islamic and Buddhist countries. These programs are considered potentially volatile by some because religion is such a divisive issue (Jabbour & Fouad, 2004). However, these religion-based public health campaigns are often less costly than others would be, and they avoid complications at the level of authority because religious leaders are key social players in the countries where they are operating. According to WHO, all religions are in a position to prohibit tobacco use, and WHO's part in religion-based interventions is traced to its inclusion of a spiritual dimension in its health strategies (El Awa, 2004).

Considering the WHO perspective, it is not surprising that an extensive review of spirituality in the health education literature reveals that in most cases, spirituality is conflated with religion, religiosity, or complementary and alternative medicine. This spiritual dimension of health remains elusive, with no standardized language of description, and is omitted from much professional literature (Perrin & McDermott, 1997). Two exceptions are research that attempts to equate spirituality with meaning making by measuring coherence in life attitude (Dennis, Muller, Miller, & Banerjee, 2004) and emerging "indigenist" models that consider how spirituality is being expressed in a particular culture (Coreil & Maynard, 2006; Walters & Simoni, 2002).

Health care professionals attempting a more academic understanding of spirituality need a clear definition in order to communicate effectively. We choose an empirically derived definition, which, like other research definitions, distinctly distinguishes spirituality from religion.

Religion is an organized community of faith that has written doctrine and codes of regulatory behavior. Spirituality, however, is more about personal belief and experience of a divine spirit or higher purpose, about how individuals construct meaning, and what they individually and communally experience and attend to and honor as the sacred in their lives. For those who were socialized in a religious tradition, spirituality and religion often are related (Tisdell, 2003, p. 29).

SPIRITUALITY AND CULTURE IN HEALTH EDUCATION

There has been much discussion in recent years about the importance of attending to cultural issues in health care and in health education (Luquis, Pérez, &Young, 2006; Shaya & Gbarayor, 2006). Given the changing demographics in society and the fact that people of color and those who are poor are more likely than other groups to lack insurance, and to lack adequate health care in general, clearly it is important for educators and health care professionals to better understand some cultural issues in health care. Further, as those concerned with cultural competence and health education suggest, it is important to have a sense of how to deal with communication issues across cultural differences as well as to understand differences in attitudes toward health and wellness across cultures.

Discussion on the role of spirituality in health care and health education has also been growing recently (Hawks, 2004; Hill, 2006). Much of the discussion specifically related to health care centers on the role of spirituality in palliative care (Puchalski, 2004); numerous studies are related to the role of religion in dealing with a particular disease (Koenig, McCullough, & Larson, 2001); to spirituality's connection to complementary and alternative medicine (Baer, 2001; Dossey, 1993, 1998; Hill, 2006); and finally, to ways in which various health practitioners such as physicians, nurses, and other health care providers can be responsive to patients' spiritual needs (McEwen, 2005). Writing more specifically from a health education perspective, Hawks (2004) notes that the field of health education has philosophically espoused the importance of attending to the multiple dimensions of health, including the physical, emotional, intellectual, social, and spiritual dimensions. However, he also observes that despite this philosophical emphasis on multidimensionality, most often in promoting health the field of health education actually gives little real attention to anything other than the physical in outlining health objectives; thus he argues that it is important for the field of health education to be proactive toward research and practice efforts that deal with the role of spirituality in health promotion and education. Perhaps toward that end, some studies have recently explored how spirituality relates to the health perceptions and behaviors of college students (Dennis, Muller, Miller, & Banerjee, 2004; Wood & Hebert, 2005).

Despite the fact that there is discussion in health education both about spirituality and about cultural competence, thus far most of the health education literature dealing with these two issues has treated them separately. Only a few authors discuss both issues together in relation to health education. Kreuter, Lukwago, Bucholtz, Clark, and Sanders-Thompson (2002), for example, discuss the importance of creating tailored approaches to health promotion that take into account the needs of particular audiences and cultural groups. They note that spirituality may be far more important to some cultural groups (and to some individuals within those groups) than it is to others. They highlight the idea that in order to be culturally responsive one must take into account not only health behaviors but also attitudes toward health and healing, and any people in that cultural group who provide different types of health and healing that might be guided by spirituality, religion, or culture.

Musgrave, Allen, and Allen (2002) make a similar point from a public health perspective, and note that spirituality has been associated with positive health outcomes for women of color, particularly for African American and Hispanic women. They argue that in considering health promotion and education for health and wellness for women of color who value spirituality, it is particularly important to attend to spirituality in order to be culturally responsive. Thus it is important to consider the role of spirituality in connection to culturally responsive education for health and wellness. Although this role is being discussed in some arenas of education for health and wellness, too often the discussions of culture and spirituality remain separate. In this chapter the intent is to connect spirituality and culture in order to explain a culturally responsive approach to education for health. This discussion begins by rooting itself in the example of an immigrant women's health conference.

SPIRITUALITY AND HEALTH: ROOTED IN EXAMPLE

A spiritually grounded and culturally responsive approach to education for health and wellness is grounded in a particular set of assumptions about the nature of health, healing, and wholeness as well as about spirituality and culture. These assumptions will be made clear in light of the following example. Picture a scene that took place at the end of an immigrant women's health conference in which both of us were involved. (This description was written immediately following the conference, on September 9, 2006.)

Vignette from an Immigrant Women's Health Conference

Ann Swartz

One hundred women of many cultures, strangers two hours earlier, are moving in a rhythmic circle dance around the room as they chant in Aramaic, to a saying that literally means "Peace be to this house." Each stops to bless with touch and visual gaze every person she passes. Energy and peace pervade the room. These women are attending a health conference for immigrant and refugee women where the theme is "creating health by nurturing inner balance." The keynote speaker, Libby Tisdell, has spoken about spirituality and culture and led them through an exercise, "Freeing Our Sacred Face," based partly on the work of David Abalos (1998). In pairs, participants talked with each other about symbols for their negative feelings, internalized oppression, and healing from their cultures of origin. In small groups we created metaphors for freeing our sacred face. My group included a Roman Catholic of Italian heritage, an Egyptian woman and her daughter who had just gained entry to the United States, and a Muslim woman from Sudan. As we introduced ourselves someone suggested we share the meaning of our names, and from this simple act our metaphor emerged. When it was our turn to share with the large group, we four women joined hands and bowed our heads as the young girl rose from the center of our circle. This expressed the combined meaning of our names: a young girl becomes a beautiful rose through wisdom, grace, and prayer.

How different from the setting in which I had met the immigrant woman who had created the organization sponsoring this conference. That was a wonderful experience that mixed refugees with refugee service workers and mental health professionals with the goal of establishing connections that would lead to improved mental health services for the population. We spent 120 hours together, learned a great deal, and met many people. But the approach tended to be cognitive and psychological, and there was no cultural or spiritual component. Our learning about those aspects of each other came during breaks and in the evening, through the sharing of food, song, dance, and family stories; but only for those who were comfortable trying to cross boundaries or question their own assumptions. Some good programs were created out of the new knowledge we gained. But distrust remained between the three groups of attendees. Would this have been so if spirituality and culture had been called to presence?

Certain assumptions we are making about the meaning of health and education for health and why they both relate to spirituality and culture are at play both in the example just presented and in the following discussion. First, health and spirituality, in the original sense of each of those terms, are intimately related. As discussed earlier, the word *health* comes from the root term *hal,* which means "to be whole." Similarly, research studies indicate that when people talk about spirituality they are most often talking about their connection to what they see as sacred, the interconnectedness of everything, and what they draw on in their journey toward wholeness (Wuthnow, 2001; Tisdell, 2003). Thus a first assumption is that to have health is to be whole, which also relates to spirituality, given that so many people describe spirituality as a journey toward wholeness. We were trying to capitalize on that sense of spirituality as a journey toward wholeness at the immigrant women's health conference.

A second and related assumption is that educating for health is about finding ways to assist people in their move toward health. Because health is interconnectedness, the movement toward it is dynamic, never ending, and cannot be described by a single or unidirectional path. A third assumption is that many people serve as educators for health (and at times, as "mis-educators") to each individual over the course of a lifetime. They include the individual's parents and other members of her home cultural community who pass on folk wisdom about ways of promoting healing, and also doctors, nurses, *curanderos,* shamans, or other health care workers who may have been part of the processes of healing at different points in her life. Religious or spiritual communities may have also provided various rituals that relate to mental, spiritual, and physical healing, and therefore they may have been important sources of health education. Thus a final assumption, based on the earlier three, is that people can find a sense of wholeness, a sense of health, partly through embracing both their culture and spirituality. Human beings always express themselves culturally—in the language they speak, in the food they eat, in the clothes they wear, in the music they make, in the art they create, and in their direct expression of what they see as sacred or as spiritual, including many of their rituals around healing (Leininger & McFarland, 2002). As a result, a culturally responsive education for health and wellness needs to honor both the spiritual and cultural dimensions of each person in her move toward health and her move toward wholeness. That's what we were trying to achieve at the immigrant women's health conference.

These assumptions about spirituality stem from the results of Libby's research on spirituality (Tisdell, 2003, 2006). They are supported by the wider body of literature and research on spirituality and health cited throughout this chapter. These findings may be summarized as follows: (1) Spirituality and religion are not the same; but for people who were socialized in a religious tradition, there is usually some overlap between the two. (2) Spirituality is always present though often unacknowledged in education and health environments. (3) Spirituality is about (a) a connection to what people experience as sacred or refer to as God, the Lifeforce, Great Mystery, or a similar term; (b) ultimate meaning making in a journey toward wholeness, healing, and the interconnectedness of all things; (c) the ongoing development of identity (including cultural identity), moving toward what many authors refer to as greater *authenticity;* or (d) the way people construct knowledge through largely unconscious and symbolic processes (as first suggested by Fowler, 1981), a process manifested in metaphor, image, symbol, music, and other expressions of creativity, which are often cultural. (4) Finally, spiritual experiences often happen by surprise. It is not always necessary to use the term *spirituality* to create experiences that people might connect to as spiritual. Rather, by drawing on multiple ways of knowing, people might experience a sense of wholeness through their own engagement and creativity; some might experience this as spiritual.

EDUCATING FOR HEALTH AND WHOLENESS IN CONTEXT

All those who educate for health and wholeness from a spiritually grounded and culturally responsive perspective do so in particular contexts. Some are health educators in specific health education contexts as identified by the discipline. Others are educators for health as health care providers or work more broadly in educating for health and wholeness in other environments. As educators, we had occasion to work together with a nonprofit organization in the community on the immigrant women's health conference. But more often we work in different contexts. Thus in this section we speak in separate voices to describe what our spiritually grounded culturally responsive approaches to educating for health and wellness look like in the contexts of our respective educational practices. We invite health educators to explore their own personal spiritual and cultural backgrounds, as these will have meaning for grounding their own practices.

Spiritually Grounded and Culturally Responsive Adult Education
Libby Tisdell

I currently teach in an adult education doctoral program, though I have occasion to do workshops with adult learners in many contexts, including the immigrant women's health conference discussed earlier. All of my work as an adult educator in any context is grounded in a belief in the importance of taking into account the multiple dimensions through which people learn, including the spiritual, the cultural, the rational, the affective, and the somatic dimensions. I attempt to find ways to address these elements of learning, though it doesn't necessarily mean that I overtly discuss all of them. Rather, it means that I try to create activities that will touch on these dimensions. Much of my work as an academic who works for the health of the society at large centers on teaching higher education classes about diversity and equity issues, and challenging systems of oppression based on race, culture, gender, or sexual orientation. I learned in my early years of teaching diversity and equity courses that it is impossible to really teach toward these goals by taking into account only rational modes of thought. Indeed, people have intensely emotional experiences of oppression and privilege based on race, culture, national origin, gender, or sexual orientation, and these experiences affect who they are and how they think. Further, many people experience recovering from these experiences and reclaiming parts of their oppressed identity in a positive way as a spiritual experience, and they often speak about it as such. This is why I eventually conducted a qualitative study exploring how spirituality informs the work of thirty-one educators of different cultural groups engaging in culturally responsive education in teaching classes about race, gender, or culture, and wrote a book about that study (see Tisdell, 2003). The results are summarized in the assumptions about spirituality in use in this chapter.

I later did another study on the ways medical educators are teaching about spirituality and complementary and alternative medicine (CAM), finding that many schools are negotiating this addition to the traditional curriculum. Educators' success in this is due in part to the general public's growing interest in these topics and the subsequent attention of grant funders. All the study participants were careful to distinguish between religion and spirituality, noting that attention to spirituality allows consideration of all the many factors that are at play in the therapeutic relationship and that contribute to healing by complementing medical intervention. The participants also specified that spirituality is separate from CAM, although CAM providers are more likely to consider it in their care. These educators are expanding the boundaries of what counts as knowledge and what constitutes healing (Tisdell, 2004). In the course of that study I also discovered the works of medical anthropologists (Baer, 2001) and academic physicians (Astrow, Puchalski, & Sulmasy, 2001; Puchalski, 2004), who have been heavily involved in dealing with spirituality in medical education. These sources remain useful in developing my education practice.

What I was trying to do in facilitating the workshop at the refugee women's health conference is what I also try to do in my doctoral-level classes that deal with culture: to draw on multiple ways that learners construct knowledge and to draw on both their culture and activities that may touch on the spiritual to facilitate learning and to facilitate healing. Obviously, doctoral students are required to read some sophisticated material and write papers that draw on theoretical concepts in educational practice, whereas those who show up at a voluntary health conference are not. But I tend to begin my courses by asking learners to explore their personal connection to the topic of the course and also their cultural connection, because most of my courses in some way deal with culture. As the educator, I also discuss my personal connection to the course and my experience of the phenomenon under study in my earlier life growing up. In so doing I am trying to make my own positionality and culture visible in order to get participants to think about what their own assumptions—growing out of the way they grew up—might be about people of a different race, culture, sexual orientation, national origin, social class, or religion. I am trying to help them look at these issues from a personal perspective. I am also trying to get them to think about this on the systemic level, to explore how these social systems of race, culture, and religion affect the education system and the knowledge production system, and to consider why certain forms of knowledge are more valued than others, particularly when they represent the interests of the dominant culture. In a variety of exercises I draw on the Hays (2001) counseling model, which codifies dominant culture in the United States according to power (white, male, moneyed, heterosexual, fully able, Euro-American born, of Christian background). Further, I try to help participants examine issues of internalized oppression—the fact that every person will have to some degree internalized the values of the dominant culture, even if he is not a member of the dominant culture and it is not in his best interest to internalize those values. At the immigrant women's health conference, even though it was not an academic setting, I did talk about the phenomenon of internalized oppression, and how the women might heal from it.

But what does this have to do with spirituality? As implied earlier, Latino writer David Abalos (1998) suggests that in order for particular cultural groups to create and sustain positive social change on behalf of themselves as individuals and on behalf of their cultural communities, they need to reclaim four *faces* of their cultural being: the personal, the political, the historical, and the sacred faces. In essence, an assumption that I make about my students is that they deal with their internalized oppression and begin to heal from it by reclaiming these four faces. People often find this reclaiming process to be a spiritual experience (Cervantes & Parham, 2005). I have found that it is by making meaning through image, symbol, and metaphor manifested in art, music, drama, or dance that people connect to their culture and deepest identity, and often to their spirituality, and this helps them to engage and free their sacred face. Thus not only do I have people in my classes do readings and write papers in order to engage the course content in rational ways, but I also encourage them to collaborate with others on projects, because knowledge by and for community use and healing is best made and given voice in a community context. Further, I try to find a way to engage their creativity by using music, metaphor, art, or dance at some point in the classroom processes, and I encourage them to do this in their own lives. Very often people do experience these creative expressions, which often also arise out of the interaction of their culture and spirituality, as an important part of their journey toward wholeness and their journey toward greater health and healing. This is also part of the way they can give expression to the knowledge that has now become embodied and anchored in them in ways beyond the rational.

As suggested earlier, I engaged these same processes in a much less detailed way in the time span of two hours at the immigrant women's health conference. My coauthor has already described her conference experience with her small group as they created and used metaphor after they had heard the cognitive explanation of internalized oppression and the importance of engaging the four faces of one's being, as described by Abalos. There was group expression and there was music and movement. Indeed, spirituality is about a journey toward wholeness, and journey connotes movement. That was why they danced!

Spiritually Grounded and Culturally Responsive Clinical Practice
Ann Swartz

My question of how to position myself as a spiritually grounded, culturally responsive health care provider was informed by my stepping outside the biomedical paradigm and considering how traditional cultures theorize about disease causation and healing. My assumptions were that even in the United States within the dominant culture, a multitude of multiethnic traditional beliefs and practices still exist and that traditional cultural beliefs of diverse ethnic groups are more similar to each other than they are to biomedicine. I hoped that by taking this perspective I could join people and their families through commonalities, share when invited whatever seemed potentially useful from biomedical knowledge, and allow others to project onto me their perception of *healer* as it made sense to them. I would hold myself accountable for remaining within my legally prescribed scope of practice. Adopting this attitude led me to work with a immigrant and refugee women's organization, in whatever way it chose to use my skills, and to find a kindred spirit in Libby Tisdell.

Histories of nursing and medical care from many cultures locate the beginnings of this care in religious settings, so the spiritual element in health care practice cannot be considered a new invention (Donahue, 1985). But spirituality often has an uncomfortable fit in the evidence-based and outcome-focused biomedicine of today. In medicine, where curing disease is paramount, the interest in spirituality has focused on belief, meditative practices, prayer as medicine, and faith and religion as related to health. Sympathetic medical researchers argue for a broader definition, relating spirituality to that which is pleasurable to the aesthetic senses (Rabin, 2003). Thus spirituality could be related to activities that regulate production of stress hormones, establishing a clinical relationship and connection with quality of life. A notable follower of this approach, Herbert Bensen (2003) has spent a career studying the *relaxation response* among followers of many faiths. He finds that practices in all faith traditions are equally effective at evoking this stress-reducing response; the words or techniques used do not matter. It is the coupling with a belief system that is necessary.

Other empirical support for spirituality as an aspect of health comes from extensive research focusing on spirituality as religious coping (Harrison, Hays, Koenig, Eme-Akwari, & Pargament, 2001). There is clearly evidence in this body of research emphasizing the individual person's traits and beliefs that a coherent belief system supports stress management and coping with challenges. Much more controversial is the study of prayer. Pioneering efforts by Dossey (1993) to study prayer as a form of nonlocal healing have progressed to randomized control trials of distant healing by strangers through prayer. Interpretations of results vary widely depending on where they are published, and systematic reviews of results remain equivocal (Roberts, Ahmed, & Hall, 2007). Research taking a more culturally grounded perspective on prayer identifies that Americans of diverse ethnicities identify prayer as both folk home remedy and spiritual practice. It is the most frequently reported home remedy (Easom, 2006).

Somewhat differently, in clinical nursing practice, where the therapeutic relationship is primary, spirituality is consistently defined as a unifying force and integrative aspect in a person, the dimension that evokes feeling and provides meaning through a transcendence and interconnectedness that manifests at many boundaries—relation to self and to others, group relations, and relation to that which is transcendent or beyond, above, or ultimate (Reed, 1992; Dossey & Guzzetta, 2000). Similarly, the nature of hope is a recurrent theme in the palliative care literature, where spirituality is emerging as a concept largely devoid of religion (Sinclair, Pereira, & Raffin, 2006). Here, where the needs for recurrent patient education are great, numerous studies show that what works is a multifaceted, personally tailored approach, using various media and activities and honoring the self (Bugge & Higginson, 2006), much like the model my coauthor, Libby, has developed for teaching.

In looking to professional literature to help define my clinical practice, I found validation in these resources. However, to avoid labeling and diagnosing spiritual needs or problems, which could open the door to transgressing religious boundaries,

I sought a less specific clinical framework than biomedicine provides and one that was consistent with my experience of spirituality in the clinical arena. The most practical help for using spirituality in a culturally responsive way has come to me from two divergent sources: family nursing research and cultural anthropology.

Family nursing theory provides an understanding of context and suggests ways to intervene. Family households, whatever their composition, produce health through a dynamic process of interactions with the complex contexts in which they are embedded. They do this in ways that are unique but also culturally consistent, using meaningful patterns of routines and rituals that can either enhance resilience or threaten well-being. Several pieces of research by Denham (1997, 1999a, 1999b, 2002) describe this in great detail. For Denham, *routines* are patterned activities that structure families through the processing of information, knowledge, and experience. *Rituals* are activities with significant meaning, satisfying symbolic forms of communication acted out over time, that relate to family identity and call upon existing strengths and resources to meet needs. Family health routines are often characterized by highly ritualized individual health practices that include patterned member interactions. Time as cycles (days, seasons, events, developmental stages) is critical to this creative process of health routine enactment. Awareness of this research should encourage health educators to reevaluate their selection of target audiences, keeping family in mind, and to consider how they might contribute to the creative development of rituals and routines that are culturally consistent but also unique to each family.

Moving to the realm of cultural anthropology, Kinsley (1996) discusses a cross-cultural perspective on health, healing, and religion. He notes that traditional cultures tend to perceive the world as filled with life and to attribute to all natural objects a soul or animating essence; human beings, especially, are believed to possess a soul or souls that underlie and define their life. Beliefs in these cultures about the ultimate causes of sickness stem from moral and theological thought. Disharmony in the relationship (broken taboos, willful or accidental offense or injury) between the sick person and another being (deity, ancestor or ghost, another living person) is posited as the ultimate cause. Therefore seeking and promoting harmonious relationships is expected to produce health. The immediate causes of sickness are seen to relate closely to the specific disease process and include soul loss, object intrusion, spirit intrusion, disease sorcery, and breach of taboo. These ideas might sound absurd to the biomedical mind, but when Kinsley (1996, p. 8) compares them to losing the will to live, germ theory, or not acting like oneself anymore, their general applicability becomes readily apparent. Dossey (1998) speaks to the same lingering on of "primitive" ideas in modern medicine in his eloquent essay about the "evil eye." Health educators need to consider the quiet presence of these enduring beliefs in populations that appear to be acculturated, even within the dominant culture. When these are quietly present as health beliefs, they will exert their power over behavioral choices even though remaining unvoiced. Astute practitioners learn to look for and identify these enduring ancient beliefs and then work with them, without ever trying to make them go away.

If remnants of these disease causation beliefs persist, what about the expectations of health care providers as healers? Often the priest and physician have been the same person, and healers are religious specialists. The most ancient and common of these healers is the shaman, followed by spirit mediums, priests or ritualists, holy persons who heal with their touch or sight, and prescriptionists who prescribe herbs, ritual, and prayers. All of these are present in the various forms of alternative and folk medicine and are argued to have correlates within Christian healing practices even today (Kinsley, 1996; Baer, 2001). Because I was not planning to become a spiritual healer, this literature did not offer me a practice prototype. But it did offer valuable information about traditional healing's central themes (Kinsley, 1996). My goal was to move past merely knowing and accepting that folk healing still occurs, so that I could allow for and support the spiritual as my patients defined it as necessary to their lives, and could create environments that would foster this process. So I wanted to address the traditional healing themes that made sense within my practice.

The themes of confession and of transference and objectification of illness (Kinsley, 1996) fell well within my previous experience, both as therapist and as one who worked with physical trauma. Much of nursing and psychotherapy is about being with a person through her unburdening and catharsis around regrettable events. This is healing if done without judgment or moralizing to enforce some level of social control. Sometimes therapeutic activities purposefully use the creation and destruction of a symbol of illness or anything negative a person wishes to move beyond. My clinical experiences with trauma patients convinced me that effective working with them involves a taking in and taking on of aspects of their experience, an almost tangible sharing of their burden, best expressed in the concepts of transpersonal psychology (Daniels, 2005).

Effective healers traditionally have prestige, confidence, and empathy (Kinsley, 1996). Prestige would be difficult to negotiate and use cross-culturally, so my personal emphasis has been on confidence and empathy. By knowing exactly what I can and cannot do and what I have to offer in a specific setting, and by showing empathy, often by revealing personal experiences of overcoming, I have found ways to operate within this theme. Sometimes just expressing genuine interest in the day-to-day lives and problems of people who never expected you to be interested is quite enough to garner a type of prestige. One of the most important themes and roles of healers is to assign meaning to illness. Relating the illness to other aspects of the patient's life and helping to restore harmony is the goal. I knew this also from experience, and knew that it requires a certain level of agreement of worldview between patient and care provider. In a multicultural context it became more important to help a person uncover how he was making such meaning, asking himself if this construction rang true within his belief system, and perhaps helping him to identify a person with a worldview more similar to his to help him with this task.

The most significant new learning about healing themes came from understanding sacred space, pilgrimage, and healing contexts, and then the importance of group solidarity in healing (Kinsley, 1996). Sacred space and sacred places have always been central to healing. Usually sacred space is established temporarily for healing and rituals. There may be aspects of drama, decoration with objects from nature or artifacts of material culture, symbolic acts, singing, chanting, and dance.

Sometimes an aspect of pilgrimage is involved. Always the person seeking healing has an active role of calling upon her own powers of healing. The family is likely to be included. Many healing rituals actually require the presence of family and community members, and they engage in ritual singing and dancing to contribute to the healing and also to strengthen interpersonal connections, which are often the source of spiritual distress. Interpersonal connection through spiritual interventions of touching, instilling hope and faith, and practicing presence requires a relationship (Achterberg, Dossey, & Kolkmeier, 1994; Anderson, 2001; McEwen, 2005). It was these aspects of healing that seemed to hold the most potential for doing something different, not offered by biomedicine, that had a chance to reach across ethnic boundaries without requiring a lot of language, and to resonate with what families naturally do to create and maintain family health.

Learning to address spirituality related to health and illness in my practice has been a nonlinear process (unlike the rational deductive diagnostic process of Western medicine). The approach to a person is a search for places to build connection, to uncover relatedness, and the "work" always has to do with his creation of meaning and, in turn, my creation of new meaning. It is a constant building through connection. The "assessment" is not of someone or of some community's "need" or "problem" as is usual in health care. It is about identifying how this person is organizing himself (or how a group is organizing itself)—and thereby creating his health—in response to various connections with other people, his family, the communities he belongs to, the Divine, and then using connection to cross a boundary and become part of that process. It is not knowledge of risk factors and evidence-based outcomes for diseases that make this possible but the elements of spiritual expression, beyond words. Therefore this may not be seen as a practical approach or one that is easily measured, but it works!

CONCLUSION

In conclusion, it is clear that there is certainly a place for spirituality in culturally responsive education for health and wellness. It is not just that there is a place for it but that it seems that if one is really concerned about healing (as opposed to curing, which is not the same thing), then it is important to consider all the pieces of the person, as she moves along her journey to greater health, or dances her way along the journey to wholeness. Spirituality is an important part of this process. Thus it is important for culturally responsive education for health.

POINTS TO REMEMBER

- WHO supports a holistic definition of health that attends to spirituality and culture.

- The field of health education espouses multidimensionality and has begun to discuss spirituality, but in practice emphasis remains on the purely physical.

■ Research supports a definition of spirituality as something different from but often connected with religion and integrally tied to culture.

■ Spiritually grounded, culturally responsive education and practice for health requires stepping beyond the biomedical model, leading by example from one's own cultural or spiritual history and current positionality, and connecting with participants through multiple ways of knowing.

CASE STUDY

You have contracted with a large, for-profit health care system to enhance the health and wellness of residents in six subsidized-housing high-rises located in both urban and suburban communities and all within a ten-mile radius. Approximately 65 percent of the group members are white and speak only English. Another 20 percent are African American. The remainder are immigrants from various Asian countries, Mexico and the Caribbean, the former Yugoslavia, and north Africa. Two-thirds of the residents are elderly. The rest are primarily middle-aged adults who are physically disabled and younger adults who are mentally or psychiatrically disabled. All are officially capable of independent living and eligible for, if not enrolled in, government health insurance programs. You are free to start by addressing the entire population, starting a test program at one building, or proceeding in any way that you choose. How will you promote health through education and clinical practice in a spiritually grounded and culturally responsive manner?

KEY TERMS

Culturally responsive	Spirituality
Education for health	Spiritually grounded

REFERENCES

Abalos, D. (1998). *La communidad Latina in the United States.* Westport, CT: Praeger.

Achterberg, J., Dossey, B., & Kolkmeier, L. (1994). *Rituals of healing: Using imagery for health and wellness.* New York: Bantam.

Anderson, M. (2001). *Sacred dying: Creating rituals for embracing the end of life.* Roseville, CA: Prima.

Astrow, A., Puchalski, C., & Sulmasy, D. (2001). Religions, spirituality and health care: Social, ethical, and practical considerations. *American Journal of Medicine, 110*(4), 283–287.

Baer, H. (2001). *Biomedicine and alternative healing systems in America: Issues of class, race, ethnicity, & gender.* Madison: University of Wisconsin Press.

Bensen, H. (2003, April). *Relaxation response.* Paper presented at the research conference "Integrating Research on Spirituality and Health and Well-Being into Service Delivery." Bethesda, MD.

Bugge, E., & Higginson, I. J. (2006). Palliative care and the need for education: Do we know how to make a difference? A limited systematic review. *Health Education Journal, 65*(2), 101–125.

Cervantes, J., & Parham, T. (2005). Toward a meaningful spirituality for people of color: Lessons for the counseling practitioner. *Cultural Diversity and Ethnic Minority Psychology, 11*(1), 69–81.

Coreil, J., & Maynard, G. (2006). Indigenization of illness support groups in Haiti. *Human Organization, 65*(2), 128–139.

Daniels, M. (2005). *Shadow, self, spirit: Essays in transpersonal psychology.* Exeter, UK: Imprint Academic.

DeHaven, M. J., Hunter, I. B., Wilder, L., Walton, J. W., & Berry, J. (2004). Health programs in faith-based organizations: Are they effective? *American Journal of Public Health, 94*(6), 1030–1036.

Denham, S. A. (1997). *An ethnographic study of family health in Appalachian microsystems.* Unpublished dissertation, University of Alabama at Birmingham.

Denham, S. A. (1999a). Family health: During and after death of a family member. *Journal of Family Nursing, 5,* 160–183.

Denham, S. A. (1999b). Family health in an economically disadvantaged population. *Journal of Family Nursing, 5,* 184–213.

Denham, S. A. (2002). *The family health model: A framework for nursing.* Philadelphia: Davis.

Dennis, D., Muller, S., Miller, K., & Banerjee, P. (2004). Spirituality among a college student cohort: A quantitative assessment. *American Journal of Health Education, 35*(4), 220–228.

Donahue, M. P. (1985). *Nursing: The finest art: An illustrated history.* St. Louis, MO: Mosby.

Dossey, B. M., & Guzzetta, C. E. (2000). *Holistic nursing practice.* In B. M. Dossey, L. Keegan, & C. E. Guzzetta (Eds.), *Holistic nursing: A handbook for practice* (3rd ed., pp. 5–26). Rockville, MD: Aspen.

Dossey, L. (1993). *Healing words: The power of prayer and the practice of medicine.* San Francisco: HarperSanFrancisco.

Dossey, L. (1998). The evil eye. *Alternative Therapies in Health and Medicine, 4*(1), 9–18.

Easom, L. R. (2006). Prayer: Folk home remedy vs. spiritual practice. *Journal of Cultural Diversity, 13*(3), 146–151.

El Awa, F. (2004). The role of religion in tobacco control interventions. *Bulletin of the World Health Organization, 82*(12), 894–895.

Fowler, J. (1981). *Stages of faith: The psychology of human development and the quest for meaning.* San Francisco: HarperSanFrancisco.

Harrison, M. O., Hays, J. C., Koenig, H. G., Eme-Akwari, A. G., & Pargament, K. I. (2001). The epidemiology of religious coping: A review of recent literature. *International Journal of Psychiatry, 13,* 86–93.

Hawks, S. (2004). Spiritual wellness, holistic health, and the practice of health education. *American Journal of Health Education, 35,* 11–16.

Hays, P. (2001). *Addressing cultural complexities in practice: A framework for clinicians and counselors.* Washington, DC: American Psychological Association Press.

Hill, F. (2006). Health promotion and complementary medicine: The extent and future of professional collaboration and integration. *Health Education, 106,* 283–293.

Jabbour, S., & Fouad, F. M. (2004). Religion-based tobacco control interventions: How should WHO proceed? *Bulletin of the World Health Organization, 82*(12), 923–927.

Kinsley, D. (1996). *Health, healing, and religion: A cross-cultural perspective.* Upper Saddle River, NJ: Prentice Hall.

Koenig, H. G., McCullough, M. E., & Larson, D. B. (2001). *Handbook of religion and health.* New York: Oxford University Press.

Kreuter, M., Lukwago, S., Bucholtz, D., Clark, E., & Sanders-Thompson, V. (2002). Achieving cultural appropriateness in health promotion programs: Targeted and tailored approaches. *Health Education & Behavior, 30,* 133–145.

Leininger, M., & McFarland, M. (2002). *Transcultural nursing: Concepts, theories, research and practice* (3rd ed.). New York: McGraw-Hill.

Luquis, R. R., Pérez, M. A., & Young, K. (2006). Cultural competence development in health education professional preparation programs. *American Journal of Health Education, 37*(4), 233–241.

McEwen, M. (2005). Spiritual nursing care: State of the art. *Holistic Nursing Practice, 19*(4), 161–168.

McSherry, W. (2006). *Making sense of spirituality in nursing and health care practice.* London: Jessica Kingsley.

Musgrave, C., Allen, C., & Allen, G. (2002). Spirituality and health for women of color. *American Journal of Public Health, 92*(4), 557–560.

Perrin, K. M., & McDermott, R. J. (1997). The spiritual dimension of health: A review. *American Journal of Health Studies, 13*(2), 90–99.

Puchalski, C. (2004). Listening to stories of pain and joy. *Health Progress, 85*(4), 20–22, 57.

Rabin, B. (2003, April). *Spirituality and psychoneuroimmunology.* Paper presented at the research conference "Integrating Research on Spirituality and Health and Well-Being into Service Delivery," Bethesda, MD.

Reed, P. G. (1992). An emerging paradigm for the investigation of spirituality in nursing. *Research in Nursing and Health, 15,* 349–357.

Roberts, L., Ahmed, I., & Hall, S. (2007). Intercessory prayer for the alleviation of ill health. *Cochrane Database of Systematic Reviews, 4,* CD000368.

Sanford, J. (1977). *Healing and wholeness.* New York: Paulist Press.

Saxena, S. (2007). *WHOQOL spirituality, religiousness and personal beliefs (SRBP) field-test instrument.* Retrieved June 10, 2007, from http://www.who.int/msa/qol.

Shaya, F., & Gbarayor, C. (2006). The case for cultural competence in health professions education. *American Journal of Pharmaceutical Education, 70,* 1–6.

Sinclair, S., Pereira, J., & Raffin, S. (2006). A thematic review of spirituality literature in palliative care. *Journal of Palliative Medicine, 9*(2), 464–479.

Tisdell, E. (2003). *Exploring spirituality and culture in adult and higher education.* San Francisco: Jossey-Bass.

Tisdell, E. (2004). The politics of medical education: Incorporating spirituality and complementary and alternative medicine (CAM) in the curriculum. In E. E. Clover (Ed.), *Proceedings of the joint international conference of the 45th annual Adult Education Research Conference and the Canadian Association for the Study of Adult Education.* Victoria, BC: University of Victoria.

Tisdell, E. (2006). Diversity, spirituality, and secular higher education: The teaching paradox. *Journal of Religion and Education, 33,* 49–68.

Walters, K. L., & Simoni, J. M. (2002). Reconceptualizing native women's health: An "indigenist" stress-coping model. *American Journal of Public Health, 92*(4), 520–524.

Wood, R., & Hebert, E. (2005). The relationship between spiritual meaning and purpose and drug and alcohol use among college students. *American Journal of Health Studies, 20,* 72–80.

World Health Organization. (1948). *Constitution.* Geneva: Author.

World Health Organization. (1998). *Health for all in the twenty-first century* (Document A51/5). Geneva: Author.

Wuthnow, R. (2001). *Creative spirituality: The way of the artist.* Berkeley: University of California Press.

CHAPTER

6

HEALTH EDUCATION THEORETICAL MODELS AND MULTICULTURAL POPULATIONS

RAFFY R. LUQUIS

LEARNING OBJECTIVES

After completing this chapter, you will be able to

- Explain cultural competence in terms of two theoretical models.
- Discuss the influence of culture, heritage, family, religion, and spirituality, among other factors, on health behaviors and practices.
- Apply culture-based models to the development of health education and promotion programs.

INTRODUCTION

In the last decade the population of the United States reached its most racially and ethnically diverse composition yet. U.S. Census Bureau (2004) projections of population growth indicate that the number of Hispanics, African Americans, Asians and Pacific Islanders, Native Americans and Alaska Natives, and members of other racial and ethnic groups will continue to grow in the next few decades. In fact, it is estimated that by 2020, the nonwhite population will have increased to 39 percent of the U.S. total (U.S. Census Bureau, 2004). (See Chapter One in this volume for a more complete description of the demographic changes taking place in the United States.)

The increasing diversification of the population confirms the health education field's need to incorporate the concepts of multicultural groups and cultural competence into every aspect of the planning, implementation, and evaluation processes of health education and promotion programs (Luquis & Pérez, 2003). It is essential that these processes incorporate theoretical models so that cultural competence and related concepts can be considered in needs assessments and in the development and implementation of culturally and linguistically appropriate health education and promotion programs. (This need is discussed in greater detail in Chapter Seven.)

Culture has been defined as the "sum of beliefs, practices, habits, likes, dislikes, norms, customs, rituals, and so forth that we learn from our families, during the years of socialization" (Spector, 2004, p. 9). To some extent, a person's cultural background defines his or her perceptions in the context of a larger group and influences how he or she behaves throughout a lifetime. Culture influences people's perceptions of their health; it also affects their health beliefs, attitudes, and actions such as diets and nutritional habits, self-care practices, communication, and health care–seeking behaviors (Nakamura, 1999). Thus it is imperative that health educators recognize the importance of and apply the concept of culture in health education and prevention interventions.

In the past health educators have relied on theories and models such as the health belief model, social cognitive theory, and the transtheoretical model, among others, to explain behavioral determinants of health. In addition, health educators have used planning models such as PRECEDE-PROCEED or MATCH to develop and implement health education and promotion programs. Although these commonly used theories and models emphasize logical and critical thinking in relation to health behaviors, they do not attend to the sociocultural determinants of health behaviors (Simon, 2006). Thus the purpose of this chapter is to describe four models that assess the role of culture in the prevention of disease and promotion of health. The first two models, Purnell and Campinha-Bacote, specifically describe the role of culture and the concept of cultural competence among health care professionals. The last two models describe two frameworks to be used when developing health promotion and disease prevention programs.

MODELS FOR ASSESSING CULTURAL COMPETENCE

The Purnell Model for Cultural Competence

The Purnell model for cultural competence provides a comprehensive, systematic, and organized framework with specific questions and a format for learning and assessing the concepts and characteristics of culture (see Figure 6.1) (Purnell & Paulanka, 2003; Purnell, 2005). With this model, health professionals across disciplines and settings can analyze the cultural data that will facilitate the development of culturally competent health promotion and illness and disease prevention programs.

The Purnell model for cultural competence is organized in a circle, with four outlying rims representing the global society, the community, the family, and the person. The interior part of the circle is divided into twelve pie-shaped sections representing cultural domains and their concepts (Purnell & Paulanka, 2003; Purnell, 2005). In the center of the model is an empty circle representing the unknown phenomena: the practices and characteristics of the individual or group of interest. This circle will expand or contract, depending on the individual user's (in this case the health educator's) level of cultural competence. The model is based on several explicit assumptions and purposes. In addition the Purnell model displays a jagged line that illustrates the nonlinear process of acquiring cultural competence. Purnell (2005) explains that an individual progresses from unconscious incompetence (not being aware of lacking knowledge about other cultures), to conscious incompetence (being aware of lacking knowledge), to conscious competence (learning and providing culturally appropriate interventions), and finally to unconscious competence (automatically providing culturally competent services). Purnell warns that it is difficult and potentially dangerous to work from unconscious competence because differences among individuals exist in every racial and ethnic group. Thus health educators must understand that cultural competence is a process and not an end point.

As stated earlier, the outside rims, or macro aspect, of this model identify global society, community, family, and person. In thinking about the global society, users of this model consider world politics and communication, conflict and welfare, natural disaster and famine, and international exchanges, among other things, and also the expanding opportunity for people to travel around the world and interact with diverse societies. World events are broadly disseminated through television, radio, the Internet, and newsprint and thus affect all societies. As a result of such events, people are forced to alter, consciously and unconsciously, their lifeways, worldviews, and acculturation patterns (Purnell & Paulanka, 2003; Purnell, 2005).

Community in this model is defined as a group of people having a common interest or identity and living in specific vicinity. Community also includes physical, social, and symbolic characteristics, such as mountains, economics, and history, that cause people to connect with one another. For example, people may define their community by their rural or urban environment or by social concepts such as politics and religion or by symbolic characteristics such as art, music, and language. *Family,* in contrast, is

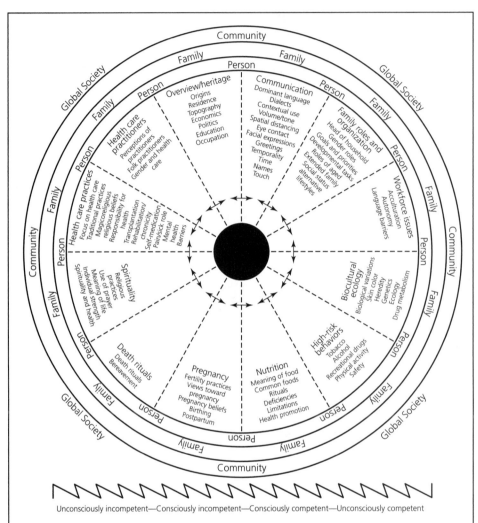

Community
Family
Person
Family
Global Society
Person
Family
Person

Overview/heritage
Origins
Residence
Topography
Economics
Politics
Education
Occupation

Communication
Dominant language
Dialects
Contextual use
Volume/tone
Spatial distancing
Eye contact
Facial expressions
Greetings
Temporality
Time
Names
Touch

Family roles and organization
Head of household
Gender roles
Goals and priorities
Developmental tasks
Roles of aged
Extended family
Social status
alternative
lifestyles

Health care practitioners
Perceptions of
practitioners
Folk practitioners
Gender and health
care

Health care practices
Focus on health care
Traditional practices
Magicoreligious
religious beliefs
Responsibility for
health
Transplantation/
chronicity
Rehabilitation/
Self-medication
Pain/sick role
Mental
health
Barriers

Workforce issues
Acculturation
Autonomy
Language barriers

Biocultural ecology
Biological variations
Skin color
Heredity
Genetics
Ecology
Drug metabolism

Spirituality
Religious
practices
Use of prayer
Meaning of life
Individual strength
Spirituality and health

High-risk behaviors
Tobacco
Alcohol
Recreational drugs
Physical activity
Safety

Death rituals
Death rituals
Bereavement

Pregnancy
Fertility practices
Views toward
pregnancy
Pregnancy beliefs
Birthing
Postpartum

Nutrition
Meaning of food
Common foods
Rituals
Deficiencies
Limitations
Health promotion

Community

Unconsciously incompetent—Consciously incompetent—Consciously competent—Unconsciously competent

Primary characteristics of culture: age, generation, nationality, race, color, gender, religion

Secondary characteristics of culture: educational status, socioeconomic status, occupation, military status, political beliefs, urban versus rural residence, enclave identity, marital status, parental status, physical characteristics, sexual orientation, gender issues, and reason for migration (sojourner, immigrant, undocumented status)

Unconsciously incompetent: not being aware that one is lacking knowledge about another culture
Consciously incompetent: being aware that one is lacking knowledge about another culture
Consciously competent: learning about the client's culture, verifying generalizations about the client's culture, and providing culturally specific interventions
Unconsciously competent: automatically providing culturally congruent care to clients of diverse cultures

FIGURE 6.1. *Purnell Model for Cultural Competence.*

Source: Purnell, 2005, p. 11. Reprinted with permission of the author.

two or more people who are emotionally connected. Family includes members of both the nuclear and extended family and close and distant blood and nonblood relatives and significant others. Family composition and roles change according to age, generation, marital status, relocation or immigration, and socioeconomic status, obligating each individual to rethink his or her beliefs and lifestyle. Finally, a *person* is a human being who is constantly biologically, psychologically, sociologically, and culturally adapting to his or her community and environment. In general, in Western culture an individual is thought of as a unique being and singular member of society; whereas in Asian culture a person is identified first as a member of a family rather than a simple element of nature (Purnell & Paulanka, 2003; Purnell, 2005).

On the micro level the model displays a framework of twelve domains and sets of concepts common to all cultures. The domains are interconnected and have implications for organizing health promotion and disease prevention interventions in a manner that respects the differences among racial and ethnic groups. The twelve domains are (1) overview/heritage, (2) communication, (3) family roles and organization, (4) workforce issues, (5) biocultural ecology, (6) high-risk behaviors, (7) nutrition, (8) pregnancy and child-bearing practices, (9) death rituals, (10) spirituality, (11) health care practices, and (12) health care practitioners (Purnell & Paulanka, 2003; Purnell, 2005).

The first domain, overview/heritage, involves concepts related to country of origin, current residence, the effect of the topographies of the country of origin and of the current residence, economics, politics, reasons for emigration, and educational status. These concepts are interconnected. For example, the social, political, and economics forces of the country of origin can often be the major reason for emigration. In addition, the value placed on education can influence the reason for emigrating among ethnic and racial groups (Purnell & Paulanka, 2003). For instance, second- and third-generation Mexican Americans have significant job skills and education; however, many current Mexican immigrants, especially from rural areas, have poor educational backgrounds and may not place a high value on education (Zoucha & Purnell, 2003). "Being familiar with the individual's personal educational values and learning modes allows health care providers, educators, and employees to adjust teaching strategies for clients, students, and employees" (Purnell & Paulanka, 2003, p.13). Thus health educators need to consider and understand these concepts as part of any health needs assessment.

The communication domain involves verbal and nonverbal interactions and considers the dominant language and use of language, dialects, paralanguage variations, eye contact, facial expression, and touch among other variables likely to be distinctive in each cultural group. Health educators must be aware of these communication patterns as they can affect the educators' interactions with members of racial and ethnic groups. (See Chapter Eight for further discussion of communication patterns.) For example, some groups may have limited English language ability; other groups may be willing to share personal thoughts and feelings only with family members and close friends and not with other people; and others may need to have their personal space respected (Purnell & Paulanka, 2003). Public health educators also need to understand that communication issues are interrelated with issues in all the other domains.

Similarly, issues in the family roles and organization domain affect other domains' issues and define what relationships will look like between insiders and outsiders. The family roles and organization domain addresses the views related to the head of the household and to gender roles; family roles including those for children, adolescents, and the elderly; and opinions about alternative lifestyles, such as single parenthood or same-sex sexual orientation (Purnell & Paulanka, 2003). For example, for many members of the Hispanic community the family is the most important institution in life and in one's cultural and social existence, as it provides a strong feeling of loyalty, reciprocity, and solidarity among its members. Health educators targeting the Hispanic community must understand the importance of family among this group as it can affect group members' decisions about health care and preventive behaviors.

The workforce issues comprise language barriers, degree of assimilation and acculturation, and matters of autonomy. Moreover, concepts from the other domains, such as gender role, cultural communication, and health care practices, affect the workforce issues in a multicultural work environment (Purnell & Paulanka, 2003). For example, Americans are expected to be punctual on the job and to use formal meetings and appointments in interacting with other workers. For individuals from cultures where time is less important, however, such timeliness and punctuality are culturally based attitudes that can cause serious worksite problems. For example, a number of researchers have suggested that Hispanics can be considered present-oriented individuals; therefore they do not demand punctuality and place more value on the quality of an interpersonal relationship than on the time during which this relationship takes place (Marín & Marín, 1991). Public health educators in administrative positions need to support cultural and diversity initiatives to diminish these possible problems.

The domain of biocultural ecology is concerned with physical, biological, and physiological variations among racial and ethnic groups. For instance, some racial and ethnic groups are more susceptible to and affected by certain illnesses and diseases than other groups are. Moreover, health care professionals treating dark-skinned people for rashes, anemia, or jaundice need to employ assessments different from those used with light-skinned people. In addition, differences among racial and ethnic groups in the way drugs are metabolized affect the prescription of medication for different groups (Purnell & Paulanka, 2003). Health educators must be educated about these variations as they will affect the health care and health promotion interventions developed for specific groups.

Understandings of high-risk behaviors such as tobacco, alcohol, and drug use; sexual practices; high-fat diets; and lack of physical activity differ among racial and ethnic groups. For example, culture, rites, and customs may influence the use of alcoholic beverages among ethnic groups. For instance, the Roman Catholic Church uses wine during the celebration of the mass, and the French ingest larger amounts of alcohol than Americans do, a fact some have related to a lower mortality rate due to cardiovascular disease in the latter population (Purnell & Paulanka, 2003). When assessing alcohol use, health professionals must place this high-risk behavior within the context of the cultural group. Likewise, the domain of nutrition looks at having adequate food, the meaning of food, common foods and rituals, food limitation and nutritional deficiencies, and the use of food for health promotion and disease prevention (Purnell & Paulanka, 2003). Cultural values and beliefs influence food choices, dietary behaviors, and the use of food for health promotion among racial and ethnic groups. For example, many racial and ethnic groups have theories that a balance of proper foods is needed for health maintenance and that selecting appropriate "hot" and "cold" foods can prevent and treat illnesses (Purnell & Paulanka, 2003; Spector, 2004). In addition, dietary patterns and food selection are closely tied to health issues such as obesity, cardiovascular disease, and diabetes. Health educators need to understand the different nutritional patterns among racial and ethnic groups to provide successful health promotion programs.

Pregnancy and childbearing practices among multicultural groups are also determined by cultural influences. This domain considers culturally sanctioned and unsanctioned fertility practices; views about pregnancy; and prescriptive, restrictive, and taboo practices used during pregnancy, birth, and after pregnancy (Purnell & Paulanka, 2003). Cultural beliefs and views regarding conception, pregnancy, and childbearing practices are passed down from generation to generation and are assimilated into each group's custom without being validated or completely understood. For example, Muslim and orthodox Jewish groups expect limited involvement of the husband during the delivery of the baby and prescribe specific steps to protect the baby from evil spirits (Cassar, 2006). Other ethnic and racial groups avoid certain foods or practices during pregnancy to prevent illness or harm to the baby (Purnell & Paulanka, 2003). Health care providers must respect cultural beliefs surrounding conception, pregnancy, and childbearing when making decisions related to the health of pregnant women.

The next two domains are interconnected with beliefs regarding life, religion, and death. Death rituals are the practices and views surrounding death and bereavement. These views are less likely than others to change over time within any cultural group and may cause concerns among health professionals (Purnell & Paulanka, 2003). For many racial and ethnic groups, rites surrounding death are connected to their beliefs about protecting the dead person and the family from evil spirits or ghosts and about preparing the dying person for his or her journey after death. For example, many groups use candles in rituals surrounding death to illuminate the way for the spirit of the deceased (Spector, 2004). Moreover, although the dominant American culture has a practice of burying the dead within few days, other cultural groups, such as the Mexicans, hold elaborate ceremonies in commemoration of the dead that may last for days. Among many groups these rituals are influenced by religious beliefs and spirituality. In the Purnell model the domain of spirituality is made up of religious practices, use of prayer, the meaning of life, and the relationship between spirituality and health care practices. For some people religious beliefs, more than cultural beliefs, direct their other beliefs, values, and practices (Purnell & Paulanka, 2003). Health educators must consider these religious and spiritual beliefs when developing health promotion programs. For example, the concept of spirituality has been used in health promotion to prevent early sexual behavior among African American adolescent girls (Doswell, Kopuyate, & Taylor, 2003) and has been associated with the development of resilience in African American children (Haight, 1998). (Given the importance of this domain among racial and ethnic groups, a chapter on spirituality and culture, Chapter Five, offers in-depth information in this topic.)

The last two cultural domains are also interconnected as they involve people's perceptions about health care practices and health care practitioners. The health care practices domain focuses on traditional, magicoreligious, and biomedical beliefs; individual responsibility for health; self-medicating; responses to pain; and views toward such medical issues as mental health and organ donation. For centuries people's health has been maintained by many different healing and medical practices. (Chapter Four is dedicated to the cultural practice of complementary and alternative medicine and holistic health and the impact of this practice on the field of health education.) In addition it is important to recognize that cultural and religious beliefs influence views on organ donation and blood transfusion. Although some racial and ethnic groups favor organ donation, others (as well as some religious organizations) are against it because of fear of medical institutions or a belief that it will result in suffering in an afterlife (Purnell & Paulanka, 2003). Health practitioners, including health educators, must explore health care practices and related beliefs among multicultural groups in order to provide culturally congruent health interventions. Finally, culture also affects people's perceptions and use of traditional health care practitioners and folk healers, and it affects views on gender in relation to health care. Cassar (2006) has noted that Muslim and orthodox Jewish women prefer a health care provider of the same sex during pregnancy and delivery. Some groups perceive older male physicians to be more knowledgeable and trustworthy than their younger counterparts; yet others consider folk and magicoreligious healers to be superior to traditional physicians or nurses (Purnell & Paulanka, 2003). Public health educators and other health professionals need to understand these perceptions among multicultural groups as they will influence people's use of traditional health prevention services.

A Culturally Competent Model of Care

Campinha-Bacote (1998, 1999, 2001, 2007) has developed a conceptual model of cultural competence that suggests that cultural competence in delivering health care services is a process.[1] This process comprises five essential constructs: cultural awareness, cultural knowledge, cultural encounters, cultural skills, and cultural desire.

Cultural awareness is the cognitive process through which the health professional becomes sensitive to the values, beliefs, and practices of different cultural groups. This process involves a honest exploration of one's own cultural background and views as well as a self-examination of one's own biases and prejudices toward other racial and ethnic groups. Moreover, this is only the first step in the journey toward cultural competence; health educators must go beyond awareness and develop other needed components of cultural competence (Campinha-Bacote, 1998, 2007).

As individuals move through the process of acquiring cultural competence, they must also go through a process of developing *cultural knowledge* in order to understand different racial and ethnic groups' worldviews. This cultural knowledge includes an understanding of the biological and sociological factors that contribute to health disparities among racial and ethnic groups. The development of cultural awareness and knowledge is essential in the preparation of health educators and promoters (Luquis & Pérez, 2003), and resources for this awareness and knowledge are increasingly available. A growing literature exists on the cultural views of racial and ethnic groups, multicultural health, and diversity. Professional organizations have been formed to promote cultural competence, and conferences are being held at which there are many opportunities to participate in workshops and presentations dealing with culture and health. In addition, a study of professional preparation programs in health education found that although most of these programs are not offering courses entirely devoted to cultural competence, they are adequately addressing content related to culture, race, ethnicity, and health in their existing courses (Luquis, Pérez, & Young, 2006). Still, because cultures are constantly evolving, becoming completely familiar with all the cultural aspects of even one group is challenging at best; thus health educators must also develop the cultural skills, encounters, and desire that allow them to obtain cultural knowledge directly from individuals.

The abilities to collect culturally relevant data and to conduct culture-specific assessments are *cultural skills*. Health educators will benefit from developing these cultural skills and applying them to develop, implement, and evaluate culturally appropriate interventions for people of diverse racial and ethnic groups (Luquis & Pérez, 2003). Developing such skills requires that health educators learn how to conduct a comprehensive cultural assessment to determine the explicit needs and appropriate intervention for the people being targeted (Campinha-Bacote, 1999, 2001). For example, Huff and Kline (1999) suggest that health educators collect cultural or ethnic group–specific demographic characteristics and cultural or ethnic group–specific epidemiological and environmental influences. Marín (1993) suggested that culturally appropriate health interventions reflect the cultural beliefs, values, cultural characteristics, and expected behaviors of members of the targeted racial or ethnic group. Thus needs assessment conducted with a multicultural population needs to include a cultural assessment as well (Luquis & Pérez, 2003). Two such cultural assessments are discussed later in this chapter.

The term *cultural encounters* describes the process of engaging in multicultural interactions with people of a racial or ethnic group (Campinha-Bacote, 1998, 2007). These interactions are opportunities for health educators to enhance their understanding and beliefs regarding that particular group. At times health educators may believe that because they have studied a specific racial or ethnic group and have interacted with three or four members of that group, they know everything they need to know about that group. However, three or four individuals may not fully represent the cultural beliefs and practices of the group. For instance, although Hispanics share many cultural values and beliefs, interaction with three or four members of the Hispanic population is not enough, as there are many Hispanic subgroups and they are culturally and socially diverse. Thus culturally competent health educators must constantly make it a priority to have cultural encounters to prevent stereotyping and to acquire the experiential knowledge needed to develop culturally relevant interventions. Every day health educators are faced with opportunities to interact with colleagues, clients, and other people with cultural backgrounds similar to and different from their own. These interactions will help individuals learn from each other as part of the process of achieving cultural competence, because learning from each other never ends. The more health educators endeavor to seek out these encounters, the better equipped they will be to provide programs to racial and ethnic groups (Luquis & Pérez, 2003).

Finally, *cultural desire* is the genuine motivating force that makes one want to work with people from diverse cultural backgrounds (Campinha-Bacote, 1998, 2007). Health educators who have cultural awareness, knowledge, skill, and encounters must also develop a true motivation to work with people from different racial and ethnic backgrounds (Campinha-Bacote, 1999, 2001). Cultural desire is not something that can be taught in a classroom but something that health educators must have within themselves or develop during their journey toward becoming culturally competent. They must be inspired to work within a multicultural society. Health educators who "want to" (as Campinha-Bacote, 1999, says) and who have the desire to work with racial and ethnic populations are doing a good service not only to the community they serve but also to the profession.

In addition to this model of cultural competence, Campinha-Bacote (1998) developed the Inventory for Assessing the Process of Cultural Competence Among Healthcare Professionals (IAPCC). In 2003, she revised this instrument (IAPCC-R) in order to add the construct of cultural desire. A sum of the scores of the five subscales shows whether a health professional is operating at a level of cultural proficiency (91 to 100), cultural competence (75 to 90), cultural awareness (51 to 74), or cultural incompetence (25 to 50). Higher scores represent a higher level of competence.

Although the process of cultural competence model and the IAPCC-R were developed to be used with health care professionals, other health professionals can use them to understand the complexity of cultural competence and measure individuals' level of cultural competence. Luquis and Pérez (2005) used a modified version of the IAPCC-R to measure the level of cultural competence among professional health educators. For their study, they defined the levels of cultural competence used in the IAPCC-R as they apply to the field of health education:

> *Culturally incompetent individuals can be described as those who lack an understanding of the difference among ethnic and cultural groups. They are at the lowest level of the cultural competence process. As they move through this process, the individual develops cultural awareness, or sensitivity to the values, beliefs and practices of different ethnic and cultural groups. Culturally competent individuals are not only culturally sensitive to the different groups, but are also able to respond appropriately to the needs of these groups. Finally, cultural proficiency can be described as the endpoint of cultural competence. An individual who is culturally competent has developed the ability to respond appropriately to groups of diverse ethnic and cultural backgrounds [p. 159].*

The results of this investigation showed that in general, health educators were operating at a level of cultural awareness. Moreover, thirty-four percent of the participants were operating at a level of cultural competence. Overall, the health educators in this study could be described as individuals who are sensitive to the values, beliefs, and practices of different ethnic and cultural groups and who would be able to respond appropriately to the needs of these groups. Study results also showed that variables such as race of the individual, encounters with diverse populations, and participation in cultural diversity educational programs influenced the level of cultural competence among health educators (Luquis & Pérez, 2005). Findings from this study demonstrate the role cultural competence education plays in developing culturally competent health educators, and they support the need for more research in this area for a better understanding of the complexity of cultural competence.

MODELS FOR DEVELOPING HEALTH EDUCATION PROGRAMS

The Cultural Assessment Framework

The cultural assessment framework (CAF), developed by Huff and Kline (1999), contains five levels of assessment that should be included when planning health promotion programs for multicultural groups. The CAF categories and subcategories suggest areas of inquiry that are race, ethnicity, and culture specific. Huff and Kline (1999) also recommend employing these areas in assessment tools such as surveys, focus groups, and other formative evaluation processes. The five major categories of assessment are (1) cultural or ethnic group–specific demographic characteristics, (2) cultural or ethnic group–specific epidemiological and environmental influences, (3) general and specific cultural or ethnic group characteristics, (4) general and specific health care beliefs and practices, and (5) Western health care organization and service delivery variables.

The cultural or ethnic group–specific demographic characteristics include age, gender, social class, education and literacy, religion, language, and acculturation, among others (Huff & Kline, 1999). The more health educators and promoters know about these factors, the better they will be at targeting health education programs toward specific ethnic and racial groups and at incorporating these characteristics into the development, implementation, and evaluation processes. For example, when developing a program for a Hispanic population it is important to note that although Hispanics as a group have some common demographic characteristics, relating to such factors as socioeconomic status, educational level, and language, there are some differences among each subgroup. When the three main Hispanic subgroups in the United States are compared, for example, Mexicans are younger, have larger families, and have less income and educational attainment than Puerto Ricans and Central Americans (Ramirez & de la Cruz, 2002). Such demographic differences need to be taken into consideration when developing programs targeting specific Hispanic subgroups.

Although most assessment models include epidemiological and environmental factors, Huff and Kline (1999) recommend that health education practitioners take a closer look at these factors. When epidemiological data are aggregated into larger categories of analysis, specific health issues in many racial and ethnic subgroups may be concealed. For example, a health educator who examines the aggregate data on the health status of Asians and Pacific Islanders might conclude that this group, as a whole, is healthy. However, a closer look at the same data by individual Asian and Pacific Islander subgroups would show that some of the subgroups have high incidences of breast, lung, and liver cancer and hepatitis B (Spector, 2004).

In addition it is important to assess environmental factors, such as the presence of advertising that might lead to use of health-damaging products and the numbers of stores that sell alcohol and fast food, as these might be associated with health disparities among racial and ethnic groups. A study by LaVeist and Wallace (2000) found that liquor stores in the Baltimore area were more likely to be located in low-income African American communities than in other communities. The findings of this study, although not conclusive, suggest that the relative prevalence of liquor stores in low-income African American communities may be associated with the disproportionate share of alcohol-related problems experienced by residents of these communities.

Throughout the health education literature, health educators (Luquis, Pérez, & Young, 2006; Luquis & Pérez, 2003; Stoy, 2000; Huff & Kline, 1999) have advocated that people in this profession need to become more culturally competent and sensitive to the racial and ethnic groups with which they work, and one level of the CAF is concerned with taking into consideration specific cultural or ethnic characteristics. These characteristics include cultural or ethnic identity, cosmology, time orientation, perceptions of self and community, social norms, values and customs, and communication patterns (Huff & Kline, 1999). As stated earlier, Spector (2004) defines culture as the beliefs, practices, habits, norms, customs, and so on, that individuals learn from their families. Culture is complex and dynamic, and although we can assume that for the most part people's concept of their culture remains constant, cultural identity can change through time (Luquis & Pérez, 2003). As individuals from different racial and ethnic groups interact with members of other groups, new environments, and new situations, their cultural identity is reshaped (Bonder, Martin, & Miracle, 2001). Cultural identity influences the individual's behavior and health choices. Consequently, it is important for health educators to begin a cultural assessment by establishing how the targeted group identifies itself (Huff & Kline, 1999), as this identity will influence other cultural characteristics of the group.

Moreover, in conducting an assessment, health educators need to be aware of specific racial and ethnic health care beliefs and practices, as these affect a group's interaction with the Western biomedical model and health promotion efforts. This level of the CAF includes assessment of a group's health and illness explanatory model, response to illness, use of Western health care and health promotion services, and health behavior practices. The Western biomedical model explains illness and disease in term of pathological agents; however, a racial or ethnic group might follow a diagnostic model that explains illness, disease, and course of treatment from a cultural point of view (Nakamura, 1999). For example, some racial and ethnic groups perceive and explain the cause of illness and disease in terms of "soul loss," "spirit possession," and "spells" (Spector, 2004). Similarly, some groups describe diseases as the consequences of an individual's personal actions or interrelationship with family and community or as related to supernatural agents (Huff, 1999); thus members of these groups would be more likely to follow a nontraditional treatment modality to deal with the disease than they would be to visit a health care provider. In addition the perceptions an ethnic group has of the Western health care system will affect access to health care and promotion services. "If target group members perceive the Western health care facility as a 'death house' where family or friends go in alive and come out dead, . . . then they will be more likely to avoid contact with this type of facility except under the most dire situation" (Huff & Kline, 1999, p. 495). Health educators must be aware of racial and ethnic groups' understanding of health and illness, their health practices, and ways that group views can be incorporated into health promotion interventions.

Finally, this model proposes an assessment of the Western health care organization and the service delivery system that provide services to multicultural groups. Although some may consider this area a separate assessment, Huff and Kline (1999) argue that the way the health care and promotion organization perceives and works with the target group plays a key role in the overall assessment process. This process must include assessment of the cultural competence and sensitivity of the agency and its staff, assessment of the extent to which organizational mission and policies enhance the process of cultural competence, and assessment of the evaluation processes in place to measure organizational efforts in this area. Although this process might be cumbersome, it is important for health promoters to understand the agency if they are to develop appropriate and effective health promotion programs.

The PEN-3 Model

The PEN-3 model was developed by Airhihenbuwa (1995) as a conceptual model for health promotion and disease prevention in African countries, specifically to guide a cultural approach to HIV/AIDS, and then it was adapted for use with African Americans. The PEN-3 model provides a functional method of addressing culture in the development, implementation, and evaluation of health education and promotion programs. Although this model draws on theories and applications in cultural studies, it incorporates existing health education models, theories, and frameworks. Initially, the PEN-3 model included three dimensions of health beliefs and behaviors: health education, educational diagnosis of health behavior, and cultural appropriateness of health behavior. The revised PEN-3 model, presented in Figure 6.2, consists of three primary domains—cultural identity, relationships and expectations, and cultural empowerment—and three components (whose initial letters spell PEN) within each domain (Airhihenbuwa & DeWitt Webster, 2004). Once health educators and practitioners have identified a health issue, they can frame relevant sociocultural issues into the nine categories displayed in Figure 6.2.

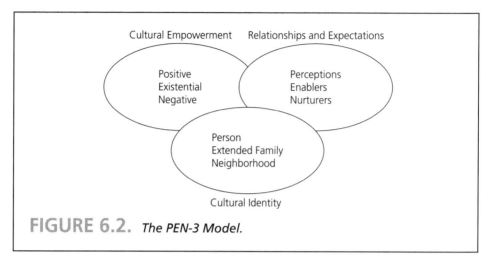

FIGURE 6.2. *The PEN-3 Model.*

Source: Airhihenbuwa, 2007, p. 38. Reprinted with permission of the author.

According to Airhihenbuwa (2007), "the PEN-3 model offers an opportunity to promote the notion of multiple truths by examining cultures and behaviors and by beginning with and identifying the positive—allowing us to examine and acknowledge the existential, which represents values that makes a culture unique—before identifying the negative" (p. 37).

The relationships and expectations domain assesses perceptions, enablers, and nurturers of behaviors from the cultural point of view. This dimension of the PEN-3 model has evolved from other theories and models, such as the health belief model (Rosenstock, 1974) and the PRECEDE-PROCEED framework (Green & Kreuter, 1999). However, this model places culture in the core of health promotion and disease prevention programs (Airhihenbuwa, 1995, 2007). Among the three components of this domain, perceptions consist of the knowledge, attitudes, values, and beliefs that exist within a cultural context and that motivate or inhibit individual or group behavioral change. For example, knowledge and cultural beliefs about breast and cervical cancer can influence cancer screening and health and health care–seeking behaviors among Hispanic women (Garcés, Scarinci, & Harrison, 2006; Luquis & Villanueva, 2006; Allison, Duran, & Peña-Purcell, 2005). Enablers are resources, institutional support, and societal or structural factors that may enhance or hinder preventive health decision and actions. For instance, the role of government policy has been noted in the low incidence or decline of new HIV cases in some African countries (Airhihenbuwa & DeWitt Webster, 2004). However, distrust of research and medical care has negatively influenced the recruitment of African American males for prostate cancer screening (Abernethy et al., 2005). Similarly, Garcés et al. (2006) have suggested that lack of information, access to care, and medications prevents Latinas from seeking health care services. Nurturers are family, friends, and community members who positively or negatively influence health beliefs, attitudes, and actions. Abernethy and colleagues (2005) identify pastors, church leaders, and community leaders as individuals who can promote prostate cancer screening among African American males. Similarly, the cultural practice of caring for a sick relative at home has become an important aspect of HIV/AIDS care in Africa (Airhihenbuwa & DeWitt Webster, 2004).

The cultural empowerment domain is an affirmation of the possibilities of cultural influences, which are positive, existential, and negative (Airhihenbuwa & DeWitt Webster, 2004). This dimension is crucial in the development of culturally appropriate health education and promotion interventions (Airhihenbuwa, 1995). As part of the development of such interventions, health educators must promote the good aspects and also recognize the unique aspects of a culture and not focus merely on its bad aspects (Airhihenbuwa & DeWitt Webster, 2004). Cultural empowerment is positive when it promotes the health behaviors of interest: for instance, the traditional healing modality for dealing with health problems such as sexually transmitted infections (Airhihenbuwa & DeWitt Webster, 2004). Similarly, eating a balanced diet, exercising, praying, and going to church are positive cultural aspects and behaviors that can be encouraged among Latinas (Garcés et al., 2006) as these behaviors will support other behaviors that help women to stay physically healthy and spiritually healthy. Existential aspects of a culture are those cultural beliefs, practices, and behaviors that are natural to a group and also have no harmful effect on health. These beliefs, practices, and behaviors should not be targeted for change and should not be blamed for the failure of the health education program. Garcés et al. (2006) describe the use of alternative and complementary healing practices, such as home remedies, as an existential behavior among Latinas. Health educators must be aware of these practices and embrace them, as they can help to produce a holistic view that can inform the development of a health education program. Finally, negative aspects are those based on values, beliefs, and relationships known to be harmful to health behaviors. Among such negative aspects are social actions that lay a foundation for inequality such as racism and differential housing and education (Airhihenbuwa & DeWitt Webster, 2004). To be successful health educators should develop programs that increase or support the naturally occurring positive behaviors while decreasing the negative behaviors and respecting the existential ones.

Finally, the cultural identity domain in the PEN-3 model seeks assessment of person, extended family, and neighborhood. It is important to understand that cultural identity, which represents an important intervention point of entry, is not defined on race and culture alone but refers to the multiple identities experienced by men and women in different cultures (Airhihenbuwa & DeWitt Webster, 2004). For example, "an African South African (such as Zulu) might out of necessity embrace the lived experiences of being Zulu (ethnicity), English (language), Afrikaans (oppressed experience) and poor person" (p. 8). Once the intervention point of entry (components of cultural identity) has been identified, the behavioral change can be addressed and promoted. It is also important to recognize that there may be multiple points of entry for addressing the social context and behaviors (Airhihenbuwa & DeWitt Webster, 2004). To promote the desired change, the individual can be provided with opportunities to acquire information and the skills needed to make quality health decisions appropriate to his or her role in his or her family and community (Airhihenbuwa, 1995). In addition health education is concerned not only with the immediate, nuclear family but also with the extended family. Family plays a key role in the lives of members of many racial and ethnic groups. For example, a husband's mother, given her influence on the expectations of the couple in such areas as sexual negotiation, might be the source of certain behaviors that need to be changed (Airhihenbuwa & DeWitt Webster, 2004). Finally, health education is committed to health promotion and disease prevention in neighborhoods and communities, as involvement of community members is critical in the provision of culturally appropriate interventions (Airhihenbuwa, 1995). For example, a community's ability to decide on billboard advertisement and communication about HIV/AIDS in its locality might be encouraged (Airhihenbuwa & DeWitt Webster, 2004). Health educators must develop interventions that target both the individual and the extended families and neighborhoods, as these are interconnected.

CONCLUSION

Today's population growth and increasing population diversity validate health educators' efforts to incorporate cultural and linguistic competence into every aspect of planning, implementation, and evaluation of health education and promotion programs. In this process it is essential to employ theoretical models that describe and explain culture and related concepts. It is vital for health educators to apply these cultural constructs in every health education, promotion, and prevention intervention targeting diverse communities. In addition to considering the four models discussed here that focus on the role of culture in the prevention of disease and promotion of health, health educators must also consider other theories discussed elsewhere in this book when addressing the needs of the multicultural population in the United States.

POINTS TO REMEMBER

- Health educators need to consider the concept of culture and cultural factors during the development and implementation of culturally appropriate health education and promotion programs.

- The Purnell model for cultural competence provides a comprehensive, systematic, and organized framework with specific questions and a format for learning and assessing the concepts and characteristics of culture.

■ Campinha-Bacote suggests that the process of cultural competence comprises five essential constructs: cultural awareness, cultural knowledge, cultural encounters, cultural skills, and cultural desire.

■ The cultural assessment framework contains five levels of racial, ethnic- and culture-specific assessments that should be conducted when planning health promotion program for multicultural groups. These assessments can also be incorporated into such tools as surveys, focus groups, and other formative evaluation processes.

■ The PEN-3 model provides a functional method of addressing culture in the development, implementation, and evaluation of health education and promotion programs. It also allows health educators to conduct culture-based research and develop effective interventions for combating illnesses in racial and ethnic groups.

CASE STUDY

As a health educator, you need to develop a community health education and promotion program for the members of a diverse community. The population of this community is 45 percent white, 35 percent African American, 10 percent Hispanic, 5 percent Asian and Pacific Islander, and 5 percent members of other ethnic groups. Preliminary data show that the African American population has a significantly higher mortality rate than the other ethnic groups for heart disease, cancer, diabetes, and HIV/AIDS and also a higher rate of infant mortality.

1. What steps would you follow to assess the health education needs of this community?

2. What cultural factors do you need to consider when developing a program?

3. What cultural factors will influence the risk behaviors among members of this community?

4. What culturally appropriate strategies will you include in your intervention?

KEY TERMS

Cultural assessment framework (CAF)
Cultural awareness
Cultural competence
Cultural desire
Cultural encounter

Cultural knowledge
Cultural skills
PEN-3 model
Purnell model

NOTE

1. For a graphical representation of this model, please see the Transcultural C.A.R.E. Associates Web site: http://www.transculturalcare.net.

REFERENCES

Abernethy, A. D., Magat, M. M., Houston, T. A., Arnold, H. L., Jr., Bjorck, J. P., & Gorsuch, R. L. (2005). Recruiting African American men for cancer screening studies: Applying a culturally based model. *Health Education & Behavior, 32*(4), 441–451.

Airhihenbuwa, C. O. (1995). *Health and culture: Beyond the western paradigm.* Thousand Oaks, CA: Sage.

Airhihenbuwa, C. O. (2007). On being comfortable with being uncomfortable: Centering an Africanist vision in our gateway to global health. *Health Education & Behavior, 34*(1), 31–42.

Airhihenbuwa, C. O., & DeWitt Webster, J. (2004). Culture and African context of HIV/AIDS prevention, care, and support. *Journal of Social Aspects of HIV/AIDS Research Alliance, 1*(1), 4–13.

Allison, K. G., Duran, M., & Peña-Purcell, N. (2005). Cervical cancer screening practices among Hispanic women: Theories for culturally appropriate interventions. *Hispanic Health Care International, 3*(2), 61–67.

Bonder, B., Martin, L., & Miracle, A. (2001). Achieving cultural competence: The challenge for clients and healthcare workers in a multicultural society. *Generations, 25*(1), 35–42.

Campinha-Bacote, J. (1998). *The process of cultural competence in the delivery of healthcare services: A culturally competent model of care* (3rd ed.). Cincinnati, OH: Transcultural C.A.R.E. Associates.

Campinha-Bacote, J. (1999). A model and instrument for addressing cultural competence in health care. *Journal of Nursing Education, 38*(5), 203–207.

Campinha-Bacote, J. (2001). A model of practice to address cultural competence in rehabilitation nursing. *Rehabilitation Nursing, 26*(1), 8–12.

Campinha-Bacote, J. (2003). *Inventory for assessing the process of cultural competence among healthcare professionals—revised (IAPCC-R).* Cincinnati, OH: Transcultural C.A.R.E. Associates.

Campinha-Bacote, J. (2007). *The process of cultural competence in the delivery of healthcare services: A culturally competent model of care* (5th ed.). Retrieved May 29, 2007, from http://www.transculturalcare.net/ Cultural_Competence_Model.htm.

Cassar, L. (2006). Cultural expectations of Muslims and orthodox Jews in regard to pregnancy and the postpartum period: A study in comparison and contrast. *International Journal of Childbearing Education, 21*(2), 27–30.

Doswell, W. M., Kopuyate, M., & Taylor, J. (2003). The role of spirituality in preventing early sexual behavior. *American Journal of Health Studies, 18*(4), 195–202.

Garcés, I. C., Scarinci, I. C., & Harrison, L. (2006). An examination of sociocultural factors associated with health and health care seeking among Latina immigrants. *Journal of Immigrant Health, 8*, 277–385.

Green, L. W., & Kreuter, M. W. (1999). *Health promotion planning: An educational and environmental approach* (3rd ed.). Mountain View, CA: Mayfield.

Haight, W. L. (1998). Gathering the spirit at First Baptist Church: Spirituality as a protective factor in the lives of African American children. *Social Work, 43*(3), 213–221.

Huff, R. M. (1999). *Cross-cultural concepts of health and disease.* In R. M. Huff & M. V. Kline (Eds.), *Promoting health in multicultural populations: A handbook for practitioners* (pp. 23–39). Thousand Oaks, CA: Sage.

Huff, R. M., & Kline, M. V. (1999). *The cultural assessment framework.* In R. M. Huff & M. V. Kline (Eds.), *Promoting health in multicultural populations: A handbook for practitioners* (pp. 481–499). Thousand Oaks, CA: Sage.

LaVeist, T. A., & Wallace, J. M. (2000). Health risk and inequitable distribution of liquor stores in African American neighborhoods. *Social Sciences and Medicine, 51*(4), 613–617.

Luquis, R. R., & Pérez, M. A. (2003). Achieving cultural competence: The challenges for health educators. *American Journal of Health Education, 34*(3), 131–138.

Luquis, R. R., & Pérez, M. A. (2005). Health educators and cultural competence: Implications for the profession. *American Journal of Health Studies, 20*(3), 156–163.

Luquis, R. R., Pérez, M. A., & Young, K. (2006). Cultural competence development in health education professional preparation programs. *American Journal of Health Education, 37*(4), 233–241.

Luquis, R. R., & Villanueva, I. (2006). Knowledge, attitudes, and perceptions about breast cancer and breast cancer screening among Hispanic women residing in south central Pennsylvania. *Journal of Community Health, 31*(1), 25–42.

Marín, G. (1993). Defining culturally appropriate community interventions: Hispanics as a case study. *Journal of Community Psychology, 21,* 149–161.

Marín, G., & Marín, B. V. (1991). *Research with Hispanic populations.* Thousand Oaks, CA: Sage.

Nakamura, R. M. (1999). *Health in America: A multicultural perspective.* Boston: Allyn & Bacon.

Purnell, L. D. (2005). The Purnell model for cultural competence. *Journal of Multicultural Nursing & Health, 11*(2), 7–15.

Purnell, L. D., & Paulanka, B. J. (2003). *Transcultural diversity and health care.* In L. D. Purnell & B. J. Paulanka (Eds.), *Transcultural health care: A culturally competent approach* (2nd ed., pp. 1–39). Philadelphia: Davis.

Ramirez, R., & de la Cruz, G. P. (2002). *The Hispanic population in the United States: March 2002* (Current Population Reports, P20-545). Washington, DC: U.S. Census Bureau.

Rosenstock, I. M. (1974). Historical origins of the health belief model. *Health Education Monographs, 2,* 328–335.

Simon, C. E. (2006). Breast cancer screening: Cultural beliefs and diverse populations. *Health and Social Work, 31*(1), 36–43.

Spector, R. E. (2004). *Cultural diversity in health and illness* (6th ed.). Upper Saddle River, NJ: Pearson Prentice Hall.

Stoy, D. B. (2000). Developing intercultural competence: An action plan for health educators. *Journal of Health Education, 31*(1), 16–19.

U.S. Census Bureau. (2004). *U.S. interim projections by age, sex, race, and Hispanic origin.* Retrieved August 16, 2004, from http://www.census.gov/ipc/www/usinterimproj.

Zoucha, R., & Purnell, L. D. (2003). *People of Mexican heritage.* In L. D. Purnell & B. J. Paulanka (Eds.), *Transcultural health care: A culturally competent approach* (2nd ed., pp. 264–278). Philadelphia: Davis.

7

DEVELOPING CULTURALLY APPROPRIATE NEEDS ASSESSMENTS AND PLANNING, IMPLEMENTATION, AND EVALUATION FOR HEALTH EDUCATION AND PROMOTION PROGRAMS

NAYAMIN MARTINEZ-COSSIO

LEARNING OBJECTIVES

After completing this chapter, you will be able to

- Identify the cultural factors that need to be taken into consideration in developing culturally appropriate health education and promotion programs.

- Recognize the best methods for conducting needs assessments and evaluations of health education and promotion programs targeting culturally diverse populations.

- Use health planning models to frame culturally appropriate health education and promotion programs.

INTRODUCTION

The literature on how to plan, implement, and evaluate health education and promotion programs is abundant (Green & Kreuter, 2005; Israel et al., 1995; Steckler et al., 1994; Centers for Disease Control and Prevention [CDC], 2005). Numerous models, theories, and methodologies are available to guide health promotion and education professionals throughout the complex process of determining a population's most relevant health problems and the most effective ways to address them. Although each model proposes different approaches, a careful review reveals that all models recommend starting with a needs assessment process that aims to identify, analyze, and prioritize the needs or problems of a given group or community. In many cases, health educators have already identified a health problem (from a previous assessment or in the mission of the organization they are working with) and just need to determine the high-risk populations. However, at other times health educators need to conduct a more extensive community assessment to analyze more than one health problem. To accomplish this, they need to collect primary and secondary data to assess the needs of the target population as well as the behavioral, social, and environmental factors associated with them (Doyle & Ward, 2001; McKenzie, Neiger, & Smeltzer, 2005).

The second step in the needs assessment process is an analysis to identify obvious differences between the current and the ideal health status of the target population. Once this analysis is done, planning models recommend different strategies to prioritize the health problem that will become the focus of the program and the basis on which goals are defined and appropriate interventions chosen. Some considerations in making this decision are (1) most significant health problems; (2) availability of resources, including enough time to address the needs; and (3) availability of suitable interventions (McKenzie et al., 2005). Planning models also address the design of the evaluation process that will measure the quality of the program and its success in reaching the expected outcomes.

Among the best-known health planning models are PRECEDE-PROCEED, MATCH, CDC-Cynergy, SMART, and intervention mapping. These models have proven to be effective tools for framing health promotion projects that target mainstream Americans (white and middle-class); however, health education professionals often find it difficult to use these best-practice models when their intended populations are culturally diverse. Among the most commonly reported problems encountered in working with a diverse population are the different subgroups' differing education levels, health beliefs, value systems, and socioeconomic conditions. Some of the challenges that health educators face given the increasing racial and ethnic diversification of the U.S. population can be illustrated by considering the following questions. When working with a subgroup of Hispanics made up of indigenous migrants from Mexico, what is the best way to collect data on this group? If official statistics on the health problems of this particular population are not available, what are the best methods for collecting primary data? What are the more effective interventions when working with a population whose first language is not English or even Spanish? How do you provide written information to a population whose native language does not have a written version?

To help health education professionals and students overcome challenges such as these, this chapter provides practical ideas for taking a culturally competent approach to designing health education and promotion programs. It also explores five of the most recognized health planning models—PRECEDE-PROCEED, MATCH, CDC-Cynergy, SMART, and intervention mapping—and provides recommendations on how to use them to understand the cultural characteristics and meet the cultural needs of diverse populations.

IDENTIFYING CULTURAL FACTORS AFFECTING HEALTH EDUCATION

When working with diverse populations, health education and promotion specialists should have an appropriate definition of culture and should have identified the aspects of culture they should take into consideration when developing health education programs (Luquis & Pérez, 2003).

Various definitions of culture have been published in the professional literature; this chapter uses one provided by Spector (1996), who defines *culture* as "the sum of beliefs, practices, habits, likes, dislikes, norms, customs, rituals and so forth that we learn from our families during the years of socialization" (p. 68). Spector's definition implies that culture is a complex and dynamic concept that encompasses many aspects of the life of a person or social group.

Given the cultural diversity in the United States, health education professionals who are in the process of planning health education and promotion programs often find it very challenging to determine what aspects of the culture of the populations they are working with they should consider to maximize the chances of program success. The following discussion offers recommendations in the areas of language and communication, health beliefs and practices, and religious practices. It is important for health education professionals to make sure that they are using appropriate communication methods—oral, written, and corporal—to educate their target population. It is equally important for them to consider the health and religious beliefs of their clients in order to plan interventions that are culturally appropriate.

Language and Communication

The primary spoken language of the target population is one of the first things to take into consideration because it is the most important means of communication; hence it plays a prominent role in the relationship that individuals establish with the professionals who are trying to maintain or restore their health. "Studies have shown that without language assistance services, such as medical interpreting and translation of written health information materials, the quality of health care for limited English proficient consumers suffers" (Bau, 2003, p. 1). Arguably, this is true not only for medical care but also for health education and promotion services, because in order for the clients to get the best out of those services they need to understand the information they are receiving. Communication between client and provider is also important in achieving compliance with any behavior modification program that may be required of the client.

Language differences are the most important obstacle that health professionals face, given the cultural diversity of the U.S. population. An illustration of the dimension of language diversity can be found in an assessment conducted in 2001 by the Instituto Nacional Indígena (National Indigenous Institute), the Mexican entity in charge of developing policies and programs targeting Mexico's indigenous population. It found that in addition to Spanish, over sixty indigenous languages are spoken by the native groups in Mexico. Members of many of these groups have migrated to the United States: Mixtecs, Zapotecs, Triquis, Chatinos, Chinantecos, Purepechas, Nahuatls, and Mayas are just the most prominent among the groups whose members have settled in California and other areas of the United States. It is also important for health educators to know that most of the languages spoken by these indigenous Mexican immigrants—along with the languages spoken by immigrants from other regions, such as the Hmong from Thailand—exist in a variety of dialects (for example, Low and High Mixtec, Zapotec del Valle, Zapotec de la Sierra, and Zapotec del Istmo), which makes communication even more difficult. Determining the specific dialect that a population speaks is crucial when the needs assessment, the intervention, or the evaluation tool requires having oral communication with the target population.

Language is also an important means of communication in its written form; however, not all languages have a written version. Furthermore, the existence of a written language does not guarantee a certain level of literacy among the population that speaks that language. Therefore, health educators must assess not only whether the language of the target population has a written version but also, if it does, whether the intended population knows how to read and write that language. Continuing with the examples of the indigenous groups from Mexico, it is important to understand that most of their indigenous languages are predominantly oral (as, for example, Chatino and Triqui are). Scholars began the work of developing written versions of some of these languages, such as Mixteco and Zapotec, less than a decade ago, and the existence of many different dialects means that this work will take time.

Complicating matters even further for health educators is the illiteracy problem among the indigenous people in Mexico. According to the 2000 census in Mexico, 5.9 million Mexicans are illiterate in Spanish, and 34 percent of this group is indigenous. Spanish illiteracy rates are three times higher among indigenous people than among mestizo Mexicans (Instituto Nacional Indigenista, 2001). Health educators working with indigenous populations with the characteristics of high illiteracy in Spanish or another major language and also the absence of a written indigenous language of their own need to take these factors into consideration at the time of developing assessment and evaluation tools and need to opt for those instruments that will allow them to overcome these communication barriers. For instance, they can select focus groups and oral interviews instead of written surveys.

Health educators should also take into consideration communication that is neither oral nor written, such as communication through body language and space orientation, because these types of communication also differ across cultures. "Sociologists say that 80 percent of communication is non-verbal. The meaning of body language varies greatly by culture, class, gender and age" (ICE Cultural and Linguistics Workgroup, 2004). For instance, whereas most European Americans interpret the lack of eye contact during a conversation as lack of respect, indigenous Mexicans show respect by lowering their heads and avoiding direct eye contact when they are talking to a stranger or someone they consider superior (Centro Binacional para el Desarrollo Indigena Oaxaqueño, 2007). Finding out the most common nonverbal ways of communicating in a given culture can help health educators avoid potentially inappropriate actions in interventions.

Health Beliefs and Practices

Culture influences the people's perceptions of their health and hence the ways and methods they pursue to maintain and restore their health. Although the predominant model is the allopathic medical model, which explains illness and disease in terms of pathological agents (Luquis & Pérez, 2003), many cultures throughout the world have nosologies (classification of diseases), etiologies (causation theories), diagnosis methods, and concepts of prevention that are markedly different from those of clinical biomedicine (Bade, 2004). For instance, Mixtecs from Mexico—along with other indigenous people from Latin America—believe that illness can occur "when a healthy individual has been exposed to a potentially disruptive force, be it physical, such as heat or cold, social, such as a relationship with a relative or neighbor, or spiritual, such as entities that occupy caves, roads and rivers" (Bade, 2004, p. 234).

Therefore, in order to plan interventions that are culturally appropriate, it is crucial that health educators take the time to assess and identify the health beliefs of their target population and the ways that population members are practicing these beliefs in the United States. Are they combining Western medicine with traditional medicine? Are they following certain rituals intended to preserve their health?

Religious Practices

Religion is one of the key cultural practices that influence the health status of individuals. Due to their religious beliefs, individuals may refuse health treatments that could extend their life span. The Hmong, for example, believe in reincarnation and therefore wish to preserve their bodies without scars for their future lives. Hmong patients who still follow their own traditions will not agree to have a surgery or amputation that will leave a scar even if that refusal puts their health in jeopardy (Bryan, 2003). Similar cases have been reported among Jehovah's Witnesses, who among other things may refuse blood transfusions. Health educators must understand a population's religious beliefs and practices in order to develop appropriate health promotion programs.

It is very important to have a good understanding of the health practices of the target population, especially when this population is composed of immigrants. Thus health educators must learn more about the socioeconomic background of this population and its health literacy level. What were these individuals' living conditions in their hometowns? Did they have access to medical care? Did they practice preventive care? How is the health care system in their home country different from the U.S. health care system? Understanding such population aspects will improve health educators' ability to plan programs that acknowledge key parts of the target population's cultural background.

CONDUCTING NEEDS ASSESSMENTS IN CULTURALLY DIVERSE GROUPS

The needs assessment is the first phase in the planning process for a health education and promotion program; this phase is also known as *community analysis, community diagnosis,* or *community assessment* (McKenzie et al., 2005). Many authors have proposed definitions of needs assessment. Gilmore and Campbell (1996) define it as a "planned process that identifies the reported needs of an individual or group" (p. 5). McKenzie, Neiger, and Smeltzer (2005) refer to it as "the process by which those who are planning programs can determine what health problems might exist in any given group of people" (p. 73). Regardless of which definition one prefers to use, the practical reality is that needs assessment is the process through which health educators can identify, analyze, and prioritize the needs or problems of the group or community that they have selected to work with.

On the surface the identification of needs might seem to be a straightforward process, but there are many issues health professionals should be aware of when using such assessments. One important fact is that they can encounter two different types of needs: *actual needs* and *perceived needs.* Actual needs are the problems that have been scientifically documented and expressed through incidence and prevalence rates. Perceived needs are the problems that the community considers to be prevalent and that do not necessarily coincide with the factual data (Green & Kreuter, 2005; Doyle & Ward, 2001). As Doyle and Ward (2001) suggest, it is important for health education professionals to find a common ground between the actual and the perceived needs or at least to attempt to increase the community's awareness of the evidence-based needs.

Through the needs assessment, health education professionals can also gain a better understanding of the characteristics of the target population, including its demographic profile, socioeconomic status, and health beliefs and practices. As mentioned earlier, assessment of health beliefs is vital, as some of these beliefs often translate into practices that influence people's health. When working with culturally diverse populations, it is important for health education professionals to recognize which practices have positive and which have negative effects and to encourage the first and try to change the second. Pregnancy-related beliefs among Oaxacan indigenous women are an example. Among other things, these women believe that taking prenatal vitamins will make them gain a lot of weight and have bigger babies and that this will increase their risk of having a C-section. Likewise, although they value maternity highly, they do not consider it necessary to have any type of prenatal care because the common practice in their hometowns is to seek the assistance of a *partera* (lay midwife) at the moment of delivery. Any health specialist attempting to develop a program targeting Oaxacan indigenous pregnant women needs to know these cultural beliefs and practices so he or she can successfully address them in the program. In this case it would be important to reinforce the positive attitudes toward maternity and to build on them to encourage women to access early prenatal care. Of equal relevance would be using information to dispel the myths that prevent indigenous women from taking prenatal vitamins.

In addition to identifying the demographic and socioeconomic characteristics and the health beliefs and practices of the target population, a needs assessment also helps health educators to recognize priority needs not being met and promising interventions not being conducted by any existing programs. Given the scarcity of resources—both human and economic—that almost all health education professionals face, it is crucial to avoid duplication of services and to ensure that new or revised health education and promotion programs will really address highly relevant needs or problems among the selected community or group.

Although some needs assessments require a comprehensive approach and a lot of resources, often health planners do not have the time or resources to conduct such comprehensive assessments. Nevertheless, they should not give in to any temptation to skip the needs assessment phase and go directly into the design of the interventions—not even if they have a theme that was selected by their funding stream or by the nature of their organization—because the information that is gathered through the needs assessment process is crucial for the success of the health promotion program. Among many other things, a good needs assessment can help health planners to avoid duplication of programs, to gain insight into the factors that will make for successful interventions, and to identify the community's priority needs and the subgroups at major risk.

One of the core tasks that health education professionals must accomplish in the needs assessment process is to collect primary and secondary data. Secondary data comprise information that has been collected by an agency, organization, or individual researchers previously. Government agencies are an important source of such information at the national and state level on issues such as population size and distribution, vital statistics, socioeconomic indicators, epidemiology of diseases, health expenditures, and health status and risks factors, to mention just the most relevant themes. Examples of some of the more common sources for these categories of information are the Statistical Abstract of the United States, the National Health Interview Survey (NHIS), the National Hospital Discharge Survey (NHDS), the Youth Risk Behavior Surveillance System (YRBSS), the *Morbidity and Mortality Weekly Report* (MMWR), and the Behavioral Risk Factor Surveillance System (BRFSS) (McKenzie et al., 2005).

Some important secondary data that are very helpful for obtaining information about minority groups and subgroups are not collected or specified by government agencies but are available from research institutes (such as the UCLA Health Center for Policy Research and the California Institute for Rural Studies); public foundations (such as the Robert Wood Johnson Foundation, the California Endowment, and the Kaiser Foundation), and voluntary health organizations (such as the March of Dimes, the American Cancer Association, and the American Heart Association). Such organizations have become an important additional source of information. The case of indigenous Mexicans from Oaxaca, a subgroup of Mexicans who have migrated massively to California since the late 1980s, is an illustration of this. Government agencies are not a good source for information on this population because government data for this group are treated as part of the data for Hispanics in general. The few studies that have been conducted to assess the living conditions of indigenous migrants in California have been produced by researchers affiliated with a nonprofit research center (the California Institute for Rural Studies) and by scholars affiliated with various universities in California (see Fox and Rivera-Salgado, 2004, for a good example of this type of research).

Primary data comprise all the information that is collected directly from the target community through a variety of methodologies, including individual assessments (surveys and Delphi technique) and group assessments (focus groups, nominal groups, and community forums). Primary data are very valuable, especially when working with diverse populations, because they provide specific information about the particular community or group that planners have selected and typically offer insights into socioeconomic characteristics and cultural practices (Doyle & Ward, 2001). The remainder of this section offers brief descriptions of the main methods of collecting primary data.

Surveys are the preferred method for collecting primary data. Surveys are very flexible tools and can be conducted through questionnaires, telephone interviews, or face-to-face interviews. Surveys can be collected through a single contact with each respondent (cross-sectional) or through a series of questionnaires administered by phone or e-mail to a group of persons considered "experts," and designed to generate consensus (Delphi technique). Surveys are a good method not only of getting a clear picture of the characteristics of the target population and of its priority needs but also of assessing program delivery preferences (McKenzie et al., 2005). Health education professionals should be aware that the quality of the information obtained from a survey depends on survey design and on considering some of the cultural aspects mentioned at the beginning of this chapter: Can the target population read and write and if so, at what level and in which language? Do cultural preferences make the target population more inclined to answer an oral interview or a written questionnaire?

The other methods of collecting primary data are group assessments conducted through a focus group, nominal group, or community forum. Focus groups consist of small groups of people (eight to twelve) who are asked preestablished questions designed to elicit their opinions, perceptions, beliefs, and attitudes about one or more topics. Nominal group technique is a structured process in which five to seven persons representing a population of interest are asked to answer questions about specific needs and to rank their responses according to what they consider the priorities for the population they represent. The community forum brings persons from the target community together to express their opinions and concerns on what they consider their priority needs or problems. In all these three qualitative methods—focus groups, nominal groups, and community forums—the discussion is guided by a trained and neutral facilitator, and all responses are recorded by other person(s); however, the results are not generalizable (Doyle & Ward, 2001; McKenzie et al., 2005). These methods are most appropriate for use with populations that are illiterate, have low levels of education, or are inclined to an oral tradition. It is important to guarantee that participants' language needs are met, that the facilitators and recorders are fluent in the language and dialects that the group speaks and are familiar with the culture and local dynamics of the target population. It is best to avoid mixed groups in which the participants speak different languages because the use of interpreters will slow down the process and also the participants might feel intimidated when they hear others speaking in another language they do not understand. When dealing with low literacy, especially in migrant populations, Pérez, Pinzon, and Luquis (1999) recommend (among other key issues) having group members who are familiar to one another, using a small group, having single rather than multiple data collection points, and selecting a homogeneous group.

Another method of collecting primary data, one often ignored by health education professionals, is to do ethnographic work with the target population. This means going out and, through direct observation and interactions, learning what the environment is in which this population lives, what the local dynamics are, who the local leaders are, and what kinds of issues affect them.

The method(s) selected will depend on the characteristics of the target population and also on the resources, time, and expertise of the health education professionals. A good general recommendation is to combine different methods and select those that can provide a clearer picture than you had previously of your target population and of its needs and also of its assets. To illustrate how this can be accomplished, the next paragraph describes selecting the best approach for conducting a needs assessment of Triqui immigrants residing on the northern California coast.

Because this population is a Mexican subgroup, using the traditional government sources of secondary data (such as the Census Bureau, BRFSS, and so forth) will not be the best approach. It will be more productive to search other types of sources, such as the research studies from such organizations as institutes and universities mentioned previously and other literature that can provide a general description of the characteristics of this population. Once the health education professionals have gained a general understanding of this target population (the language its members speak, where they come from, their sociodemographic profile, the health beliefs in their hometowns, and so forth), they need to identify where this population concentrates—which is easy because indigenous people tend to cluster in the same neighborhood—and who the local leaders are. To work with this indigenous population it is vital to gain people's trust, and one way to do this is by approaching the group's leaders. A good way to start the needs assessment is by conducting face-to-face interviews with these leaders to learn, according to their perspective, what the needs of the target population are. These leaders can facilitate the implementation of focus groups that can provide additional information on the population's perceived needs. Health education professionals should also employ a bilingual facilitator to help them overcome the language barrier. A method that can yield complementary information is conducting windshield observations of the neighborhoods where the target population lives to assess the environmental factors that affect them. Once the principal needs have been identified, health educators can conduct nominal groups to have the community prioritize these needs. Overall, the group assessments and the face-to-face interviews, rather than any written methods, will be the more appropriate methods for conducting a needs assessment of the Triqui immigrant population.

PLANNING AND IMPLEMENTING CULTURALLY APPROPRIATE PROGRAMS

The previous section explained that although the literature suggests standards for conducting a needs assessment, there are different ways to translate these standards into practice, depending on the characteristics of the target population. This is also true for the other stages of the planning and implementation of health promotion programs. Although models provide a framework to guide the work of health education professionals, it is up to these professionals to decide how to apply the models and to remember that, if necessary, it is possible to combine models to meet the needs and situations of the target population or community (McKenzie et al., 2005). In Chapter Six, two models—the cultural assessment framework (Huff & Kline, 1999) and the PEN-3 model (Airhihenbuwa, 1995)—for planning health education programs with culturally diverse populations are discussed. This chapter now describes the main premises of five other well-known health planning models—PRECEDE-PROCEED, MATCH, CDC-Cynergy, SMART, and intervention mapping—and makes recommendations on how to use them to work with culturally diverse populations (see Table 7.1 for a summary of each model).

As Table 7.1 illustrates, each model has its own way of approaching the development process of health promotion programs. PRECEDE-PROCEED prioritizes the

TABLE 7.1. Five Health Planning Models.

Model	Year of Creation	Approach	Phases
PRECEDE-PROCEED	Green and Kreuter developed PRECEDE in the 1970s and PROCEED in the 1980s (Green & Kreuter, 2005).	Ecological and educational approach	• Consists of 8 phases: PRECEDE 1. Social assessment 2. Epidemiological assessment 3. Educational and ecological assessment 4. Administrative and policy assessment PROCEED 5. Implementation 6–8. Evaluation
MATCH	Developed in 1980s.	Ecological approach	• Consists of 5 phases: 1. Goal selection 2. Intervention planning 3. Program development 4. Implementation preparation 5. Evaluation
CDC-Cynergy	Developed in mid 1990s by CDC.	Health communication model	• Consists of 6 phases: 1. Describe the problem 2. Analyze the problem 3. Plan intervention 4. Develop intervention 5. Plan evaluation 6. Implement plan
SMART	Developed in 1993 by Walsh and colleagues.	Focus on consumers to develop social marketing interventions	• Consists of 7 phases: 1. Preliminary planning 2. Consumer analysis 3. Market analysis 4. Channel analysis 5. Developing interventions 6. Implementation 7. Evaluation

(continued)

(Table 7.1 continued)

Model	Year of Creation	Approach	Phases
Intervention mapping	Developed in 2001 by Bartholomew, Parcel, Gerjo, and Gottlieb.	Ecological and social approach	• Consists of 6 steps: 1. Needs assessment 2. Matrixes 3. Theory-based methods and practical strategies 4. Program 5. Adoption and implementation plan 6. Evaluation plan

needs assessment phase, intervention mapping focuses on the development of theory-based interventions, MATCH emphasizes the implementation process, and the CDC-Cynergy and SMART models place the consumer at the center of the program design. Each model segments and names the process phases or steps differently; however, three general stages are present in all the models: (1) identification of the health problems, (2) planning and development of the intervention, and (3) implementation. The following sections describe what each of these three stages entails and how health education professionals can combine the models for a more thorough planning process.

Health Problem Identification

The five models agree that the first step in the process of creating a health promotion program must be determination of the program focus. To identify this focus, health education professionals must answer the following questions: What are the most relevant health problems? Who are these problems affecting the most? Where and when do the problems exist? What are the environmental, behavioral, and biological and genetic factors associated with the problems? How do the problems affect the quality of life of the target population? The models offer health education professionals different ways to find the answers to these questions. All the models agree that one approach is to use epidemiological data (Bartholomew, Parcel, Gerjo, & Gottlieb, 2001; Green & Kreuter, 2005; McKenzie et al., 2005). However the PRECEDE-PROCEED, SMART, and intervention mapping models are more specific and recommend conducting other types of formative research to learn more about the needs, wants, and strengths of the target population and of the subgroups within it (Bartholomew et al., 2001; Green & Kreuter, 2005; McKenzie et al., 2005).

For all the models it is also crucial to conduct a thorough analysis of the etiological factors that contribute to the health problems of the intended community (Bartholomew et al., 2001; Green & Kreuter, 2005; McKenzie et al., 2005). According to the SMART and PRECEDE-PROCEED models, it is also relevant to identify the predisposing factors (which provide motivation and rationale), reinforcing factors (which provide rewards and incentives), and enabling factors (which facilitate performance) associated with the health problems (Green & Kreuter, 2005; McKenzie et al., 2005). By identifying these factors planners gain a clearer idea of what the focus of the program can be. Before making this decision, the PRECEDE-PROCEED, intervention mapping, and CDC-Cynergy models recommend assessing the provider organization's capacity to address the problem(s) and determining whether the political context is or is not favorable. To accomplish this, CDC-Cynergy suggests conducting a SWOT analysis, that is, one that provides insight into the organization's strengths, weaknesses, opportunities, and threats (Green & Kreuter, 2005; McKenzie et al., 2005). The five models coincide in saying that health promotion programs should focus on the health problems that are most *important,* that are *serious,* and that are capable of *change.* Other factors that should be taken into account according to the CDC-Cynergy model are the availability of effective interventions, the concern of the community, and the resources (personnel, time, and money) available, to ensure selecting a manageable number of health problems (McKenzie et al., 2005).

Regardless of what model they decide to use, health education professionals need to be clear that the first step in the development of a health promotion program is to determine what the most important health problems of the community are. Reviewing the epidemiological data is one way to obtain this information but not the only way. As stated earlier, when working with minority groups and subgroups, it is always better to use a mix of methods (interviews, surveys, ethnographic research, and so forth) to make sure that you are obtaining firsthand information about the specific characteristics of the population, the most significant health problems that affect them, and the various factors associated with those health problems.

One strategy to accomplish this is to combine the PRECEDE-PROCEED and the SMART models. The first offers a thorough assessment of the health problems and of the environmental, behavioral, and risk factors related to them. The second model provides detailed information on the different segments of the population affected by the health problems, including their learning styles, readiness for change, self-efficacy, locus of control, and other factors that influence their behavior (McKenzie et al., 2005). All this is important to know when working with diverse populations. Even though minority groups are often clustered into large categories (for example Hispanics, Native Americans, Asians, and Pacific Islanders) by data collectors, each subgroup might be affected in different ways by the same problem and each might have diverse characteristics and behaviors that need special types of interventions.

Intervention Planning and Development

After identifying one or more health problems that the program will focus on, health education professionals must develop the goals, desired outcomes, and objectives that will guide their program and then determine the interventions that can be used to accomplish these desired outcomes. What is going to change after implementing the program? Who is going to be the target of the intervention? What types of interventions are more appropriate? At what level will the interventions work? What types of materials and resources are most suitable? These are the main questions that planners need to take into consideration while planning the interventions of their health promotion programs.

According to the CDC-Cynergy model, planners should develop goals, outcomes, and specific and measurable objectives for each selected health problem and then explore the most promising interventions for achieving such objectives (McKenzie et al., 2005). For the PRECEDE-PROCEED model the determinants of health and social conditions identified in the educational and ecological assessment process should become the objectives of the health program, and later those objectives must be linked to tested interventions (Green & Kreuter, 2005). Although these models recommend searching for interventions that have been tested and used effectively in other programs, it is important to remember that given the cultural diversity of the U.S. population, it is often impossible to find well-evaluated interventions that meet the needs of your specific community; therefore the best approach is to adapt interventions that have already been tested. One resource to use for this purpose is the *Guide to Community Preventive Services* (CDC, 2007), which includes a list of sixteen major health concern areas—such as alcohol, diabetes, cancer, and physical activity—and provides descriptions of population-based interventions focused on each area. It also rates the interventions (recommended, insufficient evidence, and not recommended) and describes the major findings about the utilization of the interventions. All the lists of interventions are revised periodically by the U.S. Task Force on Community Preventive Services (Bartholomew et al., 2001).

The MATCH and intervention mapping models offer guidance on how to develop interventions. The first model recommends selecting as the target for the intervention the actors that have control over the personal or environmental conditions related to the selected goals. Interventions can be designed to target individuals, groups, organizations, societies, or even governments. Depending on intervention levels and the targets selected, different types of actions—including training, teaching, counseling, policy advocacy, organizing and social action, among others—can be conducted to effect the desired changes (McKenzie et al., 2005). The intervention mapping model offers a more complex approach; it proposes the development of matrixes that specify who and what will change at each level of intervention. For each expected change, planners identify the health behavior and the environmental conditions associated with it and then write a performance objective stating how the change will take place. These objectives are then translated into theory-based methods and practical strategies that are pilot-tested with intended recipients (Bartholomew et al., 2001).

Another key element to consider during the development of the interventions is the selection of the materials, messages, and delivery channels. The consumer-focused models in particular—SMART and CDC-Cynergy—recommend that the stakeholders be involved as much as possible or, at least, that pilot tests be conducted before implementing the program to determine the most adequate materials and strategies. When making this selection, it is important to have in mind once more the characteristics of the target population, especially the factors described in the beginning of the chapter (such as language, literacy level, health beliefs and practices, socioeconomic background, and communication style), because they will determine the preferred materials (curriculums, brochures, posters, videos, pictures, flipcharts, PSAs, and so forth) and also the best channel through which to deliver the messages (individual, interpersonal, small-group, community, or organizational channels). Keep in mind that everything should revolve around when, where, and how the target audience can be effectively reached to pursue the desired change. For example, health education professionals who intend to create a program to help Mexican American pregnant women increase their access to prenatal care beginning in the first trimester—a documented public health problem among this population (Frisbie, Echevarria, & Hummer, 2001; McGlade, Somnath, & Dahlstrom, 2004)—might find it useful to use *radionovelas* (radio soap operas), a proven method of successfully providing health education to this population, which enjoys this type of entertainment. This is a way to build on materials that are culturally accepted, instead of experimenting with something that might not be attractive to a particular population.

Implementation

Implementation consists of "converting objectives into actions by the coordination of activities" (Green & Kreuter, 2005, p. 194). To accomplish this all models recommend that health education professionals develop specific plans that detail how the interventions will be executed, the actors that will be involved, and the timelines for developing the different components of the program. The consumer-focused models—CDC-Cynergy and SMART—recommend including a mechanism that obtains feedback from the program participants or recipients and then using this information to refine the program as needed (McKenzie et al., 2005).

DESIGNING CULTURALLY APPROPRIATE EVALUATIONS

The five models described here contemplate evaluation as an important component of the planning and implementation of health promotion programs. The PRECEDE-PROCEED and MATCH models recommend designing process, impact, and outcome evaluations; CDC-Cynergy calls for formative and summative evaluation; and the SMART and intervention mapping models suggest starting the evaluation process early in the planning stages and engaging all stakeholders (Bartholomew et al., 2001; Green & Kreuter, 2005; McKenzie et al., 2005). Given the relevance of this topic, the following section is dedicated to discussing why it is important to evaluate health promotion programs, identifying the different types of evaluations that exist, and examining how these evaluations are best performed when working with culturally diverse populations.

Evaluation is one of the key components of all health education and promotion for multiple reasons. It is through this process that planners learn whether a program's goal and objectives were accomplished and to what extent. Evaluation is also a way to monitor a program's standard of performance, to determine its strengths and weaknesses, and to decide whether adjustments are needed to improve it. Evaluation measures whether a program made a difference in people's lives and whether it was cost effective. Furthermore, evaluation can collect information on the target population that will allow researchers to develop hypotheses about group members' behaviors (Doyle & Ward, 2001; Taylor-Powell, Steele, & Douglah, 1996).

Health specialists should start the evaluation process at the same time they are developing the health education and promotion plan. A good way to start is by creating an evaluation plan that details the evaluation objectives, which are closely related to the program objectives, the budget assigned to the evaluation activities, and the evaluation design (Doyle & Ward, 2001). The ideal is to use only experimental designs, where you have a control group that is not receiving the intervention in addition to the group that is receiving it; with this design you can prove whether or not your intervention was the cause of observed change in people's behavior or knowledge. However this type of evaluation requires amounts of time, money, expertise, and other resources that health education professionals often cannot afford. Nevertheless, it is still desirable to make the attempt to collect information at the baseline. With baseline data for comparison, program providers can show the difference in the target population before and after the intervention, using evaluation designs that, for example, look at one group pretest and posttest or that perform static group comparisons (Doyle & Ward, 2001).

When planning the evaluation, it is important for professionals to specify what they intend to evaluate, how they will measure it, and the expected outcomes given the culture and characteristics of the target population. Oftentimes health education professionals tend to define the success of their programs in terms of standard benchmarks (such as knowledge gain or development of skills) that do not take into consideration the participants' perspectives on how the program had benefited them. One way to include participants' views is to use a *participatory evaluation approach* that involves stakeholders in planning the evaluation process, so they can describe what they would like to measure and what types of information they would like to obtain from it (Taylor-Powell et al., 1996). The following case example illustrates how relevant the target population's perspective can be for defining the indicators for measuring program success.

> *Program staff defined and evaluated their outcome of a bilingual nutrition education program as nutrition knowledge gained. An evaluation showed little, if any, gains in knowledge. Upon further probing, it was found that the participants were very satisfied with the program. For them, it had been very successful because at its conclusion they were able to shop with greater confidence and ease, saving time. Staff-defined definitions of outcomes missed some important benefits as perceived by the participants [Taylor-Powell et al., 1996, p. 6].*

Another key element in planning and conducting the evaluation is to identify the type of information that is needed to prove the effectiveness of the program and then to select collection methods and instruments that will focus on that information type. Oftentimes planners prioritize the collection of quantitative information (numerical results); however, as Green and Kreuter (2005) recommend, qualitative information should also be collected whenever possible because it can provide insights into the experiences and perceptions of the program participants and other relevant stakeholders, insights that quantitative information does not provide. In the nutrition education program described earlier, for example, evaluators learned about the program's unintended outcomes only because they had collected qualitative information about the participants' perceived benefits from the program.

The selection of methods for collecting the information depends on several factors: (1) the type of information to be collected; (2) the cultural values, capabilities, and availability of those who are being asked to provide the information; and (3) the time, resources, and expertise that evaluators have to process and analyze the information (Taylor-Powell et al., 1996). For instance, a health educator who is implementing a one-year program that aims to teach parenting skills to a group of indigenous farmworker migrants who are mostly illiterate may find that rather than conducting pre- and posttests that ask how many books they read per week to their children, it will be more appropriate to evaluate the success of this program by assessing it through face-to-face interviews with program participants and other family members and by asking, for example, whether parents are practicing their ancestral custom of storytelling with their children. It will also be important to conduct the interviews in the primary language of the target population and to use as interviewers people who are trusted by this community, such as community leaders or migrant liaisons. It will also be important when planning the interviews to consider using mostly open-ended questions, which will allow the interviews to obtain more in-depth information, and to conduct the interviews at locations and times appropriate for the target population. For these indigenous farmworkers it will be most appropriate to interview them in the evenings, or during other times when there is no farmwork, and preferably in their homes, where they can feel comfortable.

When working with culturally diverse groups it is better to be creative and to experiment with various methods than to rely only on the typical pre- and posttests and surveys. According to California evaluation consultant C. Mendoza (personal communication, February 24, 2007) information collection methods such as direct observation, focus groups, and interviews are better than other methods when the target population is illiterate or has low levels of education. However, she also warns that it is important when using these methods to ensure that the people collecting the information understand the culture of and speak the same language as the target population. One way to do this, as described earlier, is by involving persons from the target population in the evaluation process, people such as community leaders who are well known and respected. Another advantage of following this approach is that it allows health education professionals to gain the trust of the target community, a factor that is crucial when working with minority populations made up of indigenous people or Southeast Asians, because they do not open up easily to foreigners.

Most experts in evaluation methods recommend that evaluation planners save time and resources at the outset by conducting a literature review to identify tools that have already been used with populations similar to the planners' target population.

Nevertheless, as Doyle and Ward (2001) suggest, it is important to adapt those instruments to ensure that they are culturally appropriate for their new use. Here are some questions to consider when selecting an existing tool: (1) Is the tool available in the language spoken by the target population? If not, is it possible to translate it? (2) What is the readability level of the tool? Does it match the average education level of the target population? (3) Is the target population familiar with the tool's format (for example, Likert scales, multiple-choice questions, or fill-in-the-blank or open-ended questions)? The golden rule here is that whatever the tool that planners choose, it should be pilot-tested with representatives of the target population.

Regardless of the method or instrument used, once the information is collected the professionals must analyze and synthesize it. There are different methods of doing this, depending on the type of information collected. Quantitative information is usually analyzed to produce descriptive and inferential statistics; whereas qualitative information is analyzed to determine patterns or commonalities of meaning (Doyle & Ward, 2001). The final step in the evaluation process is for health education professionals to prepare an evaluation report to disseminate the findings and results. Although it is important to share this information with the funding sources, it is equally important to pass it on to the program participants and to the rest of the target population. Creativity is once again a key ingredient in accomplishing this. In addition to preparing a written report, health education professionals can also present the findings in ways that will be more meaningful and enlightening for the target population, such as videotapes, films, photo essays, displays, or Internet postings (Taylor-Powell et al., 1996).

CONCLUSION

Health educators learn early in their professional training that all their programs need to start with a solid needs assessment that captures not only epidemiological data but also information about existing resources and the identities of potential partners for the successful implementation of health promotion programs. Implicit, although not always stated, is the need to implement programs that take into account the needs of the diverse populations served by health educators. The selection of data collection methods depends on sundry factors, including the type of information to be collected; the cultural values, capabilities, and availability of those who are being asked to provide the information; and the time, resources, and expertise available to handle the information. The techniques presented in this and the other chapters of this book offer many practical methods for conducting culturally competent health education and promotion programs.

POINTS TO REMEMBER

- Acquiring cultural competence is a lifelong process that includes developing one's self-awareness as well as completing the necessary training to develop, implement, and evaluate effective health education programs designed to reach diverse populations.

- Although health education professionals currently tend to define the success of their programs in terms of standard benchmarks (such as knowledge gained or skills developed), culturally appropriate needs assessment, program planning, implementation, and evaluation require a focus on the needs of the target population and the ability and creativity to work with this population to address its members' needs.

- In addition to identifying the characteristics and the health beliefs and practices of the target population, a needs assessment should help health educators to recognize priority needs, promising interventions, and also gaps left by existing programs. Taking time to accomplish these tasks at the onset of any program will ensure successful completion of the health education and promotion activities targeting diverse audiences.

CASE STUDIES

Case One

In 2004, the U.S. government announced the arrival of thousands of refugees from Thailand, who were going to be settled primarily in several counties of the Central Valley of California. The local health departments were assigned the task of developing programs to help these families relocate and to access the main health services they needed. Each county decided to put together its own special task force, and each task force started its work by conducting a needs assessment. Using what you have learned in this chapter, answer the following questions.

1. What are the main characteristics that each task force needs to learn about in order to serve the new refugees?

2. What are the most appropriate methods of conducting the needs assessments, given what is already known about the likely characteristics of the target population?

3. Which planning model is most appropriate to use?

Case Two

The Santa Barbara Health Department identified an outbreak of active tuberculosis among a group of Mixtec men in California. Most of the infected persons rejected the treatment. One of them was incarcerated to ensure he would comply with it. Fearing that this same situation might be repeated in other parts of the state, the California TB Control Branch decided to develop a program to target Mixtec migrants and to provide them with health education on tuberculosis. Using what you learned in this chapter, answer the following questions.

1. What information does the TB Control Branch need to collect from the target population?

2. What are the most appropriate methods of collecting this information?

3. What planning model can the TB Control Branch use to frame its health education program?

4. What are the most appropriate evaluation tools in this case?

KEY TERMS

CDC-Cynergy

Culturally diverse

Evaluation

Health beliefs

Health education and promotion programs

Intervention mapping

MATCH

Needs assessment

PRECEDE-PROCEED

SMART

REFERENCES

Airhihenbuwa, C. O. (1995). *Health and culture: Beyond the western paradigm*. Thousand Oaks, CA: Sage.

Bade, B. (2004). Alive and well: Generating alternatives to biomedical health care by Mixtec migrant families in California. In J. Fox & G. Rivera-Salgado (Eds.), *Indigenous Mexican migrants in the United States* (pp. 205–244). La Jolla: University of California-San Diego, Center for U.S.-Mexican Studies.

Bartholomew, K., Parcel, G., Gerjo, K., & Gottlieb, N. (2001). *Planning health promotion programs: An intervention mapping approach* (2nd ed.). San Francisco: Jossey-Bass.

Bau, I. (2003, April). Improving access to health care for limited English proficient health care consumers: Options for federal funding for language assistance services. *Health in Brief: Policy Issues Facing a Diverse California, 2*(1), 1–8.

Bryan, N. (2003). *Hmong Americans*. Edina, MN: Abdo.

Centers for Disease Control and Prevention. (2005). *Introduction to program evaluation for public health programs: A self-study guide*. Atlanta, GA: Author.

Centers for Disease Control and Prevention. (2007). *Guide to community preventive services*. Retrieved February 11, 2008, from http://www.thecommunityguide.org.

Centro Binacional para el Desarrollo Indigena Oaxaqueño. (2007). *Oaxacan culture: Cultural competence guidebook*. Fresno, CA: Author.

Doyle, E. I., & Ward, S. E. (2001). *The process of community health education and promotion*. Mountain View, CA: Mayfield.

Fox, J., & Rivera-Salgado, G. (Eds.). (2004). *Indigenous Mexican migrants in the United States*. La Jolla: University of California-San Diego, Center for U.S.-Mexican Studies.

Frisbie, P., Echevarria, S., & Hummer, R. (2001). Prenatal care utilization among non-Hispanic whites, African Americans and Mexican Americans. *Maternal and Child Health Journal, 5*(1), 21–33.

Gilmore, G. D., & Campbell, M. D. (1996). *Needs assessment strategies for health education and health promotion* (2nd ed.). Madison, WI: WCB Brown & Benchmark.

Green, L. W., & Kreuter, M. W. (2005). *Health program planning: An educational and ecological approach* (4th ed.). New York: McGraw Hill.

Huff, R. M., & Kline, M. V. (1999). The cultural assessment framework. In R. M. Huff & M. V. Kline (Eds.), *Promoting health in multicultural populations: A handbook for practitioners* (pp. 481–499). Thousand Oaks, CA: Sage.

ICE Cultural and Linguistics Workgroup. (2004). *Better communication, better care: Provider tools to care for diverse populations*. Los Angeles: Author.

Instituto Nacional Indigenista. (2001). *Programa nacional para el desarrollo de los pueblos indigenas 2001–2006* (Plan Nacional de Desarrollo). Mexico City: Presidencia de la Republica.

Israel, B. A., Cummins, K. M., Digman, M. B., Heaney, C. A., Perales, D. P., Simons-Morton, B. G., et al. (1995). Evaluation of health education programs: Current assessment and future directions. *Health Education Quarterly, 22*(3), 364–389.

Luquis, R. R., & Pérez, M. A. (2003). Achieving cultural competence: The challenges for health educators. *American Journal of Health, 34*(3), 131–138.

McGlade, M., Somnath, S., & Dahlstrom, M. (2004). The Latina paradox: An opportunity for restructuring prenatal care delivery. *Journal of Public Health, 94*(12), 2062–2065.

McKenzie, J., Neiger, B., & Smeltzer, J. (2005). *Planning, implementing, and evaluating health promotion programs. A primer* (4th ed.). San Francisco: Pearson Benjamin Cummings.

Pérez, M. A., Pinzon, H., Luquis, R. R. (1999). Focus groups among Latino farmworker populations: Recommendations for implementation. *Migration World, 26*(3), 19–23.

Spector, R. E. (1996). *Cultural diversity in health and illness* (4th ed.). Stamford, CT: Appleton & Lange.

Steckler, A., Allegrante, J., Altman, D., Brown, R., Burdine, J., Goodman, R., et al. (1994). Health education intervention strategies: Recommendations for future research. *Health Education & Behavior, 22*(3), 307–328.

Taylor-Powell, E., Steele, S., & Douglah, M. (1996, February). *Planning a program evaluation.* University of Wisconsin Cooperative Extension. Retrieved February 24, 2008, from http:// learningstore.uwex.edu/pdf/ G3658-1.pdf.

Walsh, D. C., Rudd, R. E., Moeykens, B. A., & Moloney, T. W. (1993, Summer). Social marketing for public health. *Health Affairs,* pp. 104–119.

CHAPTER

8

COMMUNICATION AND CULTURAL COMPETENCE

MATTHEW ADEYANJU

LEARNING OBJECTIVES

After completing this chapter, you will be able to

- Describe the components of the health communication model.
- Understand the importance of communicating across cultures about health and disease.
- Understand the effects of cultural communication on personal and community health.
- Explain the similarities and differences in communication and marketing techniques.
- Understand the language barriers faced by minorities in health education practice.
- Use the guidelines for effective communication and cultural competence in planning health education programs.

INTRODUCTION

Every ethnic group has its specific cultural and communication patterns. This chapter discusses communication patterns among racial, ethnic, and other groups and the role that language plays in delivering health education programs to these population groups. The discussion focuses on historical perspectives on communication across cultures, communicating across cultures about health and disease, communication and persona and community health, communication and marketing techniques for various cultures, and communication patterns, barriers, and empowerment.

COMMUNICATION AND CULTURE

Culture is a complex concept that can be defined in many ways. It involves people's knowledge, beliefs, art, morals, laws, customs, and any other capabilities and habits that guide groups of people in their natural and immediate environments. All these capabilities can be summarized in terms of people's behavioral patterns, ideas, values, attitudes, and material objects. Culture is learned and shared. The process of acquiring culture throughout an individual's or a group's developmental life stages is called *enculturation.*

Culture is "a system of interrelated values enough to influence and condition perception, judgment, communication, and behavior in a given society" (Mazrui, 1986, p. 239). Culture is rooted in institutions such as families and schools and also in communication industries. In our daily lives, we are always making decisions about such matters as what foods to eat, what clothes to wear, how to greet others, what idiom of language to use when communicating with others, what behaviors to exhibit in a group, and how to perceive the world around us. Such decision-making processes are informed by our heritage and life experiences and these lead us to develop our own cultural identity.

Everyone comes from a culture, and individuals want to be associated with a culture. *Cultural identity* is made up of the specific and often unique ways that people think and act within the norms of their group. It encompasses a wide range of cultural influences on people's behaviors, beliefs, attitudes, and values. It is transmitted from generation to generation. Therefore cultural identity is based primarily on a shared historical, linguistic, and psychological lineage. People with a common culture live in accord with a shared set of socially transmitted perceptions about the nature of the physical, social, and spiritual world, particularly as it relates to achieving life goals (Basch, 1990).

It is paramount that planners and evaluators of health education programs and services carefully examine the differences and the similarities in groups' cultural perceptions, so that they can understand health beliefs, practices, knowledge, and attitudes more fully and hence address them appropriately within each group's particular context. Furthermore, they need to examine culture with a critical and open spirit. Culture is passed down from generation to generation. People have come before us and people will come after us. Therefore all individual moral and intellectual choices are superimposed on one's social and cultural environment and occur within a continuous, powerful, ever-evolving belief system, faith, and set of values, customs, and traditions.

Cultural education with effective communication assists us to see that knowing the world better is knowing the individual self better. Each individual person carries the cultural burden irrespective of his or her personal background. Therefore, we have to come to an understanding of the cultural weight carried by each of us and to empathize with the different loads borne by those of other cultures. This common knowledge and understanding will finally enrich us and free each one of us from our culturally repressive ideas through *intercultural communication* (communication between or among people of different cultures).

Whether a health educator is serving a client at the micro level (for example, a family or small-group unit) or working at a macro level (for example, cooperating or collaborating with another service agency or health care facility), he or she is participating in intercultural communication. Whether the desired result is knowledge gain, behavioral change, attitude change, or skill acquisition, intercultural communication skills will be needed. In fact, in health education practice, whether our client is seeking information for primary, secondary, or tertiary prevention, the ability to access information, persuade others, and participate in the selection of one's own health care protocols is essential. Intercultural communication proficiency empowers the individual or group in the decision-making processes of both personal (individual) and community (group) health.

COMMUNICATION AND CULTURAL COMPETENCE

Effective communication is the foundational building block for the health education profession. It cuts across all seven areas of responsibility for a health educator (National Commission for Health Education Credentialing [NCHEC], 2007), and it is the essential ingredient needed in conducting needs assessments and program planning, implementation, and evaluation. Effective communication is central to interacting with clients and community members and to serving as a resource person.

Cultural competence is that which allows us to develop programs in ways that are consistent with the individual's and the community's cultural framework. The 2002 report of the Joint Committee on Health Education and Promotion Terminology, for example, defined cultural competence as "the ability of an individual to understand and respect values, attitudes, beliefs, and mores that differ across cultures, and to consider and respond appropriately to these differences in planning, implementing, and evaluating health education and promotion programs and interventions" (p. 5). The concept of cultural competence goes beyond individuals' capacity to respect and tolerate values and practices different from their own. Cultural competence must also be reflected in organizational practices and policies governing the development, implementation, and evaluation of health education and promotion programs. These recommendations are similar to those contained in the standards for cultural competence for health professionals advocated by the Office of Minority Health (Luquis & Pérez, 2005).

The *communication model* involves the message, the communication medium, the sender (teller or speaker) of the message, and the receiver (listener or audience) of the message. Barriers to effective communication can arise from the sender, the message, the channel of communication (medium), and the receiver of the message. Health educators must possess the listening and speaking skills that will enable them to detect and remove these barriers. Roman, Maas, and Nisenholtz (2003) have addressed the question of obstacles that stand between the audience (the receivers of the message) and the action taken (what the receivers should do) after receiving the message. When health educators know what real or perceived barriers stand in the way of clients' taking action, they have a tremendous opportunity to develop effective communication strategies. Understanding the barriers helps health educators select either implicit or explicit action messages to which audiences are most likely to be receptive.

Communication can be verbal (spoken) or nonverbal. Nonverbal communication can involve cultural differences in the use of body gestures, eye movements, signs, touch, facial expressions, vocal qualities, silence, body distance, space, and time. All these areas of cultural difference can affect communication and self-understanding. They can serve as barriers to effective communication. For effective communication to take place there must be a strong communication strategy. A *communication strategy* describes how a message will be framed and delivered to the target audience. It is based on the thorough understanding of the audience members and their knowledge, attitude, wants, beliefs, needs, values, traditions, and the like. A communication strategy describes the target audience, the action the audience members should take, the obstacles between the audience and the action to be taken, how audience members will benefit, and how to reach them with the message. Communication plays a major role in many health education marketing efforts. Communication can be used to inform, educate, and persuade. Communication can use cultural symbols, codes, images, metaphors, or icons to frame a particular problem affecting a distinct cultural group and the solutions to such a problem.

Cultural kinetics involves communication codes, symbols, images, metaphors, meanings, and the context between the sender and the receiver. Use of cultural kinetics promotes knowledge development and comprehension. Faseke (1990) comments that an oral tradition is generally not only the heritage of the spoken or sung word; it is the heritage of the ear. Airhihenbuwa (1995), in his book *Health and Culture,* states that "people in oral tradition cultures (as in many African countries) are accustomed to learning by listening. Learning by seeing is important to the extent that what is seen is congruent with what is heard. Critical aspects of learning by listening include who was speaking, the way the words were said, and in what context" (p. 9). Furthermore, many cultures have traditional ways of communicating among the group members. In the olden days traditional news carriers were used to send messages from one place to another and to announce special events in the community. In the Yoruba culture of southwestern Nigeria, the town crier is a good example of how messages are transmitted in the community. The oral tradition, that is, the spoken word, is one of the commonest ways of transmitting information in many cultures. Symbols are also used as a medium of communication. Specific symbols mean different things. When a sender (a health educator) does not understand the culture of an audience (and hence faces a communication barrier), serious communication breakdown can occur, which then affects the message. In many cultures an oral tradition of storytelling plays an essential role in transmitting information to both children and adults alike. However, exercising cultural competence also means that the health educator is aware of the ethical and cultural incongruence of assuming the role of the storyteller without proper training or education for that role and without a thorough understanding of the cultural implications of storytelling for learning in a specific cultural context.

When a health educator is adapting a communication to a specific community, it is imperative for the sender of the message to educate himself or herself in all aspects of the communication mechanisms (for example, posters, flyers, pictorial symbols, storytelling, and so forth) within the community's culture. The educator needs to be culturally competent in the community's cultural expressions before embarking on any health education and promotion intervention program planning, implementation, and evaluation. The health educator must be aware that even when the chosen methods and materials of communicating health are appropriate, questions about when and how they should be used may still need to be addressed. As Airhihenbuwa (1995) states, "alternative methods of cross-cultural communication should be explored to ensure that the process does not dis-empower the target group" (p. 9).

A *community* is a group of individuals with a shared belief system, values, interests, or other attributes. Each cultural community has established particular codes, symbols, and strategies as methods of communication. These methods encapsulate the essence of meaning that such community groups bring to the development and acquisition of knowledge. Program planners should carefully examine these verbal and nonverbal communication methods as they relate to health behavior change processes and influence people's cultural values and beliefs. As stated earlier the power of the spoken word (oral tradition) is an ancient cornerstone of many cultures. Songs and dances too are found in the foundations of many cultures. Interpretations and decodings of the spoken word are embedded in storytelling, which may be expressed in songs and dances. Songs and dances are commonly used in different forms of rituals.

HISTORICAL PERSPECTIVES ON COMMUNICATION ACROSS CULTURES

Communication across cultures has been a dominant and recurrent theme throughout human history. Misunderstanding and mistrust among communities due to lack of effective communication can result in internal or external conflicts. This can be seen in all the wars that have taken place throughout history to the present time. Instances of deliberately misinforming people of particular cultures, as occurred during the Tuskegee Syphilis Study and in a program of sterilization of Indian women, have had long-lasting negative effects on intercultural communication and have raised awareness of ethical requirements in medical experimentation. These two cases will be further discussed later in this section.

Miscommunication between two countries of different ethnicity and cultural understandings can bring about a war. As Moroccan philosopher Mahdi Elmandjra (2003) has said, in discussing the prevention of such cultural conflicts or clashes of value systems that result in war: "We need people to communicate, to respect each other's systems and cultural diversity. The international community has no choice but to survive together" (p. 1). When a nation goes to war, the majority of its people label the people of the other nation with a single title. For example, prior to September 11, 2001, Muslims were not considered terrorists by a majority of Americans. However, since 9/11, a majority of Americans have stereotyped Muslims into the category of terrorist. It is a fact that the planners of the 9/11 catastrophe did inflict unprecedented damage to the people of the United States; however, not everybody in Afghanistan plotted to attack America. Other people's cultures need to be viewed both as wholes and as made of their own diverse parts, and also realistically, not stereotypically. And they need to be taken into consideration in order to bring about peace on Earth. Without this, we will simply be enclosed by our own borders and become our own prisoners.

A past event that has shaped the way many American Indians feel toward U.S. health care today is the sterilization of twelve thousand Indian women over the four-year period from 1972 to 1976. England (n.d.) provides an in-depth investigation of the moral issues created by the Indian Health Service (IHS) when it falsely informed Indian women about sterilization procedures. These Indian women were coerced and harassed into having the surgery and were not provided proper information beforehand. Among the things these women were told were that they were bad mothers and their existing children would be taken away from them if they did not consent, that they had enough children and it was time to stop having children, and that they could still have children after the operation. The atrocities committed by physicians on these women were inexplicable and embarrassing for our nation. The lies told to these women have given many Indians a historical perspective that warns them to mistrust U.S. health care, and they are likely to continue to carry this perspective with them for many years to come. Prior to this event, which Indians have referred to as "genocide," there were no laws concerning punishment for those involved in coercive sterilization. However, in 1979, the National Council of Churches condemned the policy of nonmedical sterilization and asked for a full investigation into the IHS parent agency, then called the Department of Health, Education, and Welfare, to find all the people responsible for this act and to determine the extent to which the IHS had integrated these actions (England, n.d.).

Another historical episode that has led to mistrust in physicians is the Tuskegee Syphilis Study. Conducted from 1932 to 1972 in Tuskegee, Alabama, this clinical study took advantage of 399 poor, illiterate African Americans (CDC, 2005). The researchers told the men who were infected with syphilis that they had "bad blood" and would receive free treatment, transportation, a hot meal, and $50 for a funeral if they were to die. They were not informed of their diagnosis, only told they had "bad blood." In reality, the researchers did not provide them with appropriate treatment, such as penicillin, but instead withheld treatment for the purpose of observing the natural etiology of the disease progression in African Americans. The study came to a halt when the press found out (CDC, 2005). However, the study should have never been conducted, because it is purely unethical to treat people in this way. Although this was an atrocious situation, some good did come out of it. It led to the writing of the Belmont Report and the creation of a national human investigation board (the National Commission for the Protection of Human Subjects of Biomedical and Behavioral Research) and of institutional review boards, which all mandate ethical standards for experiments on human subjects in the United States. Globally, the Nuremberg Code, which was established after the World War II atrocities in Nazi Germany, created a set of rules for the protection of human subjects in biomedical research (Annas & Grodin, 1995; Angell, 1989).

COMMUNICATING ACROSS CULTURES ABOUT HEALTH AND DISEASE

Most cultures have culturally specific perceptions and conceptual explanations of health and disease. Hence it is important to keep cultural sensitivities in mind in discussions across cultures about health and disease. Examples of such conceptual explanations are the demonic, celestial, phytogenic, and miasmic theories of disease causation. When taboos and myths exist for certain populations, then it is important that health educators be familiar with them in order to effectively provide health care services to these clients. There are four factors to consider when communicating across cultures: (1) the audience's degree of health literacy; (2) the audience's level of knowledge about health and disease; (3) the audience's attitudes toward health, disease, and prevention; and (4) structural obstacles.

Health Literacy

The degree of literacy, especially *health literacy* (the ability to read and comprehend health information), is important when communicating across cultures with brochures and other written educational materials, because not everybody is at the same reading level. It does not make sense to use brochures written at the high school level when the majority of the population of interest has not finished high school. Such materials would create frustration and confusion. It is crucial to provide educational materials that are targeted toward the appropriate reading and comprehension level for each cultural group. Also it is necessary to consider using different communication strategies for different cultures.

Level of Knowledge

Level of knowledge regarding health and disease is an important factor to consider when dealing with a diverse population. People from a small, rural community may be less educated than those who live in a large, urban area; therefore health educators need to communicate on the same level found among the audience for ease of comprehension. This is imperative because these less knowledgeable people are the people who need health care the most and may not be getting it due to their circumstance of health illiteracy.

Attitudes

Another consideration that must be adopted when communicating across cultures is cultural sensitivities or attitudes toward health. It is understandable that different cultures have different ways of explaining and interpreting health and disease concepts. Nonetheless, a majority of ethnic minorities have little understanding of the medical concepts of the disease process. Prevention is the key to living a healthy and quality life, and people's lack of understanding of how to prevent illness may lead to devastating health effects. Taboos are especially important factors to consider when providing health care services to clients, whether well or sick.

Structural Obstacles

Structural obstacles (barriers associated with structural issues in organizations or communities within a culture), such as limited access to health care and money and availability of translators, should be considered when dealing with a culturally diverse population. Some population groups may have to travel further to see health care providers than other population groups do. In some communities a person may travel far on foot and yet still not be able to see any health care provider, whereas others may have easy access to health care. Money and health insurance also come into play, as these are major factors for receiving health care in the United States. The majority of people who are poor and have no health insurance will not see a health care provider on a regular basis; they are more likely to get health care only when it is absolutely crucial. Prevention is the key to good health, and that message should be communicated effectively in order to prevent disease and reduce the cost of health care. Well-trained translators should be available to minorities who face language barriers.

Communicating across cultures can be difficult, but if the concepts discussed here are kept in mind, communicating with a diverse population can be easier. Knowing how a culture explains the concepts of health and disease is important in communicating effectively with people in that culture. Different communication strategies must be used to target different groups, because all groups vary to some extent in terms of their cultural, theoretical, and conceptual explanations of health and disease states.

COMMUNICATION AND PERSONAL HEALTH

Health communication is the provision of positive health information that will influence health behavior and attitudes and increase health knowledge for the prevention of disease and the promotion and protection of individual and community health. Health communication can raise individuals' awareness of health risks by informing them of potential hazards they may face. One of the seven areas of responsibility for health educators is to serve as a resource person (NCHEC, 2007). Communicating how to avoid health risks is therefore an essential role of health educators. Health risk communication is a two-way process that involves the health educator delivering a message to an interested party about the nature, significance, and management of the risk and that party receiving the message and ultimately using the information it provides for decision making about disease prevention, health protection, health promotion, and health maintenance. Both the health educator and the intended audience have responsibilities and high stakes in the avoidance of health risks. The health educator provides the health information and the clients need to comprehend the information to make informed decisions about their health. The communication must be a two-way process for any meaningful, positive health outcome to occur. It is the duty of health educators to pass along health risk communication as new data and research arise. Health educators may discuss risks one on one with a client or they may provide information through the mass media, which results in communicating with a community (Nicholson, 1999). For example, recently there have been numerous commercials telling people of warnings about and recalls of pharmaceutical products (such as Vioxx, an analgesic pain medication) due to the availability of new research and data on the adverse health effects of these products (for an example, visit www.vioxxdrugrecall .com). A health educator aware of such recall or warning information might discuss the risks in the use of such a product. The ultimate decision is for the client to make. The health educator just assists in providing available science-laden information. Additionally, the health educator can direct the client in enriching her health by promoting a better quality of life for her and preventing disease occurrence.

In communicating *personal health* (health of the individual) information, the health educator must be mindful of the influence of cultural factors on his or her client's knowledge base, attitude, and behavior. Communicating personal health information must result in changes in the individual's belief system. Knowledge and attitude changes alone will not transpose into a behavioral change. In order to change a personal health behavior, a person must have motivation to change (Glanz, Rimer, & Lewis, 2002). This has been demonstrated through the stages of the health behavior change model known as the transtheoretical model (Prochaska & DiClemente, 1983; Prochaska, DiClemente, & Norcross, 1992). This model identifies five stages that can be targeted to change a personal health behavior: precontemplation, contemplation, preparation, action, and maintenance. These stages of behavioral change are fully discussed in any general health education textbook.

Health educators are better able to motivate an individual and reduce a risk when they are able to determine which stage the person is in. For example, if a person is in the precontemplation stage, then he does not have any intention of changing within the next six months. If this is the case, having a health educator discuss with him the potential risks of not changing his behavior may move him along to the contemplation stage. Sometimes people need just a little push to get started. The health educator can apply communication strategies to give a person the little push so needed to get him started on the behavioral change path.

Health communication can help individuals find other people who are in situations similar to theirs by encouraging them to attend group therapy or other meetings. Group therapy, such as that offered through Alcoholics Anonymous, can help people overcome obstacles by providing support. Having support when in a difficult situation can enable a person to change her behavior and be less likely to slip back to where she once was. Ultimately, it will reinforce a new attitude toward changing a behavior to a healthier lifestyle. Group therapy is a very positive aspect of health communication.

Public health is constantly changing, which means the needs of individuals are changing also. One community may need a specific service, whereas another community may not. Communicating with individuals in a community can help health specialists decide what services are needed and which are not. A poor and underserved community may need assistance such as the WIC program in providing the young children in the area with nutritional foods, whereas a privileged community may not need such assistance. It is the responsibility of the health educator to serve as the resource person in assisting individuals and groups to find the needed resources for health promotion, health protection, and disease prevention.

COMMUNICATION AND COMMUNITY HEALTH

Community health refers to the health of a group of individuals with similar characteristics, common values, and shared beliefs. Community health communication can be very powerful when approached correctly. It has the ability to influence the public agenda, advocate for policies and programs, promote positive changes in the community, improve health care delivery services, and create supportive partnerships within the community.

As a community becomes more informed through health education, its members begin to recognize the health-related problems occurring in the community. When the goal is to bring changes to policies and programs, a community is much more powerful than individuals alone. A community has the ability to make its public and commercial buildings smoke free. However, it must get a majority of the community to agree with a smoking ban in order to implement that change. The only way to change the minds of the people on such a subject is to influence them through health communication. A strong community is built by strong individuals; therefore, it is important to get through to the individuals by using diffusion of innovation and mass communication theories. Among the different ways to get a message across to a large population are news releases, radio and TV commercials, newspapers, magazines, and advertisements.

Community health communication can also promote other positive changes in the community, such as changes in the physical environment. Communicating to a population about the benefits of exercise and well-being just may make people realize that their environment does not provide easy access to exercise. Some communities do not facilitate nonvehicular transportation. Successful community health education in this area could promote a change of scenery. One contemporary example of such change is building a bike path or sidewalks, which would enable people to transport themselves in more vigorous ways. One of the ways health communication can translate into advocacy is through social organization and action. *Social action* is the empowerment or mobilization of community members to take matters into their own hands, in this case for the improvement of their mutual health and the protection of their environment. The health educator is the change agent for such a mobilization, using effective communication strategies to begin and support the process.

COMMUNICATION AND MARKETING TECHNIQUES

When dealing with various cultures, it is of primary importance for health educators to first identify their target audience before proceeding to communicate and market products or ideas. Doing this first will save the health educator precious time and money. Additionally, it will enable the health educator to be more effective in communicating and marketing (more responsive to the needs, demands, and wants of the target audience) because he or she will understand the culture he or she is dealing with. There are many different techniques used in marketing public health (including health education) to promote social change (Siegel & Lotenberg, 2007). Some of the common marketing methods are brochures, mailings, advertisements (in magazines, newspapers, billboards, and so forth), commercials, and Web sites. Although these are all effective techniques, it is necessary to determine one's target audience prior to selecting a method. If marketing professionals are trying to market a health product to a poor, rural village in a developing country, using a Web site or e-mail would not be effective because the villagers most likely would not have access to these sources.

Health education professionals should realize that there are differences in the ways people learn and think. Even in the developed world, not everybody thinks the same way. Cultures are unique, and in order for health educators to be effective in communicating with the public they need to identify the differences in learning and thinking patterns among the various cultures. Making false assumptions about a culture and stereotyping (generalizing based on premature or flawed assumptions) are common phenomena. But they can negatively affect the practice of education when they are used in marketing a new product to a target population. It is important to consider not only a country's dominant culture but also its subgroup cultures. Health educators' knowledge and understanding of such subcultures can help them to plan programs that will be accepted by the desired audiences.

A given message will not be not equally effective in all cultures. In order to understand why this is so, health educators need to be aware of the different communication strategies and their uses. Communication strategies are tied to effective program planning and marketing techniques. Understanding a community's culture is one way to establish good marketing techniques for that community. This cultural understanding makes it easier to transmit information to the community. For example, Japanese audiences prefer indirect verbal communication and symbolism as the source of information, the Yoruba people of southwestern Nigeria prefer spoken words embedded in language codes, symbols, images, songs, and metaphors, and American advertising primarily relies on both spoken and written words as the source of information. Marketing techniques have strategic elements, which are often described as the four Ps: *product, price, place,* and *promotion.* In order to address cultural differences it is necessary to adjust at least one of the four Ps. The most commonly changed P is promotion, which is basically the language of the advertisement.

Symbols are also often used when marketing a product. However, using symbols is not recommended when marketing to multiple cultures. A symbol may be very meaningful in one culture and arbitrary in another. For example, in the Western world, it is gratifying to exchange gifts with visitors, and such gifts have specific meanings. In the Chinese culture, although exchanges of gifts with visitors are tolerated, visitors need to be beware of offering certain kinds of gifts. It is, for example, taboo to present a Chinese person with a clock or a green cap. In Chinese culture, a gift of a clock means that you want the recipient to die; a green cap means one is flirting with the host's wife. If one does not understand a community's culture, one can easily create a communication barrier when planning a health education program. So just as messages in translation may take on unintended and unfortunate meanings, symbols may also lead to offending the community's culture.

It is important to remember that market techniques and strategies must frequently be revised when marketing to multiple cultures (Siegel & Lotenberg, 2007). Translating a message should be entrusted only to a professional translator or advertiser. Also, as suggested earlier, symbols and icons may not have specific meanings in one culture but may have very strong meanings in another. When marketing to various cultures, keep in mind that each culture holds different values, and some strategies will not be as effective as others.

COMMUNICATION PATTERNS AND LANGUAGE BARRIERS

According to Flores (2006), 47 million people (18 percent of the population) in the United States speak a language other than English at home, and 22 million have limited English proficiency. This typically makes it difficult for these individuals to access health care, and health educators face major problems when planning, implementing, and evaluating health education services or programs for these individuals. Because of these problems these individuals' quality of care can deteriorate. The language barrier makes it difficult for the patients and health care providers to communicate effectively, and Flores (2005) found that patients who face a language barrier end up not receiving good health care. It is the responsibility of the health educator in the health care setting to ensure that proper translators are sought for such patients and optimal health care is provided.

Some studies (Peinkofer, 1994; Ponterotto, 1995; Murty, 1998; Flores, 2005, 2006; Luquis & Pérez, 2005; Velde, Wittman, & Bamberg, 2003; Wang, 2005) on the issues of communication patterns, cultural competence, and the language barriers faced by minorities in the delivery of health care in general and health education services in particular were reviewed for this chapter. Based on these reviews and the personal life experiences of the author in growing up in a developing country (Nigeria), it is deduced that language issues play a major role in the quality of all health care delivery services, including health education services. Effective communication is a cornerstone in the delivery of health care services. The importance of developing listening and speaking skills can not be overemphasized for all those involved in health care delivery services. Health care providers (including health educators) must demonstrate skill in listening, speaking, empathizing, probing, advocating, confronting, conveying immediacy, caring, and showing concern while responding to the health care needs of their clients and clients' families. They must understand the literacy levels of their clients and promote cross-cultural understanding. They should be prepared to recognize and meet the physical, social, emotional, mental, and spiritual needs of their clients.

Client confidentiality (as set out in the Health Insurance Portability and Accountability Act, or HIPAA), informed consent, and client rights are extremely important in the delivery of care. The more effective the communication that occurs between the provider and the client, the better the care provided and the healing process. To stimulate health care discussions between provider and client, a brief introduction of the provider with reference to his or her qualifications, care philosophy, cultural background, and interests and also some introduction to health topics important to the client's well-being are in order. Communication barriers impede the delivery of care and the healing process.

In order to serve culturally diverse clients, interpreters (translators) may be needed. Currently, thirteen U.S. states require reimbursement for the use of interpreters. This is one step toward fighting the communication problem faced by minority groups. It appears that the problem is now getting more national attention, but yet more needs to be accomplished. The literature reveals that more research and action are needed to address this problem (Lang, 2004). We are in the beginning steps of fighting it, and the only way to beat it is to identify and take action on each component of the problem, including communication and language patterns and barriers, health literacy, and the roles of culture, poverty, and educational opportunities.

In conclusion, the language barrier among minorities needs to be addressed. The issue is getting more attention, but it appears that rural and underserved areas and special populations in particular need help urgently. Despite the fact that this is a relatively small population, these people are the ones who need health care the most. A greater percentage of minorities live in metropolitan areas, but they are the ones mainly being targeted by existing interventions. It may seem impossible, but this issue must be addressed everywhere in the world, in large cities like New York and in small towns in rural America, Southeast Asia, Africa, and elsewhere. Additionally, efforts should be directed toward helping all minorities—whatever their difference, disability, or ethnic or racial identity—to overcome their language barriers.

CONCLUSION

The chapter highlights health educator guidelines for effective communication and cultural competence in the planning, implementation, and evaluation of health education intervention programs. Health educators working with clients whose health knowledge, beliefs, practices, and attitudes differ significantly from those of the health educator should be aware that such cultural factors influence clients' responses to health and health care services and that these clients require the development of culturally sensitive health education programs to influence their knowledge, attitudes, and behaviors. It is imperative that health educators demonstrate through their communication skills that they respect and value cultural diversity and encourage others to do so as well, while also observing unobtrusively clients' verbal and nonverbal behaviors and cues. Such behaviors and cues may be obstacles to effective communication.

Furthermore, it is crucial for health educators to exemplify how health care providers in general are supposed to communicate with different clients, demonstrating how to interact with minority clients in order to give them adequate care and how to encourage clients to actively participate in making decisions concerning their health care.

Culture-specific and sensitivity training will assist health educators to become more flexible in inferring motives or attributing meanings to other people's behavior, thereby increasing their communication effectiveness and cultural competence. They must continually advocate for effective cross-cultural communication and remember to focus on the important elements of communication, cultural sensitivity, marketing techniques, and language barriers as they carry out their roles and functions in their various practice environments.

POINTS TO REMEMBER

- Health educators should always be willing to analyze and select effective communication channels that are likely to reach and influence the program participants, that are sensitive to those participants' cultural underpinnings, and that use multicultural message strategies that are appropriate and relevant to the cultural environment.

- Health educators should institutionalize program goals and objectives within the cultural milieu of the target audience and ensure that clear and realistic health program objectives, incorporating input from the target audience, are set.

- Health educators should practice the principles of the 4 Ps of marketing by establishing a clear set of available health program *products* (intervention activities and media) that are also affordable given the target population's economic situation and acceptable costs (*price*) and that are packaged for the specific environment (*placement*). Health educators must also provide the target audience with information about how, when, and where its members can access health care information and programs (*promotion*).

- Health educators must possess active listening and speaking skills so that they will be able to remove impediments to effective communication.

CASE STUDY

Recently there was an outbreak of polio in the northern part of a West African country. There was then a massive campaign for oral polio immunization in this northern community. This community has heterogeneous ethnic groups but one major religion.

The community was skeptical about the mass immunization campaign because the vaccine was coming from the Western world. This mistrust involved a belief that the Western world was using the vaccine to control the community's population growth rate. (The religion allows polygamy.) A theory arose that a conspiracy existed between the West and the vaccine manufacturer. This conspiracy theory made one of the state governors in the north announce on television that parents should not take their children to the clinics or hospitals to be immunized against polio, and parents complied. Discuss the following questions:

1. What is polio? Expand your knowledge base on polio. Do some research about this disease.

2. How could you dispel the conspiracy theory?

3. What publicity or marketing techniques would you embark on for a successful polio immunization campaign after the governor's TV announcement?

4. Which of the seven areas of responsibility for a health educator is most relevant to a discussion of this case and the intervention to resolve it?

5. What communication and cultural competencies would serve as guidelines in your intervention planning, implementation, and evaluation?

6. What are the implications of the scenario for health education practice?

KEY TERMS

Communication model	Health literacy
Communication strategy	Intercultural communication
Community health	Language barrier
Cultural competence	Marketing
Cultural identity	Personal health
Cultural kinetics	Social action
Enculturation	Stereotyping
Health communication	Structural obstacle

REFERENCES

Airhihenbuwa, C. O. (1995). *Health and culture: Beyond the western paradigm.* Thousand Oaks, CA: Sage.

Angell, M. (1989). *New England Journal of Medicine (5 year cumulative index 1984–1988).* Waltham, MA: Massachusetts Medical Society.

Annas, G. J., & Grodin, M. A. (Eds.). (1995). *The Nazi doctors and the Nuremberg Code: Human rights in human experimentation.* New York: Oxford University Press.

Basch, P. F. (1990). *International health.* New York: Oxford University Press.

Centers for Disease Control and Prevention. (2005). *The Tuskegee syphilis timeline.* Retrieved March 15, 2007, from http://www.cdc.gov/nchstp/od/tuskegee/time.htm.

Elmandjra, M. (2003, October 20). Moroccan philosopher says cultural communication prevents war. *Asian Political News*. Retrieved October 19, 2006, from http://www.findarticles.com/p/articles/mi_m0WDQ/is_2003_Oct_20/ai_109021640.

England, C. R. (n.d.). *A look at the Indian Health Service policy of sterilization, 1972–1976*. Retrieved October 19, 2006, from http://www.dickshovel.com/IHSSterPol.html.

Faseke, M. M. (1990). Oral history in Nigeria: Issues, problems, and prospects. *Oral History Review, 18*(1), 77–91.

Flores, G. (2005). Limited English proficiency, primary language at home, and disparities in children's health care: How language barriers are measured matters. *Public Health Reports, 120*(4), 418–430.

Flores, G. (2006). Language barriers to health care in the United States. *New England Journal of Medicine, 355*(3), 229–231.

Glanz, K., Rimer, B. K., & Lewis, F. M. (Eds.). (2002). *Health behavior and health education: Theory, research, and practice* (3rd ed.). San Francisco: Jossey-Bass.

Joint Committee on Health Education and Promotion Terminology. (2002). Report of the 2000 Joint Committee on Health Education and Promotion Terminology. *Journal of School Health, 72*(1), 3–7.

Lang, Y. (2004). *Using symbols and icons in localization*. Enlaso Corporation. Retrieved October 23, 2006, from http://www.translate.com/technology/multilingual_standard/symbols_and_icons.html.

Luquis, R. R., & Pérez, M. A. (2005). Health educators and cultural competence: Implications for the profession. *American Journal of Health Studies, 20*(3), 156–163.

Mazrui, A. A. (1986). *The Africans: A triple heritage*. Boston: Little, Brown.

Murty, M. (1998). Healthy living for immigrant women: A health education community outreach program. *Canadian Medical Association Journal, 159*(4), 385–387.

National Commission for Health Education Credentialing. (2007). *Responsibilities & competencies*. Retrieved January 25, 2008, from http://www.nchec.org/aboutnchec/rc.htm.

Nicholson, P. J. (1999). Communicating health risks. *Occupational Medicine, 49*(4), 253–258. Retrieved October 20, 2006, from http://occmed.oxfordjournals.org/cgi/reprint/49/4/253.pdf.

Peinkofer, J. R. (1994). HIV education for the deaf, a vulnerable minority. *Public Health Reports, 109*(3), 390–396.

Ponterotto, J. G. (1995). A multicultural competency checklist for counseling training programs. *Journal of Multicultural Counseling & Development, 23*(1), 11–20.

Prochaska, J. O., & DiClemente, C. C. (1983). Stages and processes of self-change in smoking: Toward an integrative model of change. *Journal of Consulting and Clinical Psychology, 5*, 390–395.

Prochaska, J. O., DiClemente, C. C., & Norcross, J. C. (1992). In search of how people change. *American Psychologist, 47*, 1102–1114.

Roman, K., Maas, J., & Nisenholtz, M. (2003). *How to advertise* (3rd ed.). New York: St. Martin's Press.

Siegel, M., & Lotenberg, L. (2007). *Marketing public health: Strategies to promote social change*. Sudbury, MA: Jones and Bartlett.

Velde, B., Wittman, P., & Bamberg, R. (2003). Cultural competence of faculty and students in a school of allied health. *Journal of Allied Health, 32*(3), 189–195.

Wang, S. (2005). Developing an innovative cross-cultural strategy to promote HIV/AIDS prevention in different ethnic cultural groups of China. *AIDS Care, 17*(7), 874–891.

CHAPTER

TOWARD A CULTURALLY COMPETENT HEALTH EDUCATION WORKFORCE

EVA I. DOYLE

LEARNING OBJECTIVES

After completing this chapter, you will be able to

■ Describe the profile of a culturally competent student.

■ Name appropriate learning objectives for developing competence.

■ Describe important components of a university curriculum with a cultural competence framework.

■ Describe steps taken by leaders of a degree program (described in a case study) to address cultural competence in their curriculum.

INTRODUCTION

Recent calls for cultural competence in the health education workforce were spawned by decades of research and discussion in the health education field about appropriate terminology and training approaches. Historically, a number of evolving terms have been used to describe what health educators should understand and do to become more effective in an increasingly multicultural society. Such terms as *cultural awareness* and *cultural sensitivity* name important concepts that traditionally concerned the degree to which a health educator is equipped with the knowledge and attitudes needed for effective cross-cultural interaction. More recently these concepts have become part of a much broader paradigm that embraces measurable action as the ultimate goal. This broader paradigm is commonly referred to as *cultural competence,* which is defined by the profession as "the ability of an individual to understand and respect values, attitudes, beliefs, and mores that differ across cultures, and to consider and respond appropriately to these differences in planning, implementing, and evaluating health education and promotion programs and interventions" (Joint Committee on Health Education and Promotion Terminology, 2002, p. 4).

Under this action-oriented definition, a health educator can be deemed culturally competent if he or she possesses appropriate levels of cultural awareness and sensitivity and performs health education in ways that embody empowerment and respect for differences. This standard provides a useful framework for education and training efforts in university preparation programs and in worksite professional development efforts. Reaching the standard requires that these educational efforts include opportunities to enhance understanding and to practice measurable skills. This chapter contains an overview of practical approaches that can foster cultural competence among prospective and practicing health educators.

CULTURAL COMPETENCE AND PROFESSIONAL PREPARATION PROGRAMS

This section contains an overview of needed goals for a professional preparation program in which the targeted outcome is culturally competent students. A description of curriculum components and implementation strategies and also recommendations for effective evaluation are provided. The goal is to equip the reader with an understanding of how to design a professional health education preparation program with a strong cultural competence framework.

Clarifying Desired Performance Outcomes

Cultural competence is a developmental process that occurs over an extended period of time (Campinha-Bacote, 1994; Cross, Bazron, Dennis, & Isaacs, 1989; National Center for Cultural Competence [NCCC], n.d.). Because true cultural competence in all contexts is virtually impossible to achieve, designers of university degree programs must be patient and realistic in their expectations of students. A single course or sequenced learning experience can improve a person's cultural perspectives, but the true test of competence lies in the degree to which an individual commits to lifelong learning. Part of the profile of a culturally competent student lies in the degree to which that student is engaging in observable actions conducive to learning.

The Profile of a Competent Student. The culturally competent model of care (Campinha-Bacote, 1994) and the PEN-3 model (Airhihenbuwa, 1995), discussed in Chapter Six, can serve as a basis for a general profile of a culturally competent student in health education. Because cultural competence is an ongoing developmental process, the criteria used to gauge competence in a student must be largely based on active efforts to learn and mature in relation to these model concepts. Progress is evident when a student

- Engages in ongoing self-analysis to identify and address personal perspectives and cross-cultural biases.

- Actively seeks to view life through the eyes of others, and through that, develops a greater level of sensitivity for the values and life challenges of other groups.

- Participates in hands-on training opportunities for practice and feedback that can help him or her begin to master competent needs assessment techniques.

- Seeks opportunities to engage in cross-cultural interactions in all aspects of life.

Learning Objectives for Developing Competence. As students begin the learning process, learning objectives must guide course and program development. Exhibit 9.1 contains some objectives created by the chapter author. Though a variety of other sources (Beatty & Doyle, 2000; Doyle, Liu, & Ancona, 1996; Luquis & Pérez, 2003) were used, these objectives are based largely on the work of Luquis, Pérez, and Young (2006), who identified specific content- and skills-related program components as part of a cultural competence assessment of 157 university health education degree programs. Some of the curriculum components identified through this study have been combined, expanded, or otherwise altered in order to reflect general teaching subject areas and to fit a learning objective format.

The two categories into which the learning objectives shown in Exhibit 9.1 are divided—awareness- and knowledge-based objectives and skills-based objectives— can be readily aligned with the five process components of the culturally competent model of care (Campinha-Bacote, 1994; see Chapter Six). The awareness- and knowledge-based objectives represent learning content that a student should master when exploring personal perspectives and multiple worldviews as part of coursework. The first four objectives could be used to develop student awareness of evidence-based relationships between culture, societal factors, and health issues faced by a variety of ethnic and racial groups. Objective 5 can be used to help students understand and embrace culturally competent health promotion strategies. Objective 6 is designed to motivate students toward self-directed competency development by equipping them with learning goals and knowledge about development strategies.

EXHIBIT 9.1. Learning Objectives for University Health Education Degree Programs.

AWARENESS- AND KNOWLEDGE-BASED OBJECTIVES

The student will be able to demonstrate knowledge about and discuss the implications of

1. Common relationships between health, culture, ethnicity, religion, poverty, age, gender, and a variety of social issues.

2. Differences in health status and in health care access between minority ethnic and racial groups and the American majority.

3. Cultural beliefs and values of different ethnic and racial groups and how these cultural factors compare to personal cultural beliefs and values.

4. Health beliefs, environmental factors, and other influences on health behavior among members of different ethnic and racial groups.

5. Effective and appropriate health promotion and disease prevention strategies for different ethnic and racial groups.

6. Knowledge, perspectives, skills, and developmental approaches needed to become a culturally competent health educator.

SKILLS-BASED OBJECTIVES

The student will be able to

1. Demonstrate the ability to understand and respect the values, attitudes, and beliefs of diverse ethnic and racial groups.

2. Design instruments and methods that can be used to effectively assess needs among clients of diverse ethnic and racial backgrounds.

3. Identify resources that can be used to promote health effectively in diverse ethnic and racial communities.

4. Design culturally appropriate health education and health promotion programs for diverse ethnic and racial communities.

5. Implement health education and promotion programs in ways that empower and engage diverse ethnic and racial communities.

6. Design instruments and methods that can be used to effectively evaluate health education and promotion programs in diverse ethnic and racial communities.

7. Design media and advocacy campaigns for clients of diverse ethnic and racial backgrounds.

8. Partner with diverse ethnic and racial communities in health promotion efforts.

The skills-based objectives can serve as the basis for skills training exercises that occur in classroom settings and the cultural encounter opportunities offered through internships and in community-based projects for courses and student organizations. These objectives largely reflect the areas of responsibility for an entry-level health educator (National Commission for Health Education Credentialing [NCHEC], Society for Public Health Education [SOPHE], & American Association for Health Education [AAHE], 2006) but also contain a strong culture-based emphasis throughout. Specific curriculum design components that can be built upon these learning objectives are described in the next section.

Developing a Strong Curriculum

The ideal curriculum for health education preparation programs is one that equips students with the knowledge, sensitivity, and practical skills needed to deliver health education in a culturally competent manner. Though a variety of curricular designs can help programs achieve this goal, a well-designed degree program should include four basic components:

- Course structures and sequences that promote an integrated approach to cultural competence development

- Opportunities to examine and apply theories and models within a cultural context throughout the curriculum

- Experiential learning opportunities (hands-on, real-world experiences) specifically designed to expose students to a variety of multicultural and cross-cultural experiences

- Professors who are capable of modeling and mentoring a lifelong process of becoming culturally competent.

Course Structure and Integrated Degree Programs. In the previously mentioned study of university-based programs, Luquis et al. (2006) identified common approaches to cultural competence development. Though some form of cultural competence education was evident in most programs, few contained a course specifically devoted to cultural competence. Cultural competence was only sporadically integrated into courses that focused on health education competencies, and levels of faculty preparation to teach in-depth aspects of cultural competence were unclear. In light of these study results, the researchers recommended that the health education profession develop discipline-specific cultural competence standards that could be used by program accreditation bodies and developers of health education degree programs.

Most administrators of university health education degree programs value cultural competence and desire to infuse it into their curriculum (Luquis et al., 2006). However, both real and perceived barriers to such an infusion do exist. The need to create new courses that focus directly on cultural competence must be met within the constraints of limitations on total degree program credit hours, accreditation-related requirements for other competency-based and general education courses, and faculty work load restrictions. These factors may compel decision makers to "outsource" their cultural competence course requirements to other disciplines within their institutions. These "outside" courses often cover basic relationships between culture and social issues but may not include needed health education perspectives (Luquis et al., 2006).

Compounding the issues in the curriculum infusion discussion is the belief of some university educators that integrating cultural competence perspectives within existing courses is actually more effective than developing separate culture-based courses (Morey & Kitano, 1997). Though most health educators would support adapting existing courses to include cultural competence perspectives, problems can arise in this process. The degree to which cultural competence is truly infused and clearly evident in a course that is designed to address a health education issue (for instance, a stress management course) or health education competence (for instance, a program evaluation course) is often highly dependent on the perspectives and abilities of individual course instructors. When these instructors work independently of each other, the depth and accuracy of culture-based coverage across courses can be inconsistent.

A call for a more organized and deliberate approach to including cultural competence in university health education degree programs has been issued (Luquis et al., 2006). An important next step is to develop clear guidelines for accomplishing this goal. Figure 9.1 contains a curriculum development model that can be used to integrate cultural competence throughout a health education degree program. This model for an integrated cultural competence curriculum (IC-3 model) was created by this chapter author to help degree program designers take a deliberate approach to addressing cultural competence in their programs. It is based on recommendations from the field (Beatty & Doyle, 2000; Champagne, 2006; Doyle et al., 1996; Luquis & Pérez, 2003; Luquis et al., 2006; Redican, Stewart, Johnson, & Frazee, 1994).

The IC-3 model was designed to help degree program designers capitalize on what already exists in their current program while incorporating a clearly defined cultural competence framework into that program. The goal is to capitalize on some common degree program components: introductory, competency-based, and health topic or group-specific courses; an internship and portfolio requirement; service learning opportunities; Eta Sigma Gamma membership; other social support mechanisms (alumni e-lists, faculty-student socials); and evaluation feedback loops. Infused throughout the model is a structure that is designed to make cultural competence a salient and constant goal throughout the learning process.

The concentric circles in the IC-3 model represent progressive levels of learning that move the student from the inner circle of introductory courses outward toward a culminating internship and eventual employment. These concentric layers are presented in a progressively widening *overlay format* to illustrate integrated learning through which students apply, expand, and refine what they learn about cultural competence in the inner circles in increasingly *application-focused* learning experiences in the outer circles. The model is not intended to dictate, for instance, that competency-based

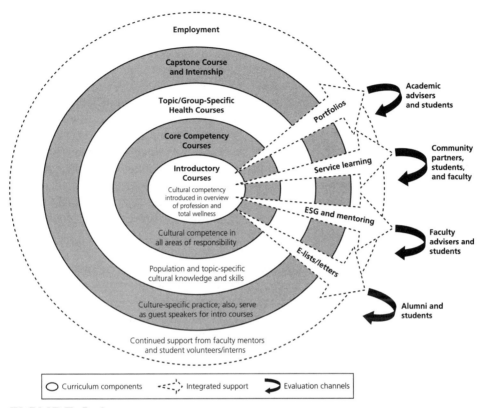

FIGURE 9.1. *Integrated Cultural Competence Curriculum (IC-3) Model.*

courses be a mandated prerequisite to health topic or group-specific courses. Instead, the model is designed as a conceptual guide for the application of competency-based perspectives to specific health issues and populations.

For example, a student could learn in an introductory course that culture, ethnicity, religion, and socialization influence the health status and practices of most populations (Spector, 2004). In competency-based courses the student could learn about culture-related aspects of needs assessment and program planning, implementation, and evaluation. In a group-specific course that focuses on "health in traditional Asian American communities," the student could be guided to apply the previously learned concepts and health education skills in order to more fully understand and address in a culturally sensitive manner such things as the cultural reasons for coining, a practice in some traditional Asian communities of scraping the skin with a coin to release "illness-causing spirits" (Spector, 2004). A student could then be placed in an internship site where the experiential application of what has been learned produces a more refined perspective.

The success of this layered learning experience depends in part on the degree to which each course contains the needed cultural competence focus. The smallest and most central circle in the IC-3 model represents the introductory course(s) of a degree program that students usually complete early in their degree plan. Instructors for these courses may introduce students to the history and evolution of the health education profession, the foundational philosophies and theories on which most health education practices are based, the skills and competencies needed for effective health education practice, and the settings and conditions in which health educators work. These introductory courses are a logical curriculum component in which to directly address the six awareness- and knowledge-based learning objectives (Exhibit 9.1) The theories and models, communication methods, and other content provided in other chapters in this book can serve as a starting point for in-class discussions and critical thinking assignments. An overview of the skills-based learning objectives (Exhibit 9.1) should also be presented in one of the introductory courses so that students will know what to expect as they progress through the degree program.

Many programs contain required competency-based courses that focus on needs assessment, program planning and implementation, evaluation, and other essential skills (NCHEC et al., 2006). These *core competency courses* in the IC-3 model (Figure 9.1) can serve as a logical avenue through which students continue to learn about the cultural competence specific to each skill set. For example, in a needs assessment course, students should be reminded of information presented in the introductory course about relationships between culture, ethnicity, social issues, and factors that contribute to health status gaps found in ethnic and racial groups. They should also learn about the specific health needs of a variety of ethnic and racial communities and the assessment instruments and methods that have been proven effective in those communities. Course projects, guest speakers, assigned readings, and class discussions should be deliberately designed to expose students to diverse assessment perspectives across a wide variety of ethnic and racial groups.

The third ring from the center of the model focuses on topic- or group-specific health courses. In some degree programs students complete health topic courses, such as stress management and human sexuality, and also population-specific courses that focus on adolescents, women, or aging populations. In these courses student should learn culture-based factors relevant to the topic areas and populations studied. Ideally, ethnicity-specific health courses (on, for example, African American health) could be added to the curriculum. However, if low resources are a barrier, carefully screened courses from other disciplines, such as sociology and anthropology, may at least be useful in presenting ethnicity-specific social issues. These courses from other disciplines should be viewed only as a supplemental component to, rather than a substitute for, cultural competence training in health education courses.

Formal internships and service learning courses that are a required component of many university health education degree programs often provide opportunities for developing culturally competent skills (Rojas-Guyler, Cottrell, & Wagner, 2006). Because fulfilling an internship is usually an integral part of course sequencing, it occupies the outer circle of the IC-3 model, just prior to graduation and employment. This ring also includes a preparation course component because, in some programs, health education majors complete either what is considered a capstone course or a small, one-credit internship preparation course, or both, as part of their final steps toward graduation (Beatty & Doyle, 2000).

The four dotted-line arrows in the IC-3 model represent integrated support components that can help students develop an integrated view of the culture-based linkages between courses and experiential opportunities for cultural encounters. A required professional portfolio that students must develop as they progress through the program can help them to visualize how each course and learning experience contributes to the overall professional development experience (Doyle & Ward, 2001). Community-based partnerships with organizations that support a variety of service learning opportunities can provide a powerfully integrated connection between students, faculty, and culturally diverse communities. A well-maintained alumni newsletter or e-mail distribution list (e-list) can serve as another valuable support component for students, who may be able to connect with alumni for diversity-based mentoring.

Effective evaluation is essential to the ongoing evolution of a dynamic degree program. The evaluation channels (curved feedback arrows) to the right of the model circles can guide the establishment of ongoing evaluation activities specific to the four integrated support components. For instance, the required portfolio can be used to document student efforts to develop cultural competence. Some examples of portfolio components are culture-specific needs assessment instruments developed in a course project, pictures of involvement in a health fair or other service project conducted in a culturally diverse setting, evidence of a poster or oral presentation containing culture-specific health information, and a certificate earned for participating in a community-based training workshop that focused on cultural competence training.

Other feedback loops can use written evaluation instruments, focus groups, and personal interviews to obtain information about the extent to which the degree program or specific integrated support components facilitate cultural competence learning. Students can write reflection papers about specific service learning activities, and faculty mentors can provide valuable feedback about project methods and observed student performance. Feedback from community partners regarding the cultural competence levels of both the students and their faculty mentors can be an important evaluation source.

Participation in Eta Sigma Gamma (ESG), a national honor society for health education majors, can provide a valuable opportunity for students from a variety of diverse backgrounds to interact outside the classroom as they work together on service projects and develop culturally competent leadership skills. More experienced and culturally competent student leaders and faculty advisers can serve as strong role models for less experienced students in this organization. Feedback from faculty and the students involved can be useful in identifying realities and perceptions related to ESG.

Another important feedback source is student alumni groups. Alumni possess useful postprogram perspectives on their learning experience. They can also provide information about real-world applications of their cultural competence training after graduation. Because alumni can serve as powerful role models and mentors for students, asking them to serve as evaluators of student competence in service learning and internship experiences can be of value. This can readily be accomplished when these alumni are working in local community organizations and, within that context, serve as internship site supervisors or partners with professors in course-based projects.

Teaching Through Models, Experiential Learning, and Mentors. Though the IC-3 model is a valuable guide for degree program development, it provides only the conceptual framework needed for connecting program components. Once the conceptual structure is in place, a careful examination of how cultural competence is taught within each course is needed. Ideally, a degree program would contain a separate course that is clearly labeled as an introduction to cultural competence (Luquis et al., 2006). However, even when a distinctively culture-based course cannot be readily developed, the basic theoretical concepts of health education can and should be introduced and thoroughly discussed within a strong cultural competence context.

The ability to apply theories and models to identify determinants of health has long been accepted as an essential health education skill. Historically, some theories encompassed a narrow, individualized framework that ignored social and environmental contexts. More contemporary theories have emerged that compel the health educator to address social and cultural influences on individual thoughts, behaviors, health status, and quality of life. However, though cultural competence is now widely accepted as having a role in health education–oriented theory, it has yet to be assigned a prominent role in many commonly used theories and models. Thus the health educator must sometimes move beyond traditional perspectives on these theories to interpret and apply them in multicultural settings (Frankish, Lovato, & Shannon, 1999). A variety of sources (DiClemente, Crosby, & Kegler, 2002; Frankish et al., 1999; Glanz, Rimer, & Lewis, 2002) that contain extensive details about theories and models common to the profession are available to health educators. (Chapter Six also contains a useful discussion of models.)

A less well known model in health education circles that can be used in the classroom for helping health education students to explore cultural competence is the model of heritage consistency (Spector, 2004). *Heritage consistency* is the degree to which a person's lifestyle reflects that person's traditional culture or cultural roots. The model assumes that all humans have cultural roots and that the values and behaviors of every individual represent and are influenced to some degree by that person's cultural heritage. According to the model, heritage consistency is influenced and characterized by one's religious beliefs and practices, ethnicity (when it is a conscious and deliberate identification); and cultural norms (habits and beliefs that may be unconsciously embraced). This model serves as an effective starting point, one that motivates students to consider their own cultural roots and how that heritage influences their worldview and interaction with individuals from other cultures.

Though models help in establishing a learning foundation, life experience is the true master teacher. Students in professional preparation programs are more likely to value and engage in learning experiences and apply what they learn through them when those learning experiences mirror or, better yet, occur within real-world settings. This is particularly true when cultural competence is the learning goal. Cross-cultural encounters are essential to helping individuals become aware of differences (cultural awareness), and multiple encounters are necessary to minimize the perpetuation of stereotypes and deepen levels of cultural understanding and skill (Campinha-Bacote, 1994). The challenge in helping students to develop cultural competence is to design learning experiences that will facilitate an appropriate progression of learning development. A natural avenue through which needed cultural encounters can occur within a university degree program is found in service learning activities.

The term *service learning* first appeared in the published literature in the late 1960s (Champagne, 2006). "Service learning in health education is designed to engage the university with the community in ways that enhance students' academic experience, and simultaneously serve the needs of the community" (Champagne, 2006, p. 97). In university settings, service learning usually entails campus-community partnerships through which students engage in experiential activities and process what they have learned through discussion and reflection.

Service learning has been deemed a highly valuable approach to training prospective health educators (Champagne, 2006; Geiger & Werner, 2004). Some benefits include enhanced satisfaction among students, faculty, and community partners with the quality of student-faculty relationships (Eyler & Giles, 1999) and with the student learning process (Berson & Youkin, 1998; Geiger & Werner, 2004; Greenberg, 2003), as well as with the service benefits to the community (Astin & Sax, 1998; Cohen & Kinsey, 1994; Geiger & Werner, 2004; Melchior, 1997). Yet despite these positive outcomes, the time needed for most projects and the low appreciation of such projects among some university administrators are barriers to an ongoing commitment to service learning. Efforts to offset these barriers and facilitate effective and widely valued service learning have been led by Health Professions Schools in Service to the Nation and Community-Campus Partnerships for Health, organizations whose goals are to foster community health, social change, and citizenship through community-campus partnerships (Champagne, 2006).

Service learning is commonly viewed as a viable mechanism through which students can develop cultural competence. Specific outcomes can include heightened cultural awareness, reduced stereotyping, and improved cross-cultural communication skills (Astin & Sax, 1998; Champagne, 2006; Geiger & Werner, 2004; Seelye, 1996). Though Champagne (2006) found that few published evaluations of service learning focused on acquired skills, the health education profession already possesses the capacity to produce skills-based evidence in support of service learning. The formal internships that are a required component of many university health education degree programs (Rojas-Guyler et al., 2006) are a readily applicable venue not only for service learning but also for skills-based evaluation of the service learning experience. The SOPHE/AAHE Baccalaureate Program Approval Committee (National Task Force on the Preparation and Practice of Health Educators, 1985), the national approval body for undergraduate health professional preparation programs, requires that health education students complete 320 internship contact hours and that the skills described in the areas of responsibility of an entry-level health educator serve as a framework for performance evaluation. Because cultural competence skills are at least mentioned in some of the responsibility areas, the evaluation of these competencies will likely become a naturally emerging component of performance evaluation.

Culturally competent mentors can also significantly influence student learning. Luquis et al. (2006) reported that the majority of health education faculty members were committed to, knowledgeable about, and comfortable with teaching cultural competence. However, upon closer inspection of specific survey responses, only 38 percent were "very" committed, 16 percent were "very" knowledgeable, and 25 percent were "very" comfortable with the subject. Perhaps even more disconcerting was that only 15 percent of faculty members were very involved with diverse ethnic, racial, and cultural groups outside of academia.

Effective leaders lead by example (Maxwell, 2001). If cultural competence is defined as a learning process, health education professors can serve as effective role models by exhibiting the same action-oriented characteristics previously described in the profile of a competent student. An important principle for professors to understand is that serving as a role model for cultural competence does not require perfection. Instead it requires a willingness to be transparent and genuine in sharing with students one's personal progress in this lifelong process. If students are to be required to take risks and submit themselves to vulnerable situations through cultural encounters and self-examination, their professors must be willing to do the same. The basic tenets of cultural competence development in the workforce that are addressed in the following section can be applied among faculty members of university degree programs.

CULTURAL COMPETENCE AND THE WORK SETTING

The quest to develop a culturally competent health education workforce does not solely rely on the abilities of university graduates who enter the job market. An additionally important component lies in the competence of those who are currently in the workforce and the organizations in which they work. The Office of Minority Health (OMH) (2004) describes cultural competence as the "capacity to function effectively as an individual and an organization within the context of the cultural beliefs, behaviors, and needs presented by consumers and their communities." Much of what has been discussed as needed for developing cultural competence among university students also holds true for health educators in the current workforce. This section of the chapter contains a profile of and recommendations for developing culturally competent organizations in which health educators can effectively work.

Organizational culture is "the collective programming of the mind that distinguishes the members of one organization from another" (Hofstede, 2001, p. 391). Sometimes referred to as *corporate cultures,* organizational cultures are socially shaped, historically influenced, and difficult to change. Whereas national cultures are characterized by shared *values,* organizational cultures are characterized by "shared perceptions about daily practices" (p. 394). These shared perceptions shape what the organization does and how the work is done. Organizational culture can enable or limit a health educator's ability to deliver services in a culturally competent manner. Health educators need to be equipped with an understanding of organizational culture and with the skills needed to perform with cultural competence within the context of accepted organizational practices.

The Profile of a Competent Organization

According to the National Center for Cultural Competence (NCCC, n.d.), cultural competence requires that organizations and their personnel "have the capacity to (1) value diversity, (2) conduct self-assessment, (3) manage the dynamics of difference, (4) acquire and institutionalize cultural knowledge, and (5) adapt to the diversity and cultural contexts of the communities they serve." This clearly defined profile of organizational competence mirrors, from the individual employee's perspective, much of what was discussed in previous chapter sections about the ongoing learning process that embodies cultural competence development.

The culturally competent model of care (Campinha-Bacote, 1994) and the recommended learning objectives in Exhibit 9.1 could be applied in professional development workshops and other training opportunities for health educators in the work setting. However, though the competence of individual employees is critical to organizational success, the full competence profile of the organization in which those employees work encompasses some broader elements that are also important. Organizational competence is dependent in part on the degree to which organizational leaders and employees understand common barriers to competence in their work environment and are committed to the institutional changes needed to overcome those barriers.

Common Barriers to Cultural Competence in the Work Environment

In a culturally competent organization, employees and clients from diverse ethnic and racial backgrounds are valued and empowered through the organization's policies and practices (Hofstede, 2001; OMH, 2001). Factors related to hiring, promotion and dismissal, salaries and rewards, supervision, and decisional control can influence an employee's perceptions about the work environment and her ability to perform at optimal levels. Though overt discrimination within most organizations is operationally defined and legally regulated, the quest for cultural competence within an organization must go far beyond the mere absence of discriminatory treatment. Even when organizational leaders desire a culturally competent work environment, institutionalized practices can negatively affect employee performance and the quality of client services.

A common barrier to cultural competence in the work environment involves institutionalized policies and procedures that revolve around time and productivity. Some health educators work with large client populations where the urgency of needed services imposes a stressful demand for time efficiency. A systems-oriented approach to organizational productivity can entail the development of time-regimented procedures such as rigid appointment scheduling and abbreviated client interviews. Though this practice often does increase the number of clients seen per day, the cultural competence of an organization and its employees can be significantly compromised when time rigidity is an institutionalized norm. In addition, differences in time orientation across cultures often result in extensive frustration and negative interactions between health educators and their clients (Spector, 2004).

An example of time orientation conflict lies in the common expectation in many health service organizations that a client will arrive on time for an appointment and must be ushered through a series of sequential procedures (sign-in, insurance confirmation, preliminary interview with a nurse, follow-up visit with a physician). If a client is "late for an appointment," it can highly stress the office personnel and cause a scheduling backlog. In addition, office personnel whose own cultural norms cause them to view a late arrival as lack of respect can feel insulted and resentful toward the client. The client, in contrast, may be operating out of an entirely different time orientation norm and may not view punctuality as a necessity and may actually feel devalued by the rushed approach to the appointment process (Spector, 2004).

Developing a Strong Professional Development Plan

The Office of Minority Health (OMH, 2001) began work in 1997 to establish national standards for *culturally and linguistically appropriate services* (CLAS) in health care. The resulting fourteen CLAS standards were designed to render health services "more responsive to the individual needs of all patients/consumers" and, ultimately, "to contribute to the elimination of racial and ethnic health disparities and to improve the health of all Americans" (OMH, 2001, p. ix). Standards 1 through 7 represent criteria for cultural competence in direct care (involving client respect, staff recruitment and training, and language access), and Standards 8 through 14 promote the organizational support (structure, policies, and processes) needed for implementing the first seven standards.

Establishing the CLAS standards was a groundbreaking effort that launched the development of practical guidelines organizations can use for implementing the CLAS standards (Salimbene, 2001), conducting organizational self-assessments (COSMOS Corporation, 2003), engaging in research (OMH, 2004), and implementing language access services (American Institutes for Research, 2005). These guidelines and other helpful documents are available for public access on the OMH, Web site (www.omhrc .gov). These resources can be used as a practical guide for enhancing the cultural competence of organizations in which health educators work. The following sections describe some models used for developing culturally competent organizations and training the employees who work in them.

Training Recommendations for Professional Development

A wide array of training approaches and topics are used throughout this country to help professionals develop cultural competence. Examples are presentations about specific cultures and overviews of culture-specific resources, use of language assistance services, development of cultural awareness and sensitivity, cross-cultural communication methods, and training specific to epidemiological and patient-centered assessments. However, evidence-based research is needed to distinguish between effective and less effective training approaches (OMH, 2004).

Doyle and Faucher (2002) reviewed the literature and compiled a list of general recommendations for health care professionals who wish to become more culturally competent in their interactions with clients. These general guidelines begin with a recommendation to become familiar with the community in which a client lives and the general cultural norms of the individual client. This can be accomplished by visiting with key informants and gatekeepers who know the community well, attending important community celebrations and other events, asking open-ended questions about community concerns and quality of life, and identifying community capacities that affect wellness in the community. Developing effective communication skills and establishing community rapport (topics addressed in more detail in Chapter Eight) are key to developing community trust. Patience, consistency, and long-term commitment to a community can serve as a platform for professional development on the job.

Luquis and Pérez (2005) used the Inventory for Assessing the Process of Cultural Competence Among Healthcare Professionals-Revised to assess the cultural competence levels of 455 health educators from across the United States. They discovered that most of the respondents were operating at a level of competence known as "cultural awareness," which is characterized by "sensitivity to the values, beliefs, and practices of different ethnic and cultural groups" (p. 159). Approximately one-third were deemed "culturally competent," which was characterized as being "culturally sensitive . . . and able to respond to the needs of other groups" (p. 159). When the sample was narrowed to only 203 school health educators (Luquis & Pérez, 2006), the results were similar except that only 20 percent of respondents scored in the culturally competent category. In analyses of both data sets, the researchers noted that respondents who had completed two degrees in health education were more culturally competent than those who had completed only one degree in health education. In addition, competence rates were higher among those who had attended cultural diversity training programs within the past three years. These findings serve as an important reminder that university health education programs in general may already contain some important diversity-oriented learning opportunities and that when cultural diversity training becomes a deliberate focus, competency outcomes increase.

CONCLUSION

Students and professionals who desire to achieve an effective level of cultural competence should avoid the pitfall of feeling overwhelmed by the task. When they characterize cultural competence as a *process* rather than an *arrival point,* then success can be defined in terms of significant steps in the processes of lifelong self-analysis, competency training, and cross-cultural interaction. Professional development programs can be designed to equip students with needed knowledge and skills along with high motivation to explore personal perspectives and multiple worldviews, understand and embrace culturally competent health promotion strategies, and engage in self-directed competency development. With appropriate levels of commitment, hard work, and patience invested in these efforts, students and the professionals who teach them will benefit from experiencing a lifelong process of becoming culturally competent.

POINTS TO REMEMBER

- Cultural competence is not an arrival point but a process of lifelong effort to continually engage in self-analysis, competency training, cross-cultural interaction, and appreciation for multiple worldviews.

- The learning objectives of a professional development program should include awareness- and knowledge-based objectives and skills-based objectives that motivate students to explore personal perspectives and multiple worldviews, understand and embrace culturally competent health promotion strategies, and engage in self-directed competency development.

- A well-designed degree program should include four basic components that promote cultural competence: an integrated approach to course structures and sequences, application of theories and models within a cultural context, experiential learning opportunities, and professors who are capable of modeling and mentoring a lifelong process of becoming culturally competent.

CASE STUDY

The bachelor's degree program in community health education (CHE) at Baylor University (www.baylor.edu) illustrates how degree program designers can deliberately infuse cultural competence into the curriculum. Leaders of this relatively new Baylor degree program have recently worked to deliberately infuse a cultural competence framework into course content and projects. In core courses the students learn about health education philosophy and theory, methodological paradigms, and professional ethics from the framework of the PEN-3 and other culture-based models. The reciprocal relationships between cultural competence, community empowerment, and quality of life are presented as critical elements when forging community partnerships to promote health. Back translation and other techniques that foster health literacy within a cultural context are presented as important skill components. The students also learn the principles of community-based participatory research (Minkler & Wallerstein, 2003) and how to work with community partners to implement culture-specific needs assessments and programs.

The students practice the principles and skills of cultural competence through community-based course projects in at least three courses. Recent project examples include needs assessment work and health promotion programming with migrant and seasonal farmworkers (predominantly Hispanics) in east Texas, with a predominantly African American housing community in south Dallas, and with a culturally diverse homeless population and a low-literacy older adult population in central Texas. As students complete these projects, they are required to write reflection papers in which they describe what they learned about themselves and their ability to serve individuals from a variety of cultures. The student feedback is often overwhelmingly positive, and students who are in the degree program but not enrolled in these specific courses often ask if they can engage voluntarily to help with these course project events.

In addition to local community-based course projects, CHE program leaders recently added an *international summer study abroad* opportunity that allows students to travel to Brazil with a health education professor and engage in learning experiences for college credit. In this program the students complete an international health education course and a cross-cultural health communication course through which they learn about global health issues, international health policies and organizational efforts that shape international health, effective health promotion strategies in international settings, and how to promote health across language and cultural barriers. The students attend classes at the program's hotel site and engage in a variety of community health projects with local Brazilian partners. Some health education majors engage in the program as international health education interns who help to develop, implement, coordinate, and evaluate the community health projects. A strong program attribute is that faculty members work side by side with their students in these projects and are willing to model and openly discuss their own personal journeys toward cultural competence. Discuss the following questions:

1. What additional steps could be taken by the leaders of this degree program to enhance opportunities for students to develop cultural competence?

2. How can the development of cultural competence among students be measured? What measurement outcomes could serve as evidence that a student has improved in the area of cultural competence?

KEY TERMS

CLAS standards	Heritage consistency
Corporate culture	International summer study abroad
Cultural competence	Organizational culture
Experiential learning	Service learning

REFERENCES

Airhihenbuwa, C. O. (1995). *Health and culture: Beyond the western paradigm.* Thousand Oaks, CA: Sage.

American Institutes for Research. (2005). *Executive summary: A patient-centered guide to implementing language access services in healthcare organizations* (Final draft). Washington, DC: U.S. Department of Health and Human Services, Office of Minority Health.

Astin, A. W., & Sax, I. J. (1998). How undergraduates are affected by service participation. *Journal of College Student Development, 39*(3), 251–263.

Beatty, C. F., & Doyle, E. I. (2000). Multicultural curriculum evaluation of a professional preparation program. *American Journal of Health Studies, 16*(3), 124–132.

Berson, J. S., & Youkin, W. F. (1998). Doing well by doing good: A study of the effects of a service learning experience on student success. Paper presented at the American Society of Higher Education conference, Miami, FL.

Campinha-Bacote, J. (1994). *The process of cultural competence in the delivery of healthcare services: A culturally competent model of care* (2nd ed.). Cincinnati, OH: Transcultural C.A.R.E. Associates.

Champagne, N. (2006). Service learning: Its origin, evolution, and connection to health education. *American Journal of Health Education, 37*(2), 97–102.

Cohen, J., & Kinsey, D. F. (1994). Doing good and scholarship: A service learning study. *Journal of Education, 48*(4), 4–14.

COSMOS Corporation. (2003). *Developing a self-assessment tool for culturally and linguistically appropriate services in local public health agencies* (Final report). Washington, DC: U.S. Department of Health and Human Services, Office of Minority Health.

Cross, T. L., Bazron, B. J., Dennis, K. W., & Isaacs, M. R. (1989). *Toward a culturally competent system of care: A monograph on effective services for minority children who are severely emotionally disturbed.* Washington, DC: Georgetown University Child Development Center, Child and Adolescent Service System Program.

DiClemente, R. J., Crosby, R. A., & Kegler, M. C. (Eds.). (2002). *Emerging theories in health promotion and practice and research: Strategies for improving public health.* San Francisco: Jossey-Bass.

Doyle, E. I., & Faucher, M. A. (2002). Pharmaceutical therapy in midwifery practice: A culturally competent approach. *The Journal of Midwifery and Women's Health, 47*(3), 122–129.

Doyle, E. I., Liu, Y., & Ancona, L. (1996). Cultural competence development in university health education courses. *Journal of Health Education, 27*(4), 206–213.

Doyle, E. I., & Ward, S. E. (2001). *The process of community health education and promotion.* Long Grove, IL: Waveland Press.

Eyler, J., & Giles, D. E. (1999). *Where's the learning in service learning?* San Francisco: Jossey-Bass.

Frankish, C. J., Lovato, W. Y., & Shannon, W. J. (1999). Models, theories, and principles of health promotion with multicultural populations. In R. M. Huff & M. V. Kline (Eds.), *Promoting health in multicultural populations: A handbook for practitioners* (pp. 41–72). Thousand Oaks, CA: Sage.

Geiger, B. F., & Werner, K. (2004). Service-learning projects to enhance preparation of professional health educators. *American Journal of Health Studies, 19*(4), 233–240.

Glanz, K., Rimer, B. K., & Lewis, F. M. (Eds.). (2002). *Health behavior and health education: Theory, research, and practice* (3rd ed.). San Francisco: Jossey-Bass.

Greenberg, J. S. (2003). A community-campus partnership for health: The Seat Pleasant-University of Maryland Partnership. *Health Promotion Practice, 4*(4), 393–401.

Hofstede, G. (2001). *Culture's consequences: Comparing values, behaviors, institutions and organizations across nations* (2nd ed.). Thousand Oaks, CA: Sage.

Joint Committee on Health Education and Promotion Terminology. (2002). Report of the 2000 Joint Committee on Health Education and Promotion Terminology. *Journal of School Health, 72*(1), 3–7.

Luquis, R. R., & Pérez, M. A. (2003). Achieving cultural competence: The challenges for health educators. *Journal of Health Education, 34*(3), 131–138.

Luquis, R. R., & Pérez, M. A. (2005). Health educators and cultural competence: Implications for the profession. *American Journal of Health Studies, 20*(3), 156–163.

Luquis, R. R., & Pérez, M. A. (2006). Cultural competency among school health educators. *Journal of Cultural Diversity, 13*(4), 217–222.

Luquis, R. R., Pérez, M. A., & Young, K. (2006). Cultural competence development in health education professional preparation programs. *American Journal of Health Education, 37*(4), 233–241.

Maxwell, J. C. (2001). *Developing the leader within you workbook.* Nashville, TN: Thomas Nelson.

Melchior, A. (1997). *National evaluation of Learn and Serve America school and community-based programs* (Interim report). Washington, DC: Corporation for National Service.

Minkler, M., & Wallerstein, N. (2003). *Community-based participatory research.* San Francisco: Jossey-Bass.

Morey, A. I., & Kitano, M. K. (Eds.). (1997). *Multicultural course transformation in higher education: A broader truth.* Boston: Allyn & Bacon.

National Center for Cultural Competence. (n.d.). *Foundations of cultural and linguistic competence: Conceptual frameworks/models, guiding values and principles.* Retrieved February 9, 2007, from http://www11.george town.edu/research/gucchd/nccc/foundations/frameworks.html#ccdefinition.

National Commission for Health Education Credentialing, Society for Public Health Education, & American Association for Health Education. (2006). *A competency-based framework for health educators—2006.* Whitehall, PA: Author.

National Task Force on the Preparation and Practice of Health Educators. (1985). *A framework for the development of competency-based curricula for entry-level health educators.* New York: National Commission for Health Education Credentialing.

Office of Minority Health. (2001). *National standards for culturally and linguistically appropriate services in health care.* Washington, DC: U.S. Department of Health and Human Services.

Office of Minority Health. (2004). *Report: Setting the agenda for research on cultural competence in health care.* Washington, DC: U.S. Department of Health and Human Services.

Redican, K., Stewart, S. H., Johnson, L. E., & Frazee, A. M. (1994). Professional preparation in cultural awareness and sensitivity in health education: A national survey. *Journal of Health Education, 25*, 215–217.

Rojas-Guyler, L., Cottrell, R., & Wagner, D. (2006). The second national survey of U.S. internship standards in health education professional preparation: 15 years later. *American Journal of Health Education, 37*(4), 226–232.

Salimbene, S. (2001). *CLAS A-Z: A practical guide for implementing the national standards for culturally and linguistically appropriate services in health care.* Washington, DC: U.S. Department of Health and Human Services. Retrieved October 13, 2006, from http://www.omhrc.gov/assets/pdf/checked/CLAS_a2z.pdf.

Seelye, H. N. (1996). *Experiential activities for intercultural learning* (Vol. 1).Yarmouth, ME: Intercultural Press.

Spector, R. E. (2004). *Cultural diversity in health and illness* (6th ed.). Upper Saddle River, NJ: Pearson Prentice Hall.

CHAPTER

10

STRATEGIES, PRACTICES, AND MODELS FOR DELIVERING CULTURALLY COMPETENT HEALTH EDUCATION PROGRAMS

MIGUEL A. PÉREZ

LEARNING OBJECTIVES

After completing this chapter, you will be able to

- Discuss and explain the definition of health education.
- Discuss and explain the role of culture in health choices.
- Define cultural competence and its application to health education.
- Discuss and apply recommendations for culturally appropriate programs.

INTRODUCTION

In one of the earliest definitions of what our field does, the Joint Committee on Health Problems in Education (1948) stated that the focus of *health education* is to provide learning experiences designed to change knowledge, attitudes, and behaviors. In 1974, the Joint Committee on Health Education Terminology identified *health education* as a *process* designed to facilitate learning and lead to behavior change. In 1992, Greenberg and Gold defined health education as a process designed to enable individuals to attain their optimal health status. One of the most recent definitions of health education has been provided by the 2000 Joint Committee on Health Education and Promotion Terminology: "Any combination of planned learning experiences based on sound theories that provide individuals, groups, and communities the opportunity to acquire information and the skills needed to make quality health decisions" (p. 6).

One of the fundamental tenets of health education is the requirement to provide current, scientifically sound, and appropriate health information in order for individuals, groups, or communities to acquire the knowledge and skills necessary to attain the highest health status they can achieve based on their biology, behaviors, and access to the health care system. This emphasis is denoted in the American Association of Health Educators' philosophy of health education, which requires health education practitioners to provide accurate and timely health-related information to their target audiences so that members of these audiences can make informed decisions that may have an impact on their health status. This philosophy is embodied in the roles and responsibilities of health educators and codified in a position statement published by the American Association of Health Educators (AAHE) (2005).

HEALTH INDICATORS

A look at the leading health indicators reveals that approximately half of the mortality indicators are related to behavioral patterns, making them powerful, yet modifiable, health determinants (Krieger, 2001; Lantz et al., 2001). A close examination of the health status of U.S. populations also reveals many health disparities related to factors such as race and ethnicity (Barnett & Halverson, 2001; Fuchs, 1974; McLaughlin & Stokes, 2002), gender (King, LeBlanc, Sanguins, & Mather, 2006), income (Kunst & Mackenbach, 1994; Polednak, 1993, 1996), educational status (Elo & Preston, 1996), social class (Diez-Roux, 2001; Kaplan & Keil, 1993), and age (Flood, & Scharer, 2006), among others. Demographic changes in the U.S. population (see Chapter One) require us to pay closer attention to the needs of an increasingly diverse population in this country.

Focus on Diversity

U.S. Census Bureau data indicate that significant shifts are occurring in the demographic characteristics of the U.S. population. According to these data the largest population increases during the last ten to twenty years have occurred among members of historically underrepresented groups, such as Hispanics (or Latinos), Asians, and

Pacific Islanders, whereas non-Hispanic whites have experienced declines as an overall percentage of the U.S. population (U.S. Census Bureau, 2004, table A-1).

Concurrent with these changes in the racial and ethnic composition of the population are changes in population age. Data from the Administration on Aging (2002) show that some thirty-three million Americans, or approximately 12 percent of the total U.S. population, are over the age of 65. This number represents a tenfold increase in this age group since the 1900s, and it makes individuals aged 65 and above one of the fastest growing population segments in the country. Population estimates also predict that the number of people aged 65 and over will double in the next three decades. In 2000, a majority of the individuals aged 65 and over (84 percent) were non-Hispanic whites, and although their majority status is expected to continue until 2050, the exact proportion of whites will also decrease in this age group.

The exact number of people who are gay, lesbian, bisexual, or transgender (transsexual) (GLBT) in the United States is difficult to ascertain, with several studies differing in their estimates. Extrapolating from data in the 2000 Census, which found some six hundred thousand households with same-gender couples in the United States, Rubenstein, Bradley Sears, and Sockloskie (2003) estimate that there are 1.2 million people who are gay and lesbian in the United States. This richly diverse group, which defies stereotypes, represents a significant proportion of the U.S. population in need of culturally appropriate health education messages. To date little research has been conducted to address the specific health education needs of this population group as well as to identify barriers they experience in accessing health care services (Clark, Landers, Linde, & Sperber, 2001; Gee, 2006; Gruskin, 1999).

Market Segmentation

As described at the beginning of this chapter, the field of health education is focused on assisting individuals to ascertain their optimal health status. Health disparities based on, among other things, race and ethnicity and the changing U.S. demographic profile provide powerful justifications for reaching different population groups with tailored health education programs. This approach requires a market segmentation that is not easily adopted by purists in the field but that is supported by the professional literature. Situational and environmental factors that may influence health educators' ability to implement a successful health education program include, but are not limited to, the target population's socioeconomic status, country of origin, English language proficiency, and acculturation.

Research has shown that in order for health education programs to be effective they must be tailored to the needs of the target population. Some authors (Acosta-Deprez & Monroe, 1996; Airhihenbuwa, 1995a; Luquis & Pérez, 2003; Pinzon & Pérez, 1997) have provided solid arguments for developing health education programs targeting members of diverse racial and ethnic groups; however, we would be derelict in our educational mission if we failed to take into account the health literacy of the members of the target population (Porr, Drummond, & Richter, 2006), their language preference

(Marín & Marín, 1991), their gender (Wyn & Solis, 2001), and their religion (Brooks, 2004; Holt & McClure, 2006). Understanding the specific needs of individuals, groups, or communities based on their demographic characteristics is key in assisting these individuals and groups to attain a positive health outcome and in avoiding coercing them to engage in activities that may run contrary to their beliefs and values.

Despite overwhelming evidence that behavior modification cannot occur without taking into account people's environment and social support networks, health educators tend to focus almost exclusively on individuals and their needs and behaviors. This approach is based on the cultural tenet that we are responsible for our own well-being but unfortunately fails to take into account differences by gender, age, and ethnic group. In this regard our approach as health educators resembles that of health care professionals who tend to focus on the pathophysiology of illness and give little regard to the individual as a whole. This shortsighted approach fails to take into account the impact of culture on the health status of individuals and may in fact diminish the impact of our scientifically sound programs (Dimou, 1995; Hall, 1990; Marmot, Siegrist, Theorell, & Feeney, 1999).

The professional literature suggests that a culturally appropriate approach to health education requires an emphasis not only on individual behavior but also on the family and the environment of the person (Airhihenbuwa, 1995a, 1995b; Anand, 2003; Casken, 1999), as each of these factors contributes to the explanatory model of health and disease as experienced by individuals and has an impact on perceptions, knowledge, attitudes, and health-related behaviors (Kleinman, 1980) and also affects the symbolism attached to an illness behavior. Recent professional literature also calls for health educators to have a good understanding of their target individuals' culture if they are to effectively work in diverse settings. For example, the following list from AAHE (1994) summarizes some differences in cultural values found among non-Western and Western cultural groups in the United States:

Cultural Values

Non-Western	Western
Fate	Personal control
Tradition	Change
Human interaction dominates	Schedules dominate
Group welfare	Individualism and privacy
Cooperation	Competition
Formality	Informality
Indirectness	Directness
Modesty	Self-confidence
Extended family	Nuclear family

In some instances culture may be perceived as an adverse partner in health education efforts. Cultural practices involving the use of alternative medicine, a different time orientation, or a family rather than an individual orientation present challenges that many health educators are ill prepared to address. Moreover, culture cannot be discounted, no matter how assimilated a target group may seem, because the health educator who fails to identify the cultural factors that shape an individual's health status may have little success in achieving the desired outcome. Furthermore, culture may in fact have a positive impact on the health status of individuals and this needs to be identified as well.

Marín and Marín (1991) address the positive impact of some cultural practices among Hispanics in the United States. Also, although the tradition of *machismo* among Hispanic men is often viewed in a negative light, it can have a positive impact on the health status of families (Ingoldsby, 1991). Similarly, cultural factors such as a diet rich in omega-3 fatty oils from fish have been identified as a contributing factor to lower rates of cardiovascular disease among the Japanese (Hino et al., 2004). And the practice among the French of ingesting wine on a daily basis has also been identified as a factor in lower rates of cardiovascular disease among that population group.

However, despite the fact that culture undoubtedly plays a positive role at times in enhancing the health status of individuals, it can also have a negative impact. Long-held beliefs and practices may prevent individuals from obtaining needed health care services or modifying behaviors that may be negatively affecting their health. Religious beliefs may also prevent people from adopting health behaviors when the behaviors conflict with those religious beliefs (Brooks, 2004). Similarly, past negative experiences with health education or the health care system may prevent people from following advice that might assist them in obtaining their optimal health status.

CULTURAL DIVERSITY AND HEALTH EDUCATION

The challenges and opportunities faced in attempts to reach diverse populations continue to be a struggle for the field of health education as a whole. For instance, none of the seminal documents in the field of health education, including the framework produced in 1985 by the Role Delineation Project (Breckon, Harvey, & Lancaster, 1998; National Commission for Health Education Credentialing, 1985; Clearly, 1997); the competencies for health education, *Standards for the Preparation of Graduate-Level Health Educators* (Society for Public Health Education, 1997); and *A Competency-Based Framework for Health Educators–2006* (National Commission for Health Education Credentialing, Society for Public Health Education, & American Association for Health Education, 2006) specifically address cultural competence.

The leading professional organizations in the field of health education have made efforts to address multicultural issues among their members. The American Association for Health Education (AAHE) has published documents concerning cultural diversity, including its 1994 publication *Cultural Awareness and Sensitivity: Guidelines for Health Educators.* In that document AAHE called for health educators to become culturally aware and sensitive in their dealings with members of diverse groups. Despite the wide dissemination of this document, there is no published evidence that the guidelines were widely adopted by health education preparation programs or by health educators in the field. Most recently, AAHE has released a position statement on cultural competency in health education (AAHE, 2006), which states that "health educators must strive to achieve cultural competency by understanding the meaning of culture, its complexity within each group, and its effect on health decisions and practices" (p. 1).

The Society for Public Health Education (SOPHE) has identified the elimination of health disparities as one of its top three advocacy priorities for 2006. As part of these efforts, two SOPHE journals, *Health Education & Behavior* and *Health Promotion Practice,* published materials based on presentations at an invitational summit titled *Health Disparities and Social Inequities: Framing a Transdisciplinary Research Agenda in Health Education.* Articles from these journals are cited throughout this book. And presentations to the SOPHE Web seminar titled "On the Road from Research to Practice: Eliminating Racial and Ethnic Health Disparities," have been made available on the SOPHE Web site (http://www.sophe.org). Results from these seminars have yielded ten consensus research questions to be addressed in the next decade (see Exhibit 10.1).

EXHIBIT 10.1. **Consensus Questions from SOPHE Web Seminars.**

1. How do economics and the built environment such as the availability of housing and sidewalks affect health, and how can we encourage the urban design and planning of communities to eliminate health disparities?

2. How does power operate in different social contexts to create and maintain disparities?

3. What factors exist in certain populations that protect them from major health issues; for example, what can we learn from African American female teens who experience less drug abuse than other teens. How can health educators and society promote such protective factors?

4. What is the impact of health literacy on health status, and how can we improve message tailoring to reach different groups?

5. How can we culturally tailor interventions to influence access to health services?

6. How do we engage and partner with policy makers in diffusing relevant research?

7. What information are consumers getting on health, and how does this information differ by race, ethnicity, socioeconomic, and cultural group?

8. Does engagement in community-based participatory research alter engagement in community structures, processes, and other attributes?

9. How can we develop more evaluation instruments that assess dynamic, changing, and social conditions such as social event history analysis?

10. How can we improve the measurement of both intended and unintended effects and outcomes in evaluation studies?

Source: Gambescia et al., 2006.

CULTURAL DIVERSITY AND HEALTH EDUCATION PROFESSIONAL PROGRAMS

The topic of cultural diversity and health education in professional programs is covered in greater detail in Chapter Nine. This chapter provides a brief summary of this information.

Bruess, Hendricks, Poehler, and Redford (1987) describe the integration of the Role Delineation Project framework into the undergraduate health education program at the University of Alabama and the resulting modifications to the curricula. Unfortunately, no similar curricular modifications seem to have been made following the release of the 1994 AAHE guidelines.

Beatty and Doyle (2000) found that professional health education program curricula did not adequately prepare health educators to work with diverse populations. In a study six years later, Luquis, Pérez, and Young (2006) found that despite a documented need for cultural training in professional health education preparation programs, most programs do not offer courses entirely devoted to cultural competence. This lack of focus on cultural competence has also been found in public health departments, denoting the need for further work in integrating cultural competence into health education coursework (Pérez, Gonzalez, & Pinzon-Pérez, 2006).

Although the health education field has been slow in integrating cultural diversity training into its professional preparation programs, and in some cases into the development and evaluation of programs, other professional areas have made great strides in this area. The federal government has been an unquestioned leader in this area. For example, the 1985 *Report of the Secretary's Task Force on Black and Minority Health* (U.S. Department of Health and Human Services, 1985) represents one of the earliest efforts to document health disparities. Although this document has been criticized for not presenting a comprehensive picture of minority health status in the United States, it represents a seminal effort to increase awareness about the health issues facing U.S. minorities.

On January 25, 2000, the U.S. Department of Health and Human Services released *Healthy People 2010,* a document designed to provide a road map for improving the health status of all Americans. The Healthy People 2010 initiative has two primary goals: increasing the quality of and extending the number of years of healthy life for individuals and eliminating health disparities among Americans. To measure the achievement of those goals, the Healthy People 2010 initiative proposed to use a series of leading health indicators that include physical activity, overweight and obesity, tobacco use, substance abuse, responsible sexual behavior, mental health, injury and violence, environmental quality, immunization, and access to health care. The integration of diversity is evident through the entire document.

CLAS STANDARDS

In 2001, the Office of Minority Health released the National Standards on Culturally and Linguistically Appropriate Services (CLAS). The fourteen standards, organized by themes, address culturally competent care (Standards 1 to 3), language access services

(Standards 4 to 7), and organizational supports for cultural competence (Standards 8 to 14). The standards can also be divided into mandates (Standards 4, 5, 6, and 7) for all recipients of federal funds, guidelines (Standards 1, 2, 3, 8, 9, 10, 11, 12, and 13) recommended for adoption by federal, state, and national accrediting agencies, and recommendations (Standard 14). All these efforts have the ultimate goal of creating cultural competence, which can translate into better services for the diverse groups in this country. Exhibit 10.2 lists all the CLAS standards.

EXHIBIT 10.2. CLAS Standards.

STANDARD 1

Health care organizations should ensure that patients/consumers receive from all staff members effective, understandable, and respectful care that is provided in a manner compatible with their cultural health beliefs and practices and preferred language.

STANDARD 2

Health care organizations should implement strategies to recruit, retain, and promote at all levels of the organization a diverse staff and leadership that are representative of the demographic characteristics of the service area.

STANDARD 3

Health care organizations should ensure that staff at all levels and across all disciplines receive ongoing education and training in culturally and linguistically appropriate service delivery.

STANDARD 4

Health care organizations must offer and provide language assistance services, including bilingual staff and interpreter services, at no cost to each patient/consumer with limited English proficiency at all points of contact, in a timely manner during all hours of operation.

STANDARD 5

Health care organizations must provide to patients/consumers in their preferred language both verbal offers and written notices informing them of their right to receive language assistance services.

STANDARD 6

Health care organizations must assure the competence of language assistance provided to limited English proficient patients/consumers by interpreters and bilingual staff. Family and friends should not be used to provide interpretation services (except on request by the patient/consumer).

STANDARD 7

Health care organizations must make available easily understood patient-related materials and post signage in the languages of the commonly encountered groups and/or groups represented in the service area.

STANDARD 8

Health care organizations should develop, implement, and promote a written strategic plan that outlines clear goals, policies, operational plans, and management accountability/oversight mechanisms to provide culturally and linguistically appropriate services.

STANDARD 9

Health care organizations should conduct initial and ongoing organizational self-assessments of CLAS-related activities and are encouraged to integrate cultural and linguistic competence-related measures into their internal audits, performance improvement programs, patient satisfaction assessments, and outcomes-based evaluations.

STANDARD 10

Health care organizations should ensure that data on the individual patient's/consumer's race, ethnicity, and spoken and written language are collected in health records, integrated into the organization's management information systems, and periodically updated.

STANDARD 11

Health care organizations should maintain a current demographic, cultural, and epidemiological profile of the community as well as a needs assessment to accurately plan for and implement services that respond to the cultural and linguistic characteristics of the service area.

STANDARD 12

Health care organizations should develop participatory, collaborative partnerships with communities and utilize a variety of formal and informal mechanisms to facilitate community and patient/consumer involvement in designing and implementing CLAS-related activities.

STANDARD 13

Health care organizations should ensure that conflict and grievance resolution processes are culturally and linguistically sensitive and capable of identifying, preventing, and resolving cross-cultural conflicts or complaints by patients/consumers.

STANDARD 14

Health care organizations are encouraged to regularly make available to the public information about their progress and successful innovations in implementing the CLAS standards and to provide public notice in their communities about the availability of this information.

Source: Office of Minority Health, 2001.

FOUR AREAS OF CULTURAL COMPETENCE

Cultural competence has been defined as "the ability of an individual to understand and respect values, attitudes, beliefs, and mores that differ across cultures, and to consider and respond appropriately to these differences in planning, implementing, and evaluating health education and promotion programs and interventions" (Joint Committee on Health Education and Promotion Terminology, 2000, p. 7). Some authors in the field group cultural competence with *cultural proficiency,* which is the highest capacity for interacting with members of diverse groups and delivering quality health education programs. Cultural competence or proficiency does not require the health educator to adopt others' racial or ethnic cultural practices nor does it require him or her to become an expert in every possible cultural group; it does require that the health educator continually develop his or her abilities in four areas—awareness, knowledge, experience, and skills—and be willing to make a commitment to a lifelong process of change.

RECOMMENDATIONS FOR WORKING WITH DIVERSE GROUPS

It should be obvious, given the discussion up to this point, that cultural competence is not an end by itself, but rather a lifelong process requiring a commitment to ongoing examination of one's cultural blinders, one's own biases, and one's desire to interact with others who are not like oneself. Cultural competence needs to constantly evolve in order to have meaning and a real-life application for health educators. Cultural competence also requires that we make a commitment to learn about our own group and avoid making assumptions about each other.

The following general recommendations, based on the professional literature and the author's personal experience, are designed to give health educators practical suggestions for dealing with different cultural groups.

- *Differentiate among culture, race, and ethnicity.* As we have seen throughout this text, the terms *culture, race,* and *ethnicity,* although used as synonyms for convenience, are not. Erroneous classifications may lead us to make erroneous assumptions about people; for instance, we might think a person to be of a given race given her skin color, but her cultural identity or ethnicity may not correspond with that color.

- *Avoid stereotypes.* Many publications, including this book, highlight some cultural health values documented in the professional literature. It is, however, important to realize that not every member of a particular group will ascribe to those generally accepted standards. Keep in mind, for example, that not everyone over the age of 65 uses a walker, and many people over 65 enjoy a satisfying social life that includes dancing and sexual activity.

- *Ascertain acculturation levels. Acculturation* has been defined as the degree to which an immigrant adopts the culture and behaviors of the host country. Income, education, and language preference are all proxies for acculturation but do not represent the complete picture. A highly educated, English proficient, first-generation immigrant may still practice alternative medicine while proficiently navigating the U.S. health care system.

■ *Be cognizant of language preference.* Generally speaking, first-generation immigrants will require translation of written materials and spoken words into their native language; less obvious is the need to provide materials in languages other than English to a number of those who are the second and subsequent generations in the United States. Meeting individuals' language preference is, however, a key factor in delivering culturally appropriate health education programs because it allows people to communicate their needs and wants in an appropriate format. Being cognizant of language preference also refers to selecting and using the terminology employed by the target population rather than the technical language health educators are used to. Finally, it also refers to having qualified personnel, regardless of cultural or ethnic background, who are proficient in the language needed. Do not assume that all Nisei speak Japanese.

■ *Be cognizant of what you do not know.* A personal experience is the most telling illustration of the point here. As a doctoral student the author of this chapter worked on the development of a culturally appropriate HIV/AIDS curriculum for migrant farmworkers. Part of the process required interviews with teachers, other school personnel, and health care professionals. The eager graduate student followed interview protocols and attempted to reach key informants in the community. Approximately halfway through the process, the graduate student was pulled from the field by his adviser, who informed him that he was obtaining only socially acceptable responses. The principle investigator took over the interviews and those interviews yielded information, some of it racist, that could not have been obtained by the graduate student who was a member of the target ethnic group. This story serves to illustrate that even in today's society people may hide their true feelings and instead provide socially acceptable responses.

■ *Be clear about your objectives.* One of the easiest ways to lose an educational opportunity is to be insufficiently organized. Your goals and objectives need to be clear, well articulated, and developed in conjunction with the target population—this is part of the empowerment process (Anspaugh, Dignan, & Anspaugh, 2000).

■ *Remember family dynamics.* Health educators tend to focus on individuals rather than on the social networks individuals share. This process, although expedient, goes against the basic cultural values of some groups health educators may be called on to work with. Family members are a powerful and strong source of support to many cultural and ethnic groups in the United States. This may be a residual of having once lived in communities less affluent than their current home, communities where, as Casken (1999) points out, "The ties to the family ensure that no one goes hungry or homeless" (p. 408). Family ties continue to be a primary source of support to minority members especially those living in medically underserved areas in the United States (Baffour, Jones, & Contreras, 2006).

■ *Create strong coalitions.* Successful programs incorporate a group's strengths and explore ways to make weaknesses into opportunities. This can be accomplished only when members of the target group are deeply involved in the planning and implementation process. The creation of strong coalitions not only increases the chances for a successful program but also almost guarantees that the program will become institutionalized.

■ *Develop trust.* Target population members may show deference and respect given a health educator's title and institutional affiliation, but that does not mean they trust the health educator. This issue may be further compounded by feelings of betrayal or apathy, or concerns about racism in the health education or the health care system. The health educator needs to become familiar with the target population, participate in community events, and be accepted into the everyday life of the community before trust can be achieved. The health educator needs to become a familiar face in the community and to participate in activities other than his or her own programs.

■ *Select communication methods carefully.* Many entry-level health educators feel comfortable with developing written material and distributing it among the target population, with little if any regard for people's language preference and literacy level. Although written materials are well accepted in the majority culture, not everyone can read or likes to get printed materials, as this approach may be perceived to be too clinical. This issue is further compounded when the materials are poorly developed and show, among other problems, spelling errors.

■ *Incorporate cultural assessments.* One of the first things that we need to do as health educators is to include a cultural assessment in all our program needs assessments.

■ *Incorporate cultural values, beliefs, and practices into programs.* Health education interventions that have no relevance to the target community will not succeed. Along with information gathered from Western-style medicine, we need to include information that is relevant to the community. Whenever possible provide a contrast between the Western and non-Western approaches to health and illness, beliefs, and practices (Kim, McLeod, & Shantzis, 1992). Be careful not to show reverence for one and disdain for the other.

■ *Involve members of the target group in the planning and decision-making process.* These participants may include healers, informal leaders, and community organizers.

■ *Accommodate different learning styles.* As health educators we cannot afford to forget that not everyone learns in the same manner. Some people like to read, others to explore on their own, and others to be shown. Be sure to incorporate activities that address the different learning styles that are likely to be found in your target group.

■ *Make a commitment to multiculturalism.* No one can ask you to change your beliefs any more than you can ask someone else to change his or hers. In working with diverse groups, however, it is important to have a good handle on one's own culture, stereotypes, and in some cases prejudices. Only when we can be honest with ourselves can we reach members of other ethnic groups or in some cases members of our own ethnic group who do not fit our personal socioeconomic profile (Airhihenbuwa, 1995a).

■ *Work within existing social networks.* Needs assessment data should yield information about existing groups and support in the community. Involve as many of them as possible, making it easier to work *with* the community, not *on* the community.

■ *Bring information back to the target audience.* One of the greatest, and accurate, criticisms of university-based health educators is that they use people and then retreat to their ivory tower. Although it is important to share the knowledge gained through our interventions with the scientific community, it is just as important to share the findings with the target community. These findings must be presented in a way that is useful to the community and that furthers the empowerment process.

■ *Understand traditional health beliefs.* Each of us, regardless of cultural heritage, holds numerous health beliefs. In North America we tend to recommend that people who have flu-type symptoms eat chicken soup and get plenty of rest. Members of the Hmong culture perceive that epilepsy is caused by ancestral spirits entering the body, and some Hispanic groups strongly adhere to the theory of "hot" and "cold" foods to understand and treat certain illnesses. Understanding and respecting those beliefs will make the practice of health education in a multicultural setting much easier.

■ *Respect religious beliefs.* Several researchers (Pinzon & Pérez, 1997) describe the health beliefs of Latin Americans, including concepts such as *susto*. The Kahuna Lapa'au in Hawaiian traditions helps people heal with the aid of a helping spirit known as the Akau (Mokuau & Tauili'ili, 1992). Similarly, Confucian ideology, Buddhism, and Taoism influence some Asian cultures (Hoylord, 2002). Although most of us in the United States value a separation of church and state, several groups do not make that distinction. We must be careful not to offend or contradict the religious beliefs held by the target population.

■ *Make it easy for the target audience to participate.* This applies the principle of the "golden rule," which requires health educators to make their programs as user friendly as possible. Bring the program to the residences of the target audience, employ bilingual experts, hold the program after hours. Each of these little steps shows respect and will increase your ability to reach the target audience.

■ *Seek to empower the target population.* The idea of empowerment is not new (Freire, 1992; Laverack, 2006) and has in fact been criticized in some health education fields. However, if health educators are to ensure a lasting impact from short-term interventions, they must not only involve the target populations through culturally competent needs assessments (Arizona Department of Health Services, 1995) but also provide these populations with the tools necessary to enact change in their environments.

CONCLUSION

The field of health education is predicated on the delivery of accurate and timely health information so that individuals may make informed decisions to enhance their health status. The diversification of the U.S. population, however, requires health educators to modify their approaches, philosophies, and techniques to reach a variety of diverse population groups. This transformation requires changing long-held practices and beliefs to take into account the needs of different groups; in essence, it requires the development of cultural competence. It should be noted, however, that acquiring cultural competence is a lifelong process and not a destination in and of itself. Cultural competence requires respect for others' beliefs, modification of practices, and the development of new language skills in order to reach others.

POINTS TO REMEMBER

- The fourteen CLAS standards
- The continuing need to incorporate the knowledge and skills related to cultural competence into health education
- The recommendations for working with diverse groups

CASE STUDY

Imagine the following interaction between a health educator and a monolingual person with no education. The female health educator, who is fluent in the language spoken by the client, attempts to convey the necessity of performing a monthly breast self-examination (BSE) as a tool in the early detection of breast cancer. The client, in awe at the health educator for bringing up such a sensitive subject, cannot suppress a look of confusion when the health educator asks her if she performs breast self-exams. "Me, touch my own breasts?" asks the client, giving a response she believes the health educator wants to hear. The astute health educator, realizing that the client may not realize the importance of a BSE, proceeds to show her, using an anatomically correct model, the correct procedure for a BSE. Pretty soon the client remembers she has another commitment and must leave now, but not before promising to get back to the health educator on the progress of her newly developed skill. To analyze this situation, please discuss the following questions:

1. Do you think this is an example of a good health education intervention?

2. What additional steps might be needed to make this an effective health education effort?

3. What did the health educator do correctly?

4. What could she have done differently?

5. On what do you base your answer to question 4?

Construct your own scenario. How would you change the interaction described here in light of your own experience and the concepts presented in this chapter?

KEY TERMS

CLAS standards
Cultural competence
Diversity

Health education
Health indicators

REFERENCES

Acosta-Deprez, V., & Monroe, D. (1996). Preservice teachers' awareness and attitudes towards multicultural health education. *Wellness Perspectives: Theory, Research and Practice*, *12*(4), 212–220.

Administration on Aging. (2002). *A profile of older Americans: 2002*. Retrieved June 24, 2005, from http://www.aoa.gov/prof/statistics/profiles2002.asp.

Airhihenbuwa, C. O. (1995a). *Health and culture: Beyond the western paradigm*. Thousand Oaks, CA: Sage.

Airhihenbuwa, C. O. (1995b). Culture, health education, and critical consciousness. *Journal of Health Education*, *26*(5), 317–319.

American Association for Health Education. (1994). *Cultural awareness and sensitivity: Guidelines for health educators*. Reston, VA: Author.

American Association for Health Education. (2005). *Philosophy of health education*. Retrieved September 15, 2006, from http://www.aahperd.org/aahe/template.cfm?template=publications-position.html.

American Association for Health Education. (2006). *Cultural competency in health education*. Retrieved September 15, 2006, from http://www.aahperd.org/aahe/template.cfm?template=publications-position.html.

Anand, R. (2003). *Cultural competency in healthcare: A guide for trainers* (3rd ed.). Washington, DC: National Multicultural Institute.

Anspaugh, D., Dignan, M., & Anspaugh, S. (2000). *Developing health promotion programs*. Long Grove, IL: Waveland Press.

Arizona Department of Health Services. (1995). *Cultural competence needs assessment*. Phoenix: Arizona Department of Health Services, Center for Minority Health.

Baffour, T. D., Jones, M. A., & Contreras, L. K. (2006). Family health advocacy: An empowerment model for pregnant and parenting African American women in rural communities. *Family & Community Health*, *29*(3), 221–228.

Barnett, E., & Halverson, J. (2001). Local increases in coronary heart disease mortality among blacks and whites in the Unites States, 1985–1995. *American Journal of Public Health*, *91*(9), 12–20.

Beatty, C. F., & Doyle, E. I. (2000). Multicultural curriculum evaluation of a professional preparation program. *American Journal of Health Studies*, *16*(3), 124–132.

Breckon, D. J., Harvey, J., & Lancaster, R. B. (1998). *Community health education: Settings, roles, and skills for the 21st century* (4th ed.). Boston: Jones & Bartlett.

Brooks, N. (2004). Overview of religions. *Clinical Cornerstone, 6*(1), 7–16.

Bruess, C. E., Hendricks, C. M., Poehler, D. L., & Redford, J. (1987). Application of the Role Delineation Project "framework" to a professional preparation program. *Journal of School Health, 57*(5), 183–185.

Casken, J. (1999). *Pacific Islander health and disease: An overview.* In R. M. Huff & M. V. Kline (Eds.), *Promoting health in multicultural populations: A handbook for practitioners* (pp. 397–417). Thousand Oaks, CA: Sage.

Clark, M. E., Landers, S., Linde, R., & Sperber, J. (2001). The GLBT health access project: A state-funded effort to improve access to care. *American Journal of Public Health, 91*(6), 895–896.

Clearly, H. P. (1997). *The credentialing of health educators: An historical account, 1970–1990.* Allentown, PA: National Commission for Health Education Credentialing.

Diez-Roux, A. V. (2001). Investigating neighborhood and area effects on health. *American Journal of Public Health, 91,* 1783–1789.

Dimou, N. (1995). Illness and culture: Learning differences. *Patient Education and Counseling, 26,* 153–157.

Elo, I., & Preston, S. (1996). Educational differentials in mortality: United States 1979–85. *Social Science and Medicine, 42*(1), 47–57.

Flood, M., & Scharer, K. (2006). Creativity enhancement: Possibilities for successful aging. *Issues in Mental Health Nursing, 27,* 939–959.

Freire, P. (1992). *Pedagogy of the oppressed.* New York: Continuum.

Fuchs, V. (1974). *Who shall live?* New York: Basic Books.

Gambescia, S. F., Woodhouse, L. D., Auld, M. E., Green, B. L., Crouse, S., & Airhihenbuwa, C. O. (2006). Health disparities and social inequities: A road map for SOPHE action. *Health Education & Behavior, 33*(4), 532–537.

Gee, R. (2006). Primary care health issues among men who have sex with men. Journal of the American Academy of Nurse Practitioners, 18(4), 144–153.

Greenberg, J., & Gold, R. (1992). *The health education ethics book.* Dubuque, IA: Wm. C. Brown.

Gruskin, E. (1999). *Treating lesbians and bisexual women: Challenges and strategies for health professionals.* Thousand Oaks, CA: Sage.

Guiachello, A. (1995). *Cultural diversity and institutional inequality.* In D. L. Adams (Ed.), *Health issues for women of color: A cultural diversity perspective.* Thousand Oaks, CA: Sage.

Hall, S. (1990). *Cultural identity and diaspora.* In J. Rutherford (Ed.), *Identity: Community, culture, difference.* London: Lawrence & Wishart.

Hino, A., Adachi, H., Toyomasu, K., Yoshida, N., Enomoto, M., Hiratsuka, A., et al. (2004). Very long chain N-3 fatty acids intake and carotid atherosclerosis: An epidemiological study evaluated by ultrasonography. *Atherosclerosis, 176*(1), 145–149.

Holt, C. L., & McClure, S. M. (2006). Perceptions of the religion-health connection among African American church members. *Qualitative Health Research, 16*(2), 268–281.

Hoylord, E. (2002). Health-seeking behaviors and social change: The experience of the Hong Kong Chinese elderly. *Qualitative Health Research, 12*(6), 731–750.

Ingoldsby, B. B. (1991). The Latin American family: Familism vs. machismo. *Journal of Comparative Family Studies, 22*(1), 57–62.

Joint Committee on Health Education Terminology. (1974). New definitions: Report of the 1972–1973 Joint Committee on Health Education Terminology. *Journal of School Health, 44*(1), 33–37.

Joint Committee on Health Education and Promotion Terminology. (2000). Report of the 2000 Joint Committee on Health Education and Promotion Terminology. *Journal of School Health, 72*(1), 3–7.

Joint Committee on Health Problems in Education. (1948). *Health education.* Washington, DC: National Education Association.

Kaplan, G., & Keil, J. (1993). Socioeconomic factors and cardiovascular disease: A review of the literature. *Circulation, 88*(4), 1973–1998.

Kim, S., McLeod, J., & Shantzis, C. (1992). *Cultural competence for evaluators working with Asian American communities: Some practical considerations*. In M. A. Orlandi, R. Weston, & L. G. Epstein (Eds.), *Cultural competence for evaluators*. Rockville, MD: U.S. Department of Health and Human Services, Office for Substance Abuse and Prevention.

King, K. M., LeBlanc, P., Sanguins, J., & Mather C. (2006). Gender-based challenges faced by older Sikh women as immigrants: Recognizing and acting on the risk of coronary artery disease. *Canadian Journal of Nursing Research, 38*(1), 16–40.

Kleinman, A. (1980). *Patients and healers in the context of culture*. Berkeley: University of California Press.

Krieger, N. (2001). Theories for social epidemiology in the 21st century: An ecosocial perspective. *International Journal of Epidemiology, 30*, 668–667.

Kunst, A., & Mackenbach, J. (1994). International variation in the size of mortality differences associated with occupational status. *International Journal of Epidemiology, 23*(4), 742–750.

Lantz, P. M., Lynch, J. W., House, J. S., Lepkowski, J. M., Mero, R. P., & Musick, M. A. (2001). Socioeconomic disparities in health change in a longitudinal study of US adults: The role of health-risk behaviors. *Social Science & Medicine, 53*(1), 29–40.

Laverack, G. (2006). Improving health outcomes through community empowerment: A review of the literature. Journal of Health, Population, and Nutrition, 24(1), 113–120.

Luquis, R. R., & Pérez, M. A. (2003). Achieving cultural competence: The challenges for health educators. *Journal of Health Education, 34*(3), 131–138.

Luquis, R. R., Pérez, M. A., & Young, K. (2006). Cultural competence development in health education professional preparation programs. *American Journal of Health Education, 37*(4), 233–241.

Marín, G., & Marín, B. V. (1991). *Research with Hispanic populations*. Thousand Oaks, CA: Sage.

Marmot, M., Siegrist, J., Theorell, T., & Feeney, A. (1999). *Health and the psychosocial environment at work*. In M. Marmot & R. G. Wilkinson (Eds.), *Social determinants of health* (pp. 105–131). New York: Oxford University Press.

McLaughlin, D., & Stokes, C. (2002). Income inequality and mortality in US counties: Does minority racial concentration matter? *American Journal of Public Health, 92*(1), 99–104.

Mokuau, N., & Tauili'ili, P. (1992). *Families with Native Hawaiian and Pacific Island roots*. In E. W. Lynch & M. J. Hanson (Eds.), *Developing cross-cultural competence: A guide for working with young children and their families*. Baltimore: Brookes.

National Commission for Health Education Credentialing. (1985). *A framework for the development of competency-based curricula for entry-level health educators*. New York: Author.

National Commission for Health Education Credentialing, Society for Public Health Education, & American Association for Health Education. (2006). *A competency-based framework for health educators—2006*. Whitehall, PA: Author.

Office of Minority Health. (2001). *National standards for culturally and linguistically appropriate services* (CLAS). Retrieved September 15, 2006, from http://www.omhrc.gov/templates/browse.aspx?lvl=2&lvlID=15.

Pérez, M. A., Gonzalez, A., & Pinzon-Pérez, H. (2006). Cultural competence in health care systems: A case study. *California Journal of Health Promotion, 4*(1), 102–108.

Pinzon, H. L., & Pérez, M. A. (1997). Multicultural issues in health education programs for Hispanic/Latino populations in the United States. *Journal of Health Education, 28*(5), 314–316.

Polednak, A. (1993). Poverty, residential segregation, and black/white mortality ratios in urban areas. *Journal of Health Care for the Poor and Underserved, 4*, 363–373.

Polednak, A. (1996). Segregation, discrimination, and mortality in US blacks. *Ethnicity and Disease, 6*, 99–108.

Porr, C., Drummond, J., & Richter, S. (2006). Health literacy as an empowerment tool for low-income mothers. *Family and Community Health, 29*(4), 328–335.

Rubenstein, W. B., Bradley Sears, R., & Sockloskie, R. J. (2003). *Some demographic characteristics of the gay community in the United States.* The Williams Project, UCLA School of Law. Retrieved September 15, 2006, from http://www.law.ucla.edu/williamsinstitute/publications/GayDemographics.pdf.

Society for Public Health Education. (1997). *Standards for the preparation of graduate-level health educators.* Washington, DC: Author.

U.S. Census Bureau. (2004). *Current population survey* (Table A-1). Retrieved January 25, 2005, from http://www.census.gov/population/socdemo/school/tabA-1.pdf.

U.S. Department of Health and Human Services. (1985). *Report of the Secretary's Task Force on Black and Minority Health.* Washington, DC: Author.

U.S. Department of Health and Human Services. (2000). *Healthy people 2010.* Washington, DC: Government Printing Office.

Wyn, R., & Solis, B. (2001). Women's health issues across the life span. *Women's Health Issues, 11*(3), 148–159.

CHAPTER

AGING AND HEALTH EDUCATION

Partners for Learning

CAROLINA AGUILERA
WILLIAM H. DAILEY JR.
MIGUEL A. PÉREZ

LEARNING OBJECTIVES

After completing this chapter, you will be able to

- Describe the characteristics of the aging population.

- Name model programs that enhance health among older people.

- Understand the importance of providing primary prevention programs for the older population.

- Understand why health promotion efforts and priorities for aging populations should be developed through interactive collaboration.

- Understand the importance of culturally competent programs for aging population cohorts.

- Identify the components of quality of life that assist in maintaining independence, mental health, and overall well-being among older populations.

INTRODUCTION

In the last couple of decades, significant resources have been devoted to examining the social, health, and economic impacts of what some have called the "graying of America." Despite increasing research on this topic, most people continue to view aging as a mysterious and fearsome process, one that is enshrined in myths and stereotypes extending from health to economics and, especially in the United States, an almost universal fear of getting old. Regardless of how we define aging or when we believe it to start, there is one truth we cannot escape: everyone is bound to experience what Walt Whitman poetically romanticized as one of the four seasons in our lives. This chapter presents an overview of the older population's demographics, a brief summary of the health status of its members, and a review of successful health intervention programs focused on older adults.

DEMOGRAPHIC CHARACTERISTICS OF OLDER AMERICANS

According to the Profile of Older Americans (Administration on Aging, 2005), some 36.8 million Americans, or approximately 14 percent of the total U.S. population, are over the age of 65. This number represents a tenfold increase in this age group since the 1900s (see Figure 11.1), and it makes individuals aged 65 and above one of the fastest growing population segments in the United States. Population estimates also predict that the number of people aged 65 and over will double in the next three decades.

Current and future demographic changes in the older adult population require an examination of the racial and ethnic composition of that population group. In 2000, a majority of the individuals aged 65 years and over (84 percent) were non-Hispanic whites (see Figure 11.2). Population estimates predict that by 2050 that trend will continue, albeit at a smaller rate. The ethnic group with the smallest number of individuals in the 65 and older category is the American Indian and Alaska Native group.

As might be expected, the older adult population is not evenly distributed over the fifty states. In 2000, the states of Florida, West Virginia, Pennsylvania, Iowa, and North Dakota reported comparatively high proportions of older adults in their populations. In California, individuals aged 65 and over accounted for about 10 percent of the total population (Wallace, Pourat, Enriquez-Haass, & Sripipatana, 2003).

One of the reasons for the large number of individuals in the age 65 and older category is the increase in life expectancy for U.S. residents. For instance, a person born in 2000 can expect to live an average of twenty-nine years longer than someone born in 1900. Better access to health care, advances in medical science, and less dangerous occupations account for the increases in life expectancy. One thing that has not changed much since the turn of the century, however, is the difference

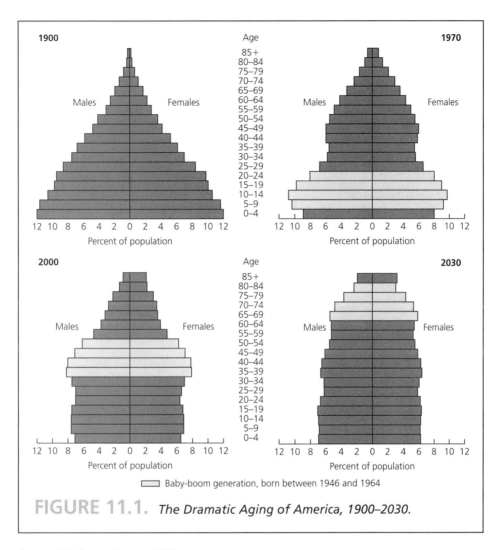

1900

Age

1970

85+
80–84
75–79
70–74
65–69
60–64
55–59
50–54
45–49
40–44
35–39
30–34
25–29
20–24
15–19
10–14
5–9
0–4

Males   Females

Males   Females

12 10 8 6 4 2 0 2 4 6 8 10 12
Percent of population

12 10 8 6 4 2 0 2 4 6 8 10 12
Percent of population

2000

Age

2030

85+
80–84
75–79
70–74
65–69
60–64
55–59
50–54
45–49
40–44
35–39
30–34
25–29
20–24
15–19
10–14
5–9
0–4

Males   Females

Males   Females

12 10 8 6 4 2 0 2 4 6 8 10 12
Percent of population

12 10 8 6 4 2 0 2 4 6 8 10 12
Percent of population

☐ Baby-boom generation, born between 1946 and 1964

FIGURE 11.1. *The Dramatic Aging of America, 1900–2030.*

Source: U.S. Census Bureau, 2002.

by gender. In general, women tend to live longer than men (51 years on average in 1900 and 80 years in 2000 for females, and 48 years in 1900 and 74 years in 2000 for males). Population projections by the U.S. Census Bureau suggest that future generations' pyramids will appear rectangular, representing the progressive growth of the proportion of older individuals in our society (Federal Interagency Forum on Aging-Related Statistics, 2000; He, Sengupta, Velkoff, & DeBarros, U.S. Census Bureau, 2005).

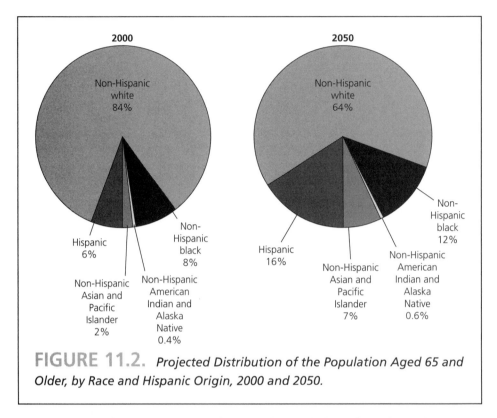

FIGURE 11.2. *Projected Distribution of the Population Aged 65 and Older, by Race and Hispanic Origin, 2000 and 2050.*

Note: Data are middle-series projections of the population. All data refer to the resident U.S. population. Hispanics may be of any race.

Source: U.S. Census Bureau, 2002.

ISSUES FACING THE OLDER ADULT POPULATION

Ageism refers to negative stereotypes and discrimination based on age (Bahr, 1994; Moody, 2006; Stallard, Decker, & Sellers, 2002). When directed toward older adults it tends to be based on negative assumptions about the expected biological slowdowns that occur naturally with advancing age. Ageism tends to be experienced mostly by aging populations but is also exhibited toward the teenage population (Hagestad & Uhlenberg, 2006).

Contrary to popular misconceptions, findings from the National Health Interview Survey show that a majority of Americans aged 65 and over report having good to excellent health (Schiller & Bernadal, 2004). This trend is supported by older individuals' increasing years of active life, increasing participation in prevention activities, and fewer complications from previously fatal health conditions (Bernstein et al., 2003; Centers for Disease Control and Prevention [CDC], 2004, n.d.). Generally speaking, non-Hispanic whites are more likely than Hispanics and African Americans to report good health.

The research literature suggests that the major issues facing older people in the United States today are loss of independence, loss of economic or social position, changes in marital status including loss of a spouse, and changes involving loss of family members and friends. Additional challenges to *healthy aging* are a higher likelihood of developing chronic diseases and the limited availability of affordable transportation resources, housing options, health care options, and personal care to help people remain independent (Bernstein et al., 2003; Hogson & Cai, 2001).

One group within the older adult population that requires specific discussion is the baby boomer population, which as it ages will markedly affect the proportions of the elderly and the "oldest old" in the total population (Eggebeen & Sturgeon, 2006). As a result of baby boomer aging, it is projected that one in five people will be 65 years old or older by 2030 (Federal Interagency Forum on Aging-Related Statistics, 2006). In fact, it has been suggested that the impact of the baby boom generation will be equal to that of immigration during the first part of the twentieth century.

The majority of health educators seem ill-equipped for dealing with these demographic changes affecting the U.S. population. Furthermore, few if any health educators complete any formal education in how to design, implement, and evaluate health promotion programs targeting the older adult population. Moreover, some health educators might not wish to work with the older adult population due to fears of facing their own aging process (Hogson & Cai, 2001). This disconnect reveals the need for health educators to become more educated in strategies designed to reach the older population. One strategy to achieve this goal seeks to address the health literacy of the older adult population.

HEALTH LITERACY AMONG OLDER ADULTS

Health literacy may be defined as "a multidimensional issue encompassing the ability to read, understand, and use health information to make appropriate healthcare decisions and follow instructions for treatment that allow patients to manage their health and improve the quality of their lives" (Brown et al., 2004, p. 150). It is a key issue to be considered when dealing with elderly populations because it influences patient-provider interactions, including compliance with treatment (Greene, Hibbard, & Tusler, 2005; National Institute on Aging [NIA], 2006; Osborne, 2005).

Results from the 2003 National Assessment of Adult Literacy (NAAL) show that 29 percent of the adult population 65 years old and older had a health literacy proficiency of 30 percent and were at the basic level, 38 percent were at the intermediate level, and only 3 percent of the participants were at the proficient health literacy level (Kutner, Greenberg, Jin, & Paulsen, 2006; NIA, 2006). According to these findings, adults 65 and older have the lowest health literacy level when compared to the average level of the other age groups (Kutner et al., 2006; NIA, 2006).

According to a study by Lee, Gazmararian, and Arozullah (2006), older adult populations with low health literacy tend to be comparatively isolated from the society in which they live; therefore they obtain less social support and their health tends to diminish as a consequence. Similarly, findings from the NAAL indicate that adults categorized as being in the "below basic" range of health literacy have difficulties reading documents, filling in medical forms, and navigating the health care system (Osborne, 2005; Powell, Hill, & Clancy, 2007).

Osborne (2005) discusses the importance of considering a person's background before starting to convey information. For example, the health educator should be aware of people's personal health, such as the presence of chronic illnesses, complications, and medications, because this knowledge will facilitate the implementation of health promotion programs. Health educators can meet the needs of older adults by determining the health literacy of the target population and then employing improved communication skills and well-written instructions that are at the appropriate level for the older adult population they seek to reach.

Osborne (2005) suggests that information presented to an older adult population should be limited to a few important points, adjusted according to the audience attention span, and repeated. Nakasato and Carnes (2006) suggest that health promotion programs targeting older adults address three key needs of these individuals: (1) to maintain a low risk of experiencing disease and disease-related disabilities, (2) to maintain a mentally and physically active lifestyle, and (3) to maintain their engagement in life. The following strategies can be applied in these health promotion programs:

- *Create a shame-free learning environment.* Group participants can be encouraged to draw from their vast experiences and to share their lifelong learning about health. Health educators can work to "update" the information clients have when it does not conform to established scientific standards.

- *Create an environment conducive to learning and good communication* with large visual aids, well-lit rooms, and quiet spaces to talk. Culturally apt and age-appropriate graphics that are easy to read and follow can facilitate the learning process. Health educators working with older adult populations need to be mindful of their voice projection to ensure they can be heard without shouting or sounding condescending.

- *Make spoken information concrete and concise.* As just mentioned, voice projection is important in delivering information to and discussing issues with older adult populations. Health educators should also seek to decrease their use of *jargon,* technical language that may not be understood by their target audience. Examples too should be placed within a context that can be experienced by the target population.

- *Engage in short trips "down memory lane."* Older adults enjoy recalling facts they have learned and the experiences they have had and the people with whom they shared these experiences.

- *Incorporate social activities into health education and promotion programs.* Active learning must be encouraged and promoted throughout health promotion programs.

CULTURAL COMPETENCE WITH OLDER ADULTS

Betancourt, Green, Carrillo, and Ananeh-Firempong (2003) find that health care can be considered culturally competent when it is based on an evident understanding of the ways in which patients' society and culture influences their health behaviors and health beliefs. Health education practitioners can build cultural competence with aging populations by using the Core Curriculum in Ethnogeriatrics, a model developed in 1999 and 2000 by the Collaborative on Ethnogeriatric Education. The collaborative has noted that there are flaws and limitations in the U.S. Census data that affect our ability to learn about cultural and demographic groups (Yeo, 2000).

Demographic data and ethnic and cultural perspectives affect the educational community programs developed to meet the needs of our growing population of older adults. Acknowledging ethnogerontological educational resources may provide the context for better collaborative efforts among aging populations and health education practitioners and thus better learning outcomes.

A study in rural Florida, where 772 physicians were surveyed regarding their opinion toward the aging population, found that even physicians showed ageist perceptions, especially toward people 85 years of age and older and those living in nursing homes (Gunderson, Tomkowiak, Menachemi, & Brooks, 2005). Health promotion programs need to reduce this type of discrimination. This can be achieved by creating culturally competent programs with linguistically appropriate educational materials. Also, the implementation of cultural competence training at the organizational, structural, and clinical levels can help in the transition to less ageist views.

Figure 11.3 depicts the ethnogeriatric context for working with older adult populations. It emphasizes that interrelations exist between health, transcultural health, and healthy as well as productive aging.

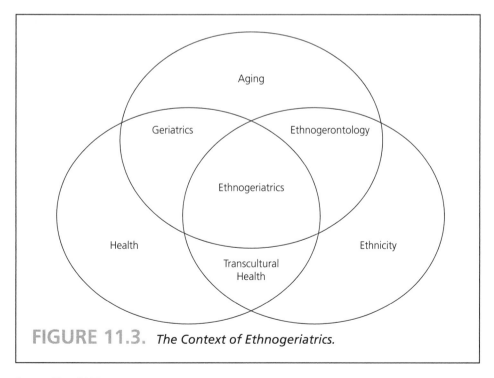

FIGURE 11.3. *The Context of Ethnogeriatrics.*

Source: Yeo, 2000.

HEALTHY AGING AND HEALTH EDUCATION

The expected economic impact on the nation's health care system resulting from population increases among individuals aged 65 and over demands that additional prevention services be developed and implemented among and specifically for that population group (Wallace, 2005). Health care expenditures on the elderly account for approximately 38 percent of all today's health care expenditures. It is expected that the projected increase in the 65 and older population will translate into even higher levels of health care service demands and expenditures for this population group (CDC, 2004). In fact, government estimates project a 25 percent increase in health care expenditures by 2030 as a result of the increase in the overall age of the population (CDC, n.d., p. 2). Given the toll this will take on economic as well as personal resources, it is not surprising that public health professionals are being called on to assist older adults to improve their quality of life and prevent or avoid debilitating and expensive treatments.

The expected increased demand for health care services and subsequent increased costs is partially due to the fact that approximately one out of every three older adults has at least one chronic condition affecting his or her ability to function (Lang, Moore, Harris, & Anderson, 2005). Individuals in the older age group are also more likely to be hospitalized than younger individuals (Lewin Group, 2001).

Given the population shifts described previously, it is not surprising that the CDC has identified three specific areas that need to be addressed in our attempts to reach the elderly in the United States with health education. Attention to these areas improves the likelihood of the happy and functional transition from our working years to our retirement age that most of us look forward to (Atchley & Barusch, 2004; Hillier & Barrow, 2007). Specially, the CDC has recommended additional efforts in the areas of (1) the adoption of a healthy lifestyle, one that incorporates physical activity, proper nutrition, and avoidance of tobacco products; (2) the early detection of diseases, including the use of diagnostic exams such as sigmoidoscopy, colonoscopy, and tests for colorectal cancer; and (3) the use of specific immunizations, such as flu shots.

The U.S. Department of Health and Human Services (2000), while establishing new guidelines for health promotion and disease prevention through *Healthy People 2010,* notes that a major focus of these goals is increasing functional life expectancy.

The challenges for partnerships in learning and collaborative efforts to develop effective educational venues involve dealing with cultural limitations, social and economic constraints, health care access, and transportation barriers. Older adults' participation in and acceptance of community endeavors involves additional considerations, such as their willingness to accept community support, their personal financial constraints, and their lack of previous knowledge about community resources available to them.

Health promotion programs targeting the elderly should be designed to promote well-being in old age and, more specifically, to promote productive, robust, and *successful aging.* To meet these criteria health promotion and education programs should take into account cognitive changes experienced as part of the aging process and physiological changes and limitations, as well as expected outcomes on the part of program participants (Flood & Scharer, 2006; also see Hooyman & Kiyak, 2005). Programs should promote an early focus on disease prevention, injury and disability prevention, mental health, and physical health and should also encourage social engagement activities (Nakasato & Carnes, 2006).

The road we must take to reach the older adult population travels up a long learning curve. Appendix D lists a variety of resources available on the Internet that will help you access methodologies and community of practice and other innovative possibilities for health education practitioners focused on bringing together new ideas and concepts to make a difference in the lives of older adults.

CONCLUSION

The ongoing growth of the population of older adults is creating challenges and opportunities for aging and health education practitioners (Atchley & Barusch, 2004; Hillier & Barrow, 2007).

Building a working foundation of partnerships between health educators and health practitioners specializing in aging in order to meet the challenges of living longer, adopting healthier lifestyles, and remaining active will allow the development of new ideas, programs, and services that promote the concepts of managing chronic diseases, promoting well-being in old age, and maintaining a perspective of productive, robust, and successful aging. Resourceful strategies from health educators and aging practitioners throughout our life journey can bring together life experiences and emerging options and opportunities to serve today's older adults. Successful health education for older adults will promote disease prevention, injury and disability prevention, mental health, physical health, and social engagement. At the same time health educators and practitioners have to take into consideration "the biological realities of aging" and tailor interventions to adequately serve the increasing and culturally diverse older population (Nakasato & Carnes, 2006).

POINTS TO REMEMBER

- Thanks to medical advances, an increase in health care access, and a decrease of danger in the workplace, the life expectancy of Americans went up by an average of 29 years between 1900 and 2000. Yet many public health professionals are not adequately prepared to provide preventive services to older Americans.

- Issues faced by the elderly include ageism, loss of family and friends, reduction in socioeconomic status, loss of independence, and experiencing one or more chronic diseases.

- Health educators should familiarize themselves with education techniques especially designed to reach the aging population. In particular they should be prepared to overcome low levels of health literacy.

- Non-Hispanic whites are currently a majority of the older population, but the proportions of other ethnic and racial groups are growing rapidly. Health educators working with older adults need to become culturally competent.

- The context of the ethnogeriatrics model (Figure 11.3) relates ethnicity, aging, and health and thus provides a structure for building cultural competence for working with older adults. Ethnogeriatric materials intend to contribute to the attainment of the *Healthy People 2010* goal to increase functional life expectancy.

- Health promotion and prevention programs for older adults may be best carried out by partnerships among public health departments, agencies with a focus on aging, and voluntary organizations.

CASE STUDY

During her first week at work at a large metropolitan hospital, Chris discovers that the majority of people in her sleep apnea group are individuals aged 65 and older. The majority of these people appear to be healthy, and none of them have any experience with health education programs. Most seem uncomfortable with having a "young" person dictate to them what they have to do; this sleep apnea group is turning into just another example in the long list of one-sided conversations they have had with the health care system. Discuss the following questions:

1. How can Chris involve these older patients in seeking hospital resources for help with nutrition, exercise, and medication?

2. Do you think it would be beneficial for Chris to obtain medical histories that she could use to check her assumptions about the health status of these elderly individuals?

3. Would information about these older adults' previous experiences with the hospital setting help Chris to increase their participation?

4. Would Chris benefit from working with a professional in aging to broaden her views and assumptions about older adults and the kinds of interactions she can have with them?

KEY TERMS

Ageism	Healthy aging
Health promotion	Successful aging

REFERENCES

Administration on Aging. (2005). *A profile of older Americans: 2005*. Retrieved October 22, 2007, from http://www.aoa.gov/PROF/Statistics/profile/2005/2005profile.pdf.

Atchley, R. C., & Barusch, A. S. (2004). *Social forces and aging: An introduction to social gerontology*. Belmont, CA: Wadsworth.

Bahr, R. T. (1994). *An overview of gerontological nursing*. In M. O. Hogstel (Ed.), *Nursing care of the older adult* (3rd ed., pp. 2–25). Albany, NY: Delmar.

Bernstein, A. B., Hing, E., Moss, A. J., Allen, K. F., Siller, A. B., & Tiggle, R. B. (2003). *Health care in America: Trends in utilization*. Hyattsville, MD: National Center for Health Statistics.

Betancourt, J. R., Green, A. R., Carrillo, J. E., & Ananeh-Firempong, O. (2003). Defining cultural competence: A practical framework for addressing racial/ethnic disparities in health and health care. *Public Health Reports, 118*, 293–302.

Brown, D. R., Ludwig, R., Buck, G. A., Durham, D., Shurmard, T., & Graham, S. S. (2004). Health literacy: Universal precautions needed. *Journal of Allied Health, 33*(2), 150–155.

Centers for Disease Control and Prevention. (2004). *Healthy aging for older adults*. Retrieved June 24, 2004, from http://www.cdc.gov/aging.

Centers for Disease Control and Prevention. (n.d.). *Healthy aging: Preventing disease and improving quality of life among older Americans, 2004*. Atlanta, GA: Author.

Eggebeen, S., & Sturgeon, S. (2006). *Demography of the baby boomers*. In S. K. Whitbourne & S. L. Willis (Eds.), *The baby boomers grow up: Contemporary perspectives on midlife* (pp. 45–71). Mahwah, NJ: Erlbaum.

Federal Interagency Forum on Aging-Related Statistics. (2000). *Older Americans 2000: Key indicators of well-being*. Retrieved June 24, 2004, from http://agingstats.gov/chartbook2000.

Federal Interagency Forum on Aging-Related Statistics. (2006). *Data sources on older Americans, 2006*. Hyattsville, MD: National Center for Health Statistics.

Flood, M., & Scharer, K. (2006). Creativity enhancement: Possibilities for successful aging. *Issues in Mental Health Nursing, 27,* 939–959.

Greene, J., Hibbard, J., & Tusler, M. (2005, June). *How much do health literacy and patient activation contribute to older adults' ability to manage their health?* Washington, DC: AARP Public Policy Institute.

Gunderson, A., Tomkowiak, J., Menachemi, N., & Brooks, R. (2005, July-September). Rural physicians' attitudes toward the elderly: Evidence of ageism? *Quality Management in Health Care, 14*(3), 167–176.

Hagestad, G. O., & Uhlenberg, P. (2006, November). Should we be concerned about age segregation? Some theoretical and empirical explorations. *Research on Aging, 28*(6), 638–653.

He, W., Sengupta, M., Velkoff, V. A., & DeBarros, K. A., U.S. Census Bureau. (2005). *65+ in the Unites States: 2005*. Retrieved September 22, 2007, from http://www.census.gov/prod/2006pubs/p23-209.pdf.

Hillier, S. M., & Barrow, G. M. (2007). *Aging, the individual and society* (8th ed.). Belmont, CA: Wadsworth.

Hogson, T. A., & Cai, L. (2001). Medical care expenditures for hypertension, its complications, and its comorbidities. *Medical Care, 39*(6), 599–615.

Hooyman, N. R., & Kiyak, H. S. (2005). *Social gerontology: A multidisciplinary approach*. Boston: Pearson Education.

Kutner, M., Greenberg, E., Jin, Y., & Paulsen, C. (2006). *The health literacy of America's adults: Results from the 2003 National Assessment of Adult Literacy* (NCES 2006483). Hyattsville, MD: National Center for Education Statistics.

Lang, J. E., Moore, M. J., Harris, A. C., & Anderson, L. A. (2005). Healthy aging: Priorities and programs of the Centers for Disease Control and Prevention. *Generations, 29*(2), 24–29.

Lee, S., Gazmararian, J. A., & Arozullah, A. M. (2006). Health literacy and social support among elderly Medicare enrollees in a managed care plan. *Journal of Applied Gerontology, 25*(4), 324–337.

Lewin Group. (2001). *AHA Trend Watch, 3*(3).

Moody, H. R. (2006). *Aging: Concepts and controversies* (5th ed.). Thousand Oaks, CA: Pine Forge.

Nakasato, Y. R., & Carnes, B. A. (2006, April). Health promotion in older adults: Promoting successful aging in primary care settings. *Geriatrics, 61*(4), 27–31.

National Institute on Aging. (2006). *Working with your older patient.* Retrieved September 20, 2006, from http://www.nia.nih.gov/HealthInformation/Publications/WorkingwithYourOlderPatient/default.htm.

Osborne, H. (2005). *Health literacy from A to Z: Practical ways to communicate your health message.* Boston: Jones & Bartlett.

Powell, C. K., Hill, E. G., & Clancy, D. E. (2007, January/February). The relationship between health literacy and diabetes knowledge and readiness to take health actions. *The Diabetes Educator, 33*(1), 144–151.

Schiller, J. S., & Bernadal, L. (2004, May). Summary health statistics for the US population: National Health Interview Survey, 2002. *Vital and Health Statistics, 10*(220), 1–110.

Stallard, J. M., Decker, I. M., & Sellers, B. J. (2002, April-June). Health care for the elderly: A social obligation. *Nursing Forum, 37*(2), 5–15.

U.S. Census Bureau. (2002). Elderly Americans. *Population Bulletin, 56*(4), 1–10.

U.S. Department of Health and Human Services. (2000). *Healthy people 2010.* Washington, DC: Government Printing Office.

Wallace, S. P. (2005, Summer). The public health perspective on aging. *Generations, 29*(2), 5–10.

Wallace, S. P., Pourat, N., Enriquez-Haass, V., & Sripipatana, A. (2003). *Health of older Californians: County data book.* Los Angeles: UCLA Center for Health Policy Research.

Yeo, G. (Ed.). (2000). *Curriculum in ethnogeriatrics.* Stanford Geriatric Education Center. Retrieved February 7, 2007, from http://www.stanford.edu/group/ethnoger/leftf.html.

CHAPTER

CULTURE AND SEXUAL ORIENTATION

KAY WOODIEL

KATE BRINDLE

LEARNING OBJECTIVES

After completing this chapter, you will be able to

- Acknowledge the diversity within the gay cultures.

- Recognize health risks and common health concerns specific to lesbians and bisexual women, gay and bisexual men, transgender individuals, and racially and ethnically diverse LGBT people.

- Increase awareness of and sensitivity to health issues relevant to the LGBT culture.

- Demonstrate cultural competence when working with and addressing the LGBT culture.

INTRODUCTION

There are some who might argue against including the lesbian, gay, bisexual, and transgender (LGBT) community in a multicultural health education book. Indeed, they might argue that LGBT individuals do not constitute a cultural group. This argument would narrowly confine culture to race and ethnicity. Restricting culture to race, ethnicity, or heritage narrows its scope and breadth. Culture involves behaviors and beliefs characteristic of a particular social, ethnic, or age group. Culture can go beyond behaviors and beliefs and present a dynamic set of shared values, customs, communication patterns, and norms often influencing the behaviors and action of the group (Campinha-Bacote, 1999; Smith, 1998). Indeed culture can guide people's behavior along shared paths.

These shared behavioral paths can become the shared attributes of a group of people and then their culture. People, particularly the LGBT community, can share a culture regardless of their race or ethnicity, in the same way that workers in the automobile industry share a culture regardless of race or ethnicity. So it is important for health educators to extend their definition of culture beyond race and ethnicity to include socioeconomic status, physical abilities and limitations, religious beliefs, and political affiliation, as well as sexual orientation. The LGBT culture is an undeniable fact, as evidenced by the symbol of the rainbow flag, pride parades, and drag queens.

All health educators and health professionals should strive to provide culturally competent services. Yet the majority of LGBT people do not feel they are receiving culturally competent care (Meyer, 2001). The high profile assigned to human immunodeficiency virus (HIV) and acquired immunodeficiency syndrome (AIDS) has led many health educators and health professionals to conclude that this is the only health issue affecting the LGBT community. There is a lack of knowledge and appreciation for the extent of the problems facing this unique cultural group. This lack is further complicated by the fact that as previously discussed, certain segments of the U.S. population do not wish to recognize LGBT people as a cultural group. It is imperative that health educators and professionals recognize that the *gay* culture is made up of a collective of LGBT populations that are as diverse as their members.

Members of the LGBT community have significant health disparities in areas such as substance abuse, teen suicide, health care access, and hate-crime violence (Dean et al., 2000). The most significant health disparity is the comparative lack of research. Information about transgender health is extremely limited and on some issues completely absent. Several well-recognized health agencies have acknowledged the inadequate research on LGBT health. The National Institute of Mental Health, the Centers for Disease Control and Prevention, the American Medical Association, the American Public Health Association, and the Institute of Medicine have all released reports indicating that health care research in lesbian, gay, bisexual, and transgender communities is largely inadequate (Shankle, 2006). Despite the need for increased research among this population group, federal research dollars remain narrowly focused on HIV and AIDS.

This chapter addresses the health behaviors of the LGBT community. We will explore cultural factors and myths, offering culturally sensitive information for health educators and health professionals who will work with the community. We have included a table of definitions for the key terms in this chapter to enhance the reader's knowledge and understanding of the LGBT community (see Table 12.1). We hope this information will assist in decreasing the common confusion surrounding terminology for this culture.

TABLE 12.1. Definitions of Key Terms.

Bisexual	A man or a woman with a sexual and emotional orientation toward people of both sexes (U.S. Department of Health and Human Services [USDHHS], Office on Women's Health, 2000).
Coming out	The process by which LGBT people acknowledge that they are not exclusively heterosexual. It may involve two phases, coming out to oneself and then coming out to others. This may occur over a short, intense period or gradually over time. Coming out is extremely influenced by the person's comfort level and both internal and external influences.
Gay	Most commonly refers to men whose primary emotional and sexual attraction is to men, but may also be used to refer to a homosexual person of either sex. Some lesbians identify as gay (Gay and Lesbian Medical Association [GLMA] et al., 2001).
Gender identity	A person's sense of self as being either male or female. Gender identity does not always match biological sex. Unlike sex, which is biologically determined, gender is considered a social construct (USDHHS, Substance Abuse and Mental Health Services Administration [SAMHSA], 2000; Peterkin & Risdon, 2003).
Heterosexism	Belief that heterosexuality is the only "natural" sexuality and that it is inherently healthier than or superior to other types of sexuality (Shankle, 2006).
Homophobia	Irrational fear or hatred of lesbian, gay, bisexual, or transgender people (GLMA et al., 2001).
Homosexual	An outmoded term used primarily for diagnostic purposes, meaning *same-sexual* (Peterkin & Risdon, 2003).

(continued)

(Table 12.1 continued)

Lesbian	A woman whose primary emotional and sexual attraction is to other women (GLMA et al., 2001).
LGBT	Acronym for *lesbian, gay, bisexual,* and *transgender.* (The preferred order of these four terms may vary, resulting in other acronyms in other books or articles.)
Queer	Once a derogatory term for gays and lesbians, this term is now being used with a sense of pride by members of the LGBT community, especially those born after 1970 (Peterkin & Risdon, 2003).
Sexual identity	A chosen mode of self-presentation, based on social identity, sexual behavior, or both. A person may choose to publicly identify with a term that does not strictly conform to his or her sexual behavior (a self-termed "bisexual" woman may be intimate only with women). How one identifies is a personal choice (Peterkin & Risdon, 2003).
Sexual orientation	A person's innate sexual desires and attractions. This term should replace *sexual preference,* which implies that these desires are a matter of choice rather than a result of one's nature (Peterkin & Risdon, 2003).
Transgender	A person whose gender identity or gender expression is not congruent with his or her biological sex. This term is sometimes used as an umbrella term encompassing transsexuals and cross-dressers (GLMA et al., 2001).
Transphobia	Irrational fear or hatred of transgender or transsexual individuals (GLMA et al., 2001).
Transsexual	An individual whose gender identity is that of the biologically opposite sex. There are female-to-male and male-to-female transsexuals. A transsexual may or may not have had sex reassignment surgery (GLMA et al., 2001).

THE LGBT CULTURE

According to various studies, roughly 5 to 10 percent of the U.S. population is lesbian, gay, bisexual, or transgender (National Coalition for LGBT Health & Boston Public Health Commission, 2002). It is thought that these percentages are in reality higher, because people completing studies are sometimes fearful or reluctant to classify themselves as lesbian, gay, bisexual, or transgender. Further, the LGBT community is an extremely diverse group of people. They vary in sociodemographic characteristics such as ethnic or racial identity, age, education, income, and place of residence (Meyer, 2001).

This diversity extends to the degree to which they may or may not self-identify with the community. As a result, the community is referred to by a myriad of names. Terms such as *LGBT* and *GLBT* and *queer, homosexual, gay,* and *lesbian* are often used interchangeably. The terminology chosen will be specific to the individual's own personal identity and politics (Ferris, 2006). It is crucial that health educators and public health professionals not assume that any one term captures everyone who identifies as LGBT. For example, some lesbians may prefer the term *gay* to the term *lesbian.* Some members of the LGBT community, especially those born after 1970, may be very comfortable with the term *queer,* whereas many other member of the community find the term extremely offensive (Peterkin & Risdon, 2003). Although terminology is certainly not the foundation of any community, it can be relevant and helpful as health educators and health professionals attempt to address and target a community for disease prevention and health promotion (Ferris, 2006).

HEALTH ISSUES OF THE LGBT COMMUNITY

Heterosexism and *homophobia* are the two most obvious social health issues for the LGBT community. Studies show that lesbian, gay, bisexual, and transgender populations have the same basic health needs as the general population but experience health disparities and barriers related to *sexual orientation* and *gender identity* or expression. Many individuals avoid or delay care or receive inappropriate or inferior care because of perceived or real homophobia and discrimination by health educators and health care professionals (Shankle, 2006).

Sadly, literature regarding health education and sexual orientation is extremely limited. Obviously, this area is controversial, and policymaking specific to sexuality education and especially programs involving sexual orientation has become increasingly politicized (Rienzo, Button, Sheu, & Li, 2006). Lack of sensitive curricula and program policies forces many gay youths to become the invisible minority (Anderson, 1997). Moreover, the limited research that has been done supports the existence of homophobia and heterosexism among health educators in the schools, which increases the invisibility of gay youths. It is impossible for gay youths to feel emotionally safe in schools if they first are invited to feel invisible (Woodiel, Angermeier-Howard, & Hobson, 2003).

For example, one study revealed that one-third of health teachers indicated gay and lesbian rights are a threat to the American family and its values (Telljohann, Price, Poureslami, & Easton, 1995). Additionally, more than half of the health teachers indicated that gay and lesbian support groups would not be supported by their school administrator (Telljohann et al., 1995). Another study looked at physical educators' confidence in teaching health education content areas and revealed that they felt least confident teaching about sexual orientation (Larson, 2003). In another study, students who identified as gay or lesbian reported that the subject of homosexuality was virtually absent from classroom instruction. The same study revealed strong support for sexuality education, but homosexuality was the least-supported subject in the survey (Lindley & Reininger, 2001).

HEALTH ISSUES COMMON TO ALL LGBT GROUPS

One of the biggest issues common to LGBT communities is substance abuse, including smoking tobacco, drinking alcohol, and using drugs. According to one study, LGBT people are 40 percent more likely to smoke than their heterosexual counterparts (Ryan, Wortley, Easton, Pederson, & Greenwood, 2001). Several factors contribute to this high rate of smoking, including participating in the "bar scene" in order to be part of an LGBT community and using smoking to deal with the stress of homophobia, transphobia, and LGBT discrimination and oppression (GLMA et al., 2001).

Peterkin and Risdon (2003) found that along with higher rates of smoking, lesbians and gay men have higher rates of alcohol consumption than heterosexual people do. Most of the research in this area has focused on lesbians and gay men; there is little research about the alcohol consumption rates of bisexual and transgender people. As in the general population in the United States, substance abuse in the LGBT community is associated with a myriad of challenges, including HIV and AIDS, sexually transmitted diseases (STDs), violence (of particular concern are acts committed by and against the LGBT community), and chronic disease conditions, such as cirrhosis of the liver.

LGBT youths use alcohol and other drugs for many of the same reasons as their heterosexual peers do: to experiment and assert independence, to relieve tension, to increase feelings of self-esteem and adequacy, and to self-medicate for underlying depression or other mental health problems (GLMA et al., 2001). Although alcohol consumption has decreased in these communities throughout the past two decades, there is still widespread alcohol use among young gay and lesbian communities (GLMA et al., 2001).

Depression and mental health issues also affect LGBT people at a higher level than found among heterosexual people. Although homosexuality is no longer characterized by the American Psychiatric Association as a mental disorder, gender identity disorder (GID) is listed in the *Diagnostic and Statistical Manual of Mental Disorders, Volume Four* (*DSM-IV*). Simply stated, GID is the condition of significant discomfort with one's assigned gender (Peterkin & Risdon, 2003).

Therefore, in order to receive health services, some transgender people are forced to identify themselves as having a mental illness. This is not true for lesbian, gay, and bisexual people who do not identify as transgender. Regardless, studies show cases of depression among LGBT populations (GLMA et al., 2001). Like substance abuse, this depression can be directly related to individuals' LGBT identification, which can involve navigating through the threat of hate crimes and violence, homophobic and transphobic laws and procedures, and coming out to family members, friends, and coworkers.

In addition to depression and substance abuse, domestic violence is also problematic in LGBT communities. According to a 2001 study, 2,183 LGBT persons reported domestic violence to the National Coalition Against Domestic Violence. Forty-three percent of the domestic violence survivors were lesbians, 49 percent were male, and 4 percent identified as transgender (National Coalition Against Domestic Violence, 2003). Although domestic violence centers on power and control in LGBT relationships, as it does in heterosexual relationships, it also has unique elements when it occurs in LGBT relationships. One of the major ways abusers control victims is through the victims' fear that their abusers will "out" them (disclosing their LGBT identity to family, friends, coworkers, and so forth). This results in LGBT people not reporting domestic violence. Another reason that LGBT people do not report domestic violence is fear of a homophobic and transphobic legal system, where same-sex relationships are not afforded the same legal rights as opposite-sex relationships. This can become a tool used by the batterer, who may repeatedly tell the victim that he or she will never be helped by the legal system. There are several institutional barriers to obtaining domestic violence services as well. For example, crime victims' compensation (CVC) programs provide services only to legally married couples. Because LGBT people cannot legally marry in the majority of the states in the United States, they are often denied these services (Baernstein et al., 2006).

Along with domestic partner violence, external anti-LGBT violence and hate crimes also harm the health of LGBT people. It is estimated that up to 80 percent of hate crimes toward LGBT individuals are never reported to authorities (Public Health—Seattle and King County, 2004). Violence resulting from hate crime, domestic violence, suicide, and other forms of physical, sexual, emotional, and environmental violence takes a heavy toll on the LGBT population. Between one-quarter and one-third of all LGBT individuals have experienced domestic violence. LGBT individuals are more than four times as likely as the general population to have attempted suicide (Public Health—Seattle and King County, 2004).

Additionally, not all state reporting systems use sexual orientation and gender identity as reporting categories for hate crimes. Therefore it is hard to get accurate statistics about hate-crimes rates. However, we know that anti-LGBT crimes do exist and that the threat of hate crimes can affect people's stress levels and mental health. This issue goes beyond the LGBT community and becomes everyone's responsibility. Hate crimes affect the mental health of the victim, his or her family, and all societal members.

HEALTH ISSUES OF LGBT YOUTHS

Adolescence is a difficult time regardless of sexual orientation; however, a growing body of research on LGBT youths indicates that they have health problems and needs that are different from those of heterosexual youths (Lock & Steiner, 1999). The most prevalent health and social problems for gay teens are depression, family rejection, suicide, substance abuse, running away, homelessness, prostitution, truancy, victimization, violence, STDs, high-risk sexual behavior, and poor health maintenance (Peterkin & Risdon, 2003). Additionally, compared to risk behaviors among heterosexual youths, these risk behaviors are more prevalent, begin earlier, and are more frequently clustered together (Hunter, Cohall, Mallon, Moyer, & Riddle, 2006).

Moreover, LGBT youths often have had negative experiences with health professionals (Garofalo & Katz, 2001). When LGBT youths fear rejection, stigmatization, lack of confidentiality, and embarrassment, they will be reluctant to seek health services, will avoid health education altogether, or will not reveal their sexual identity to the health professionals (Ginsberg et al., 2002). Homophobia and heterosexism play a distinct role in their rejection of health care and health education.

Sadly, issues surrounding LGBT youths provide fuel for controversy in the schools, and for LGBT students nationwide, discrimination and harassment have become the rule, not the exception (Woodiel et al., 2003). Homophobia and heterosexism create a hostile environment that does not invite support from other students and teachers. Therefore it becomes difficult for heterosexual students and teachers to be informed and supportive about the special health issues of gay youths (Rienzo et al., 2006).

For instance, one report revealed that Boston's lesbian, gay, and bisexual youths were more likely than their heterosexual counterparts to be threatened or injured with a weapon in school. They were also found to be much more likely than heterosexual high school students to carry a gun or weapon and to be involved with a gang (National Coalition for LGBT Health & Boston Public Health Commission, 2002). The average high school student hears twenty-five antigay slurs each day. One out of three LGBT youths in Chicago had had an object thrown at him or her and one out of five had been kicked, punched, or beaten because of his or her sexual orientation (Hunter et al., 2006).

HEALTH ISSUES OF LESBIAN AND BISEXUAL WOMEN

The health care needs of lesbians and bisexual women are similar to those of all women. However, homophobia and heterosexism can mean that lesbian and bisexual women will experience additional risk factors and barriers to education and care, and these can affect their health status. We will discuss some health conditions that disproportionately affect lesbians and bisexual women and conditions that affect lesbian women differently than they do heterosexual women. However, not enough research has focused solely on the concerns of both lesbian and bisexual women. The majority of the research in this field focuses on lesbian women, and there is a definite lack of information about the health concerns of bisexual women (Baernstein et al., 2006).

Among the main issues affecting lesbian and bisexual women are reproductive cancers. Although there is nothing biological to suggest that lesbian and bisexual women are more at risk than heterosexual women, lesbians are less likely to receive regular gynecological care, including regular pap smears and breast exams (Matthews, Brandenburgh, Johnson, & Hughes, 2004). Lesbians and bisexual women avoid regular visits to the gynecologist due to past negative experiences, placing them at higher risk of late diagnosis of cervical, ovarian, and endometrial cancers. Fewer pregnancies and decreased use of contraceptives also contribute to increased rates of ovarian and endometrial cancer, and human papillomavirus (HPV) (which is associated with cervical cancer) can be transmitted by unclean sex toys (Baernstein et al., 2006).

According to the U.S. Department of Health and Human Services (USDHHS, Office on Women's Health, 2000), another reason lesbians are likely to receive inadequate treatment is that some health care providers falsely believe lesbians are immune to certain reproductive cancers and therefore do not conduct the proper tests to screen for cancer. Still, lesbian and bisexual women, like all women, need regular gynecological care and breast and STD screenings.

Along with cancer risks, lesbians and bisexual women are also at risk for obesity and heart disease. There is evidence that lesbians are more likely to be overweight than their heterosexual counterparts, possibly because of cultural norms within the lesbian community and because lesbians may relate differently to, not accept, or not internalize mainstream notions of ideal beauty and thinness (Aaron et al., 2001). On average, lesbians have been found to have higher BMIs (body mass indexes), and higher BMIs have been found to predict health status in regard to obesity (Baernstein et al., 2006).

HEALTH ISSUES OF GAY AND BISEXUAL MEN

Like other LGBT people, gay and bisexual men make up a diverse group of people who identify as different races, ethnicities, nationalities, and religions and who represent multiple socioeconomic classes from various areas in the United States. These identities directly affect the health issues facing gay and bisexual men. However, we will focus on issues we see as the most common and relevant and as sometimes overlooked in gay and bisexual men's communities.

The use of *club drugs,* such as crystal methamphetamine (often referred to as *crystal meth*) and ecstasy appears to be increasing in gay and bisexual men's communities (GLMA et al., 2001). Crystal methamphetamine can cause erratic, violent behavior among its users. Effects also include suppression of appetite, interference with sleeping behavior, mood swings, tremors, convulsions, and an irregular heart rate. The long-term effects of the drug can include coma, stroke, and death (Partnership for a Drug-Free America, 2006). Additionally, crystal methamphetamine, which is highly addictive, can increase the risk of HIV transmission, as it lowers users' inhibitions, which can result in unsafe sex practices (Reuters, 2004). Crystal methamphetamine is especially popular in rural and economically depressed areas, as it is produced easily and inexpensively (Reuters, 2004).

Eating disorders and negative body image also affect gay and bisexual men. Research indicates that eating disorders occur more often among gay men than among heterosexual men (Meyer, Blissett, & Oldfield, 2001). Eating disorders, such as anorexia (characterized by self-starvation) and bulimia (characterized by binging and purging food), can lead to kidney damage, cardiovascular disorders, dental damage, and in severe cases, even death. Although women with eating disorders still outnumber men with eating disorders, men's eating disorders often develop at a later age. One study suggests that for the general population, the average age for men developing an eating disorder is 21, compared to an age of 17 for women (Braun, Sunday, Huang, & Halmi, 1999).

HEALTH ISSUES OF TRANSGENDER COMMUNITIES

Transgender individuals remain the most misunderstood and underrepresented members of the LGBT communities. Transgender patients also have unique health care needs. Unlike nontransgender lesbian, gay, and bisexual people, transgender people may want or need medical intervention in order to obtain hormone therapy or sex reassignment surgery.

One of the biggest barriers to obtaining adequate health care services for transgender people is lack of health insurance or having health insurance without allowable "trans" health services. There are very high rates of unemployment and poverty in transgender communities, especially in transgender communities that are racially and ethnically diverse (Amnesty International USA, 2007). As a result, transgender people often do not see health care providers regularly to screen for cancers, high blood pressure, sexually transmitted diseases, and other illnesses. Transgender health services (including hormone therapy and sex reassignment surgery) are rarely covered by insurance providers. These procedures are very expensive and put transgender people in the difficult position of trying to obtain them illegally when they are not affordable (National Coalition for LGBT Health, 2004).

In order to receive services from a lot of health care providers, transgender patients must admit to having gender identity disorder (GID). This presents problems on several levels. First, it requires that transgender people admit they have a psychiatric disorder, as GID is still classified as such by the American Psychiatric Association. Also, there is a rather lengthy evaluation system that accompanies diagnoses of GID. Therefore transgender people must often wait for extended periods of time before they can obtain services. Mental health providers then make decisions about who can obtain hormone therapy and sex reassignment surgery and who cannot. This lengthy process and fear of being judged by mental health care providers often puts transgender people in the position of either not taking advantage of services at all or going to the street to obtain hormones or surgery.

Often the lack of access to health care options results in the practice of dangerous procedures. Many transgender women participate in injection silicone use (ISU for short). This means that they inject silicone (or have someone else inject it) directly into their breasts. Studies in cities across the United States have indicated that as many as 33 percent of transgender women have reported participating in ISU (Reback, Simon, Bemis, & Gatson, 2001). There are several health risks associated with ISU, including the spread of viral infections (such as HIV and hepatitis). It can also lead to systemic illness and disfigurement and even death in some cases. The use of hormones acquired illegally on the street is also extremely dangerous (National Coalition for LGBT Health, 2004).

Along with not obtaining health care because of lack of insurance or not wanting to be diagnosed with GID, there are other reasons why transgender people do not obtain health care. Health educators and professionals may be transphobic in addition to homophobic. Additionally, not all transgender people are aware of the health needs that are important for them to address, given their identity and whether or not they have used hormones or had surgery. (Table 12.2 summarizes transgender health needs.)

HEALTH ISSUES OF LGBT RACIALLY AND ETHNICALLY DIVERSE COMMUNITIES

In this section we will focus primarily on African American and Latino (or Hispanic) lesbian, gay, bisexual, and transgender people. Although these ethnic and racial groups do not represent all of the LGBT racially and ethnically diverse communities, the majority of the research in this field is focused on African Americans and Latinos. Fourteen percent of the U.S. population is Latino and 13 percent is African American (Berstein, 2007). If we use the more conservative estimate of the LGBT percentage in a community and say that 5 percent of ethnic and racial populations are LGBT, this could translate to as many as 2 million Latino and 2 million African American people who are LGBT (National Coalition for LGBT Health & Boston Public Health Commission, 2002).

Racially and ethnically diverse LGBT people have some significant cultural factors contributing to their identity. Cultural factors influencing identity for African

TABLE 12.2. **Cultural Alert: Transgender Health Needs.**

	Always Applicable	Prehormones Presurgery	After Hormones	After Surgery
Male to female (MTF)	Prostate exams Sigmoidoscopies	Routine testicular exams	Breast exams Mammograms	Clinical vaginal exams
Female to male (FTM)	Breast exams Mammograms Sigmoidoscopies	Uterus and ovaries exams	Blood pressure, cholesterol Heart health	Pap smear Breast exams (though not as often) Clinical penis exams

Source: Long, 2005. Reprinted with permission of the author.

American and Latino LGBT individuals include the importance of family and of traditional gender roles, conservative religious values, and widespread homophobia (Rosario, Scrimshaw, & Hunter, 2004). All of these factors would influence the formation of an LGBT identity and the coming out process.

Another issue that primarily affects African American and Latino LGBT communities is the interaction between homophobia and racism. A case study in Boston found that African American and Latino LGBT people often encounter several forms of oppression and discrimination (National Coalition for LGBT Health & Boston Public Health Commission, 2002). The study addresses the specific combination of homophobia and racism and how it can lead to negative outcomes, such as violence. For example, in the year 2000, a disproportionate number of victims of reported LGBT hate crimes were African American or Latino.

African American and Latino LGBT people face unique issues in the health care system. Research has shown that they are more likely to have poor health than other LGBT populations (Kirby, 2001; Lisotta, 2004). A significant reason for this gap is lack of access to health care. A case study conducted in Washington, D.C., found that 47 percent of African American transgender people were without health insurance (Xavier, 2000). Additionally, Latina and non-Hispanic white lesbian and bisexual women in Jamaica Plain, Massachusetts, about twice as likely to be without health insurance as their heterosexual female counterparts (National Coalition for LGBT Health & Boston Public Health Commission, 2002). Health care costs are not affordable. Not having health insurance hinders access to preventive health care services and means that LGBT individuals do not see health care providers regularly.

Other issues that affect African American and Latino LGBT communities are cardiovascular diseases, diabetes risks, and HIV/AIDS. According to a Los Angeles–based case study, African American and Latina lesbian and bisexual women are much more likely to be overweight than heterosexual African American and heterosexual Latina women. Obesity can lead to cardiovascular disease and diabetes. Additionally, women who are overweight or obese are less likely to be tested for breast and cervical cancer by their primary health care provider (Mays, Yancey, Cochran, Weber, & Fielding, 2002). HIV and AIDS affect racially and ethnically diverse LGBT people at a disproportionate rate as well. According to a seven-city survey, the new HIV infection rate is substantially higher for young African American gay and bisexual men than it is for their gay and bisexual white and Latino counterparts (Centers for Disease Control and Prevention, 2000). In another study conducted in San Francisco, 63 percent of African American male-to-female transgender participants were living with HIV (Clements-Nolle, Guzman, & Katz, 2001).

INCREASING CULTURAL SENSITIVITY TOWARD THE LGBT COMMUNITY

Initially, health educators may be invited to believe that the health care needs of the LGBT community are no different from those of the general population. Indeed, everyone needs age-appropriate health education and treatment as well as information about preventive measures for his or her health. However, the LGBT community has specific health needs that should be recognized and addressed. Studies show that LGBT populations, in addition to having the same basic health needs as the general population, experience health disparities and barriers related to the expression of their sexual orientation or their gender identity (Kaiser Permanente National Diversity Department, 2004). Many avoid or delay care or receive inappropriate or inferior care as a result of perceived or real homophobia and discrimination on the part of health professionals and institutions.

In spite of the many differences that separate them, the members of the overall LGBT community have similar experiences of discrimination, rejection, shame, and violence. There are numerous ways that health educators and health professionals can reduce homophobia and heterosexism in their daily work. It is vital that all of us who are health educators and practitioners strive to provide a welcoming, supportive, and inclusive environment as we address health promotion and disease prevention for the LGBT community.

We must *address our own attitudes and behaviors* about gender identity and sexual orientation (Matthews, Lorah, & Fenton, 2006). Failure to be authentically affirming and accepting will invite the continuation of shame among this community. Consider the health educator who says things intended to show that he is affirming and accepting but who also immediately increases the physical space between himself and his LGBT client. LGBT people will readily read such negative nonverbal and verbal cues and will feel validated in their distrust of the health educators and professionals.

We need to provide a *physically welcoming environment.* Members of the LGBT community will immediately scan our environments for clues that invite them to feel comfortable with a health care experience. Simple symbols such as rainbow flags, pink triangles, and LGBT–friendly stickers can be placed in offices, restrooms, or waiting areas (Dinkel, 2005). In addition, health educators and health professionals should consider using posters or brochures that display racially and ethnically diverse same-sex couples or transgender people. We can visibly display and provide a written copy of a nondiscrimination policy that addresses gender identity and expression along with age, race, ethnicity, physical ability or attributes, religion, and sexual orientation (GLMA, 2006). And we can advocate for gender-inclusive (unisex) restrooms, as they are safer and more comfortable for transgender people than single-sex restrooms.

We should use *culturally sensitive language.* Forms, assessments, and conversation should employ inclusive choices such as *partner* instead of *spouse* and *relationship status* instead of *marital status.* Adding the option of *transgender,* with selections for *male-to-female* and *female-to-male,* will invite immediate acceptance. We can use the same language that the transgender person does to describe self, sexual partners, relationships, and identity. Remember that an individual may not define herself through a sexual orientation label, yet she may have sex with persons of the same sex or gender or with persons of both sexes. For example, men who have sex with men, especially African American and Latino men, may identify as heterosexual and have both female and male partners (GLMA, 2006).

We should *not make assumptions* about past, current, or future sexual behaviors. The fact that a woman identifies as a lesbian does not mean that she has never had a male sexual partner or never had children. We should include questions on violence as part of the screening or intake process. LGBT people are not exempt from intimate partner and other domestic violence. However, the circumstances surrounding the violence and the process of helping the victim can be different because of LGBT individuals' fears of being "outed" to employers and/or family.

Health educators and other health professionals are encouraged to participate in LGBT cultural competence training. The Sexuality Information and Education Council of the United States (SIECUS) works with the Centers for Disease Control and Prevention's Division of Adolescent and School Health to provide one-day training ("culturally competent HIV prevention and sexuality education") for health educators. SIECUS also offers free self-guided training modules to assist health educators in exploring culture and sexual health. (These modules are available on the SIECUS Web site at http://www.siecus.org/school/trainingModules/index.html.)

All of us can best achieve competence in this area by acquiring and applying skills in both simulated and actual settings. Training should be skill based and "practiced" with actual LGBT people. Empathy training could be a part of the work, so that we all come to better understand the stigmas and discrimination faced by LGBT people.

Finally, we can increase our knowledge of *gay-affirming resources* in our communities. Find and visit the resources that exist in your community.

CONCLUSION

The *American Journal of Public Health* devoted its June 2001 (Vol. 91, No. 6) issue to LGBT health issues. The demand was so great that this issue sold out—the first time in the journal's history that an issue had sold out With this increase in knowledge, have health educators and the health care profession responded with more culturally sensitive care for LGBT people? The experiences of the majority of LGBT people and scholarly evidence indicate that we are not yet offering our services in the most competent or culturally sensitive way. LGBT people are in our families, communities, and workplaces and are valuable and contributing members of our society. As health educators it is imperative that we be nonjudgmental and strive to develop culturally sensitive skills to address the health issues of the LGBT community effectively and assist in eliminating the health disparities experienced by this underserved culture. We are one human family, and our charge as human beings is to help other human beings.

POINTS TO REMEMBER

- Health educators and health professionals should acknowledge the LGBT community as a culture, one with health disparities similar to those associated with race, ethnicity, socioeconomic status, and gender.

- Health educators and health professionals should recognize and accept that there are more differences among the individuals within a culture than there are between cultures. For example, there is more diversity within the LGBT community than there is difference between the LGBT community and other cultural identity groups.

- When health educators and health care professionals deliver services to the LGBT community, it is important for them to remember that LGBT individuals may have experienced real or perceived homophobia and discrimination from others, including people in the field of health.

- Health educators and health professionals are encouraged to look for ways to provide a welcoming environment for the LGBT community. This includes, but is not limited to, using culturally sensitive language, not making assumptions, and respecting self-identity. For example, behavior does not always dictate identity. Men who have sex with men may not identify as gay.

- It is vital that health educators and health professionals explore their own homophobia, transphobia, and heterosexism, and consider participating in trainings and workshops to increase their awareness and skills.

CASE STUDY

Jason is a 25-year-old female-to-male transsexual. Jason came out as transgender and began living as a male at age 22. For the past six months, Jason has been taking transgender hormone therapy (THT). Jason's insurance does not cover this hormone therapy, and he is currently saving out of pocket for "top" surgery (many female-to-male transgender individuals choose breast removal only, with no vaginal surgery). Jason has continued needs for annual gynecological exams and is concerned about selecting a health care provider because he needs someone who will be sensitive to his transitioning needs. The hormones have successfully produced significant facial hair, and Jason can now readily "pass" as a male. Please discuss the following questions (refer to Table 12.2 as needed when considering Jason's health care needs).

1. What are some real fears that Jason might have about making this appointment?

2. What major concerns should Jason address before making this appointment with a gynecologist?

3. What could a gynecologist do to make his or her office a more physically welcoming environment for Jason?

4. What culturally sensitive language could the gynecologist and the office staff use to make Jason more comfortable?

5. What assumptions might Jason find that the professionals at this office are making about him and his current or past health behaviors?

6. What resources or referrals might be appropriate for Jason?

KEY TERMS

Bisexual	LGBT
Coming out	Queer
Gay	Sexual identity
Gender identity	Sexual orientation
Heterosexism	Transgender
Homophobia	Transphobia
Homosexual	Transsexual
Lesbian	

REFERENCES

Aaron, D. J., Markovic, N., Danielson, M. E., Honnold, J. A., Janosky, J. E., & Schmidt, N. J. (2001). Behavioral risk factors for disease and preventive health practices among lesbians. *American Journal of Public Health, 91*(6), 972–975.

Amnesty International USA. (2007). *Transgender day of remembrance.* Retrieved March 30, 2007, from http://www.amnestyusa.org/outfront/transgender_remembrance.html.

Anderson, J. D. (1997). Supporting the invisible minority. *Educational Leadership, 54*, 65–68.

Baernstein, A., Bostwich, W. B., Carrick, K. R., Dunn, P. M., Goodman, K. W., Hughes, T. L., et al. (2006). In M. D. Shankle (Ed.), *The handbook of lesbian gay, bisexual, and transgender public health: A practitioner's guide to service* (pp. 87–117). New York: Harrington Park Press.

Berstein, R. (2007). Minority population tops 100 million. Retrieved February 15, 2007, from http://www.census.gov/Press-Release/www/releases/archives/population/010048.html.

Braun, D. L., Sunday, S. R., Huang, A., & Halmi, K. A. (1999). Sexual orientation and eating psychopathology: The role of masculinity and femininity. *International Journal of Eating Disorders, 25*(4), 415–423.

Campinha-Bacote, J. (1999). A model and instrument for addressing cultural competence in health care. *Journal of Nursing Education, 38*(5), 203–207.

Centers for Disease Control and Prevention. (2000). HIV incidence among young men who have sex with men–Seven U.S. cities, 1994–2000. *Morbidity and Mortality Weekly Report, 50*(21), 440–444.

Clements-Nolle, K., Guzman, R., & Katz, M. (2001). HIV prevalence, risk behaviors, health care use, and mental health status of transgender persons: Implications for public health intervention. *American Journal of Public Health, 91*(6), 915–921.

Dean, L., Meyer, I. H., Robinson, K., Sell, R. L., Sember, R., Vincent, M. B., et al. (2000). *Lesbian, gay, bisexual, and transgender health: Findings and concerns* (GLMA-Columbia University white paper). Retrieved January 30, 2008, from http://www.glma.org/_data/n_0001/resources/live/Columbia-GLMA%20White%20Paper.pdf.

Dinkel, S. (2005). Providing culturally competent care to lesbians. *The Kansas Nurse, 80,* 10–12.

Ferris, J. (2006). *The nomenclature of the community: An activist's perspective.* In M. D. Shankle (Ed.), *The handbook of lesbian gay, bisexual, and transgender public health: A practitioner's guide to service* (pp. 3–10). New York: Harrington Park Press.

Garofalo, R., & Katz, K. E. (2001). Healthcare issues of gay and lesbian youth. *Current Opinions in Pediatrics, 13*, 298–302.

Gay and Lesbian Medical Association. (2006). *Guidelines for care of lesbian, gay, bisexual, and transgender patients.* Retrieved September 9, 2006, from http://ce54.citysoft.com/_data/n_0001/resources/live/GLMA%20guidelines%202006%20FINAL.pdf.

Gay and Lesbian Medical Association et al. (2001). *Healthy people 2010 companion document for lesbian, gay, bisexual, and transgender (LGBT) health.* San Francisco: Gay and Lesbian Medical Association.

Ginsberg, K. R., Winn, R., Rudy, B. J., Crawford, J., Zhao, H., & Schwarz, D. R. (2002). How to reach sexual minority youth in the health care setting: The teens offer guidance. *Journal of Adolescent Health, 31,* 407–416.

Hunter, J., Cohall, A. T., Mallon, G. P., Moyer, M. B., & Riddle, J. P. (2006). Health care delivery and public health related to LGBT youth and young adults. In M. D. Shankle (Ed.), *The handbook of lesbian gay, bisexual, and transgender public health: A practitioner's guide to service* (pp. 221–245). New York: Harrington Park Press.

Kaiser Permanente National Diversity Department. (2004). *A provider's handbook on culturally competent care: Lesbian, gay, bisexual, and transgender populations* (2nd ed.). Oakland, CA: Kaiser Permanente.

Kirby, D. (2001, March 27). Coming to America to be gay—Migration to United States of gay Latin Americans. *The Advocate,* p. 29. Retrieved March 30, 2007, from http://find.galegroup.com/ips/infomark.do?&contentSet=IAC-Documents&type=retrieve&tabID=T003&prodId=IPS&docId=A72050601&source=gale&userGroupName=lom_emichu&version=1.0.

Larson, K. L. (2003). Physical educators teaching health. *Journal of School Health, 73*(8), 291–292.

Lindley, L., & Reininger, B. (2001). Support for instruction about homosexuality in South Carolina public schools. *Journal of School Health, 71*(1), 17–22.

Lisotta, C. (2004). Homophobia of all hues. *The Nation, 278*(19), 15–17.

Lock, J., & Steiner, H. (1999). Gay, lesbian and bisexual youth risks for emotional, physical and social problems: Results from a community-based survey. *Journal of American Academic Child and Adolescent Psychiatry, 38*(3), 297–304.

Long, E. (2005). Transgender: A health transition. *4 Our Health, 3*(1), 2.

Matthews, A. K., Brandenburgh, D. L., Johnson, T., & Hughes, T. L. (2004). Correlates of underutilization of gynecological cancer screening among lesbian and heterosexual women. *Preventive Medicine, 28,* 105–113.

Matthews, C. R., Lorah, P., & Fenton, J. (2006). Treatment experiences of gays and lesbians in recovery from addiction: A qualitative inquiry. *Journal of Mental Health Counseling, 28,* 111–122.

Mays, V. M., Yancey, A. K., Cochran, S. D., Weber, M., & Fielding, J. E. (2002). Heterogeneity of health disparities among African American, Hispanic, and Asian American women: Unrecognized influences of sexual orientation. *American Journal of Public Health, 92*(4), 632–639.

Meyer, C., Blissett, J., & Oldfield, C. (2001). Sexual orientation and eating psychopathology: The role of masculinity and femininity. *International Journal of Eating Disorders, 29*(3), 314–318.

Meyer, I. H. (2001). Why lesbian, gay, bisexual and transgender public health? *American Journal of Public Health, 91,* 856–859.

National Coalition Against Domestic Violence. (2003, March 24). *Domestic violence among the gay, lesbian, bisexual and transgender communities.* Retrieved September 15, 2006, http://www.ncadv.org.

National Coalition for LGBT Health. (2004, August). *An overview of U.S. trans health priorities: A report by the Eliminating Disparities Working Group.* Retrieved September 30, 2006, from http://www.spectrumwny.org/info/HealthPriorities.pdf.

National Coalition for LGBT Health & Boston Public Health Commission. (2002, June 28). *Double jeopardy: How racism and homophobia impact the health of black and Latino lesbian, gay, bisexual, and transgender (LGBT) communities.* Retrieved September 21, 2006, from http://www.lgbthealth.net/downloads/research/BPHCLGBTLatinoBlackHealthDispar.doc.

Partnership for a Drug-Free America. (2006). *Crystal meth.* Retrieved September 28, 2006, from http://www.drugfree.org/Portal/drug_guide/Crystal_Meth.

Peterkin, A., & Risdon, C. (2003). *Caring for lesbian and gay people: A clinical guide.* Toronto: University of Toronto Press.

Public Health—Seattle and King County. (2004, March 22). *Gay, lesbian, bisexual, transgender health: Safety and hate crimes.* Retrieved August 20, 2006, from http://www.metrokc.gov/health/glbt/hatecrime.htm.

Reback, C., Simon, P., Bemis, C., & Gatson, B. (2001). *The Los Angeles transgender health study: Community report.* Los Angeles: University of California, Los Angeles.

Reuters. (2004, June 7). *Crystal meth linked to AIDS in New York.* Retrieved September 29, 2006, from http://www.msnbc.msn.com/id/5158153.

Rienzo, A. A., Button, J. W., Sheu, J., & Li, Y. (2006). The politics of sexual orientation issues in American schools. *Journal of School Health, 76*(3), 93–97.

Rosario, M., Scrimshaw, E. W., & Hunter, J. (2004). Ethnic/racial differences in the coming-out process of lesbian, gay, and bisexual youths: A comparison of sexual identity development over time. *Cultural Diversity and Ethnic Minority Psychology, 10,* 215–228.

Ryan, H., Wortley, P. M., Easton, A., Pederson, L., & Greenwood, G. (2001). Smoking among lesbians, gays, and bisexuals: A review of the literature. *American Journal of Preventive Medicine, 21*(2), 142–149.

Shankle, M. D. (Ed.). (2006). *The handbook of lesbian, gay, bisexual and transgender public health: A practitioner's guide to service.* New York: Harrington Park Press.

Smith, L. S. (1998). Concept analysis: Cultural competence. *Journal of Cultural Diversity, 5,* 4–10.

Telljohann, S. K., Price, J. H., Poureslami, M., & Easton, A. (1995). Teaching about sexual orientation by secondary health teachers. *Journal of School Health, 65*(1), 18–22.

U.S. Department of Health and Human Services, Office on Women's Health. (2000, November 2). *Lesbian health fact sheet.* Retrieved September 28, 2006, from http://www.4woman.gov/owh/pub/factsheets/lesbian1.pdf.

U.S. Department of Health and Human Services, Substance Abuse and Mental Health Services Administration. (2000). *A provider's introduction to substance abuse treatment for lesbian, gay, bisexual, and transgender individuals.* Rockville, MD: Author.

Woodiel, K., Angermeier-Howard, L., & Hobson, S. (2003). School safety for all: Using the coordinated school health program to increase safety for LGBTQ students. *American Journal of Health Studies, 18*(2/3), 98–103.

Xavier, J. M. (2000). *The Washington transgender needs assessment survey: Final report for phase two.* Washington, DC: Administration for HIV/ AIDS of the District of Columbia.

CHAPTER

13

CULTURAL COMPETENCE AND HEALTH EDUCATION

Challenges and Opportunities for the Twenty-First Century

RAFFY R. LUQUIS
MIGUEL A. PÉREZ

LEARNING OBJECTIVES

After completing this chapter, you will be able to

- Understand and explain the importance of cultural and linguistic competence in health promotion and education.

- Discuss ways to integrate cultural and linguistic competence into health promotion and education programs.

- Discuss strategies to promote cultural and linguistic competence in order to work effectively with the individuals or communities served by your organization and to address their health needs successfully.

231

INTRODUCTION

As described in the first chapter of this book, the U.S. population is becoming more racially and ethnically diverse. In addition, demographic estimates suggest that U.S. racial and ethnic populations, such as the populations of African Americans, Hispanics, Asians, Pacific Islanders, and others, will continue to grow in the next few decades. Consequently, it is estimated that by 2050 the percentage of non-Hispanic whites will be only half of the total U.S. population (U.S. Census Bureau, 2004). As proposed throughout this book, and especially Chapter One, this increasing racial and ethnic diversification of the U.S. population is making it essential to incorporate the concept of cultural and linguistic competence into every aspect of the planning, implementation, and evaluation processes of health education and promotion programs (Luquis & Pérez, 2005, 2006; Luquis, Pérez, & Young, 2006; Marín et al., 1994; Pérez, Gonzalez, & Pinzon-Pérez, 2006). Moreover, leading public health organizations, including the Institute of Medicine (2004) and the Office of Minority Health (2000), have advocated for a workforce capable of delivering culturally competent and linguistically appropriate services to an ever more diverse U.S. population.

What do these changes have to do with health educators? The field of health education is predicated on the belief that providing health information and skills through planned learning experiences will enable the individuals, groups, and communities receiving that education to make informed choices that will assist them in making quality health decisions and attaining their optimal health status. Similarly, health promotion is based on the belief that providing a combination of educational, political, environmental, regulatory, and organizational mechanisms can support actions and conditions of living conducive to the health of individuals, groups, and communities. However, these foundational beliefs often fail to address the reality that given the current diversity of the population in the United States, health education and promotion interventions found to be effective in one racial or ethnic group might not be equally effective with another group. Thus, in order to be effective, health education and prevention strategies must address each group's unique culture, experiences, language, age, gender, and sexual orientation and be culturally and linguistically appropriate.

The purpose of this chapter is to provide some final thoughts on the importance of cultural and linguistic competence and to discuss how to integrate these concepts into health education and health promotion programs. This chapter will also discuss some strategies for promoting cultural and linguistic competence that can assist health education specialists in working with individuals or communities effectively and addressing their health needs successfully. Finally, this chapter will discuss standards to promote cultural and linguistic competence in health education.

UNDERSTANDING THE NEED FOR CULTURAL AND LINGUISTIC COMPETENCE

The professional literature discussed in the previous chapters reveals that nonwhites in the United States are less likely than their non-Hispanic white counterparts to have access to health insurance and to take advantage of preventive services, and are also more likely to postpone obtaining health services until it may be too late for effective treatment. These differences have been called *health disparities.* Moreover, the need to decrease health disparities has been documented in the professional literature. For example, the Racial and Ethnic Approach to Community Health (REACH) project found that members of minority populations were more likely to report being in a condition of poor health and were less likely to seek health care than non-Hispanic whites were (Centers for Disease Control and Prevention [CDC], n.d.). Special efforts are needed to reach underrepresented groups that have traditionally had lower levels of education and income and that are more likely to be poor than members of the white population are.

One of the two goals presented in *Healthy People 2010* is the elimination of health disparities among the different segments of the population, including disparities that occur by race or ethnicity, gender, disability, or sexual orientation, among others (U.S. Department of Health and Human Services [USDHHS], 2000). *Healthy People 2010* and its health indicators provide a clear mandate for improving the health status of underrepresented groups in the United States.

Although several studies have provided excellent suggestions for improving the health status of underrepresented groups, *Healthy People 2010* is the first document of the new millennium that challenges us to better incorporate prevention and treatment into health promotion and health care services and thereby not only improve the health status of the U.S. population but also help to decrease soaring health care costs.

Nonetheless, the elimination of health disparities is a challenge as there is no one single cause of the problem (Health Resources and Services Administration [HRSA], HIV/AIDS Bureau, 2002). Health disparities are caused by a myriad of factors including lack of health information, lack of health insurance, individuals' beliefs and attitudes about accessing health care, a shortage of diverse health care providers, comorbidity involving other serious health problems such as addiction and mental illness, and poverty (HRSA, HIV/AIDS Bureau, 2002). There are, however, also several broadly applicable and unifying factors that have been identified in the literature, including income, race or ethnicity, and language competence. An overwhelming amount of evidence suggests that both cultural and linguistic competence could play a significant role in decreasing health disparities. For example, the lack of background information about different ethnic groups, the lack of culturally competent health care providers and health educators, the small percentage of racial and ethnic minorities working in the health care and health promotion fields, the inadequate number of health professionals with skills for working with diverse groups, and the fact that current health care services are culturally biased toward the majority population have all been identified as detrimental factors for the health status of nonwhite populations (Brach & Fraser, 2000; USDHHS, 2003; Diversity Rx., 2003; King, Sims, & Osher, n.d.). Thus culturally and linguistically competent health interventions have been described as an approach to achieve the second goal of *Healthy People 2010* (Denboba, Bragdon, Epstein, Garthright, & Goldman, 1998; National Center for Cultural Competence [NCCC], 2002), to eliminate health disparities among segments of the population (USDHHS, 2000).

Similarly, the National Center for Cultural Competence (NCCC) (Cohen & Goode, 1999, revised by Goode & Dunne, 2003) has suggested a variety of reasons why cultural and linguistic competence are required at the health provider and patient level. For example, people's beliefs about health and their perceptions of disease and illnesses vary by their cultural groups. Individuals' cultural groups also influence their help-seeking behaviors and their attitudes toward health care providers, and play a role in their use of traditional and complementary healing practices. Exhibit 13.1 displays six of the salient reasons identified by the NCCC that highlight the critical importance of cultural and linguistic competence in health care.

The recommendations listed in Exhibit 13.1 for incorporating cultural and linguistic competence into health care practice apply to health educators just as much as they do health care providers. Our work is an essential ally of health care services, and if

---

EXHIBIT 13.1. Six Reasons Why We Need Cultural and Linguistic Competence in Health Care and Health Education.

1. *To respond to current and projected demographic changes in the United States.* As stated previously in this chapter and throughout this book, significant population increases are occurring among racially, ethnically, and culturally and linguistically diverse groups in the United States. Health care organizations and programs must implement systemic change in order to meet the health needs of this diverse population.

2. *To eliminate long-standing disparities in the health status of people of diverse racial, ethnic, and cultural backgrounds.* Although there has been progress in the overall health of the nation, African Americans, Hispanics, Native Americans, Asians, and Pacific Islanders still have poorer health in many areas than the U.S. population as a whole does. In response to these disparities the federal government has aggressively targeted and committed resources to six areas: cancer, cardiovascular disease, infant mortality, diabetes, HIV/AIDS, and child and adult immunizations (see CDC, n.d.).

3. *To improve the quality of services and health outcomes.* The delivery of accessible, effective, cost-efficient, and high-quality primary health care calls for health care practitioners who have a deep understanding of the sociocultural backgrounds of their patients and their patients' families and who are also aware of the environments in which their patients live. Culturally and linguistically competent health services facilitate encounters with more favorable outcomes, enhance the potential for a more rewarding interpersonal experience, and increase the satisfaction of the individual receiving health care and disease prevention services.

4. *To meet legislative, regulatory, and accreditation mandates.* Title VI of the Civil Rights Act of 1964 mandates that "no person in the U.S. shall, on ground of race, color, or

national origin, be excluded from participation in, be denied the benefits of, or be subjected to discrimination under any program or activity receiving Federal financial assistance." In addition, in 2000, the federal Office of Minority Health published the final national standards on culturally and linguistically appropriate services (CLAS) in health care. Accreditation bodies such as the Joint Commission on Accreditation of Healthcare Organizations, the Liaison Committee on Medical Education, and the National Committee for Quality Assurance support these standards.

5. *To gain a competitive edge in the marketplace.* The current health care environment is concerned with issues such as health care cost and quality, the cost effectiveness of services delivery, and the marketing of such services. Health care organizations that incorporate culturally competent policies, structures, and practices into their services for people with diverse ethnic, racial, cultural, and linguistic backgrounds are well positioned in the current marketplace and for the future as the diversity of the U.S. population continues to increase.

6. *To decrease the likelihood of liability or malpractice claims.* Lack of awareness about racial, ethnicity, and cultural differences and failure to provide culturally and linguistically appropriate services may result in liability under tort principles in several ways. For example, health care organizations might potentially be challenged with claims that the failure on the part of their health care providers to understand and appropriately respond to the beliefs, practices, and behaviors of patients breaches professional standards of care. In addition, the practices of offering effective communication in languages other than English and addressing the communication needs of persons with disabilities and those with low or no literacy have been shown to be effective in reducing the likelihood of malpractice claims.

Source: Adapted from Cohen & Goode, 1999, revised by Goode & Dunne, 2003.

that work is to fulfill all its functions we must join forces with health care and allied health professionals to eliminate health disparities and to accomplish the goals enumerated in *Healthy People 2010.*

ACHIEVING CULTURAL COMPETENCE

To become culturally competent, health educators and health promoters need to understand the complexity of cultural competence. Recall that *cultural competence* is defined by the 2000 Joint Committee on Health Education and Promotion Terminology as "the ability of an individual to understand and respect values, attitudes, beliefs, and mores that differ across cultures, and to consider and respond appropriately to these differences in planning, implementing, and evaluating health education and promotion programs and interventions" (p. 5). Although this definition provides a basic understanding of the concept, it does not go beyond defining the capability of the individual to work with the existing racially, ethnically, and culturally diverse population. Some of the chapter authors for this book have provided other definitions of cultural competence. Here is another definition, from Cross, Bazron, Dennis, and Isaacs (1989), who define cultural competence as "a set of congruent behaviors, attitudes, and policies that come together in a system, agency, or among professionals that enables this system, agency, or those professionals to work effectively in cross-cultural situations" (p. 4). Thus, in keeping with these definitions, Luquis and Pérez (2003) have suggested that in the field of health education we define cultural competence as "the capacity of an individual and organization to understand, behave, and respect the values, attitudes, and beliefs of different cultural groups, and to incorporate these differences in the development and implementation and evaluation of policies and health education and promotion programs" (p. 113).

Health educators must also realize that the process of becoming culturally competent does not happen overnight; it is a lifelong journey. At the organizational level the process of acquiring cultural competence requires a comprehensive and coordinated plan that specifies interventions at many levels: policymaking, infrastructure building, program administration and evaluation, the delivery of service and enabling support, and the individual (Goode & Sockalingam, 2000). At the personal level, the individual must examine both his or her own cultural values and his or her awareness and acceptance of the cultural values and beliefs among other diverse groups. In addition the individual must make a commitment to honor and respect the beliefs and values of other cultures. Working toward cultural competence must also include acquiring the ability to develop, adapt, and implement practices and skills that fit the cultural context of the individuals being served. Therefore, given the cultural diversity of the United States, developing cultural competence must be seen as a complex process rather than an end point, and it is unrealistic for an organization to expect to serve all cultural groups in a competent manner; rather, it must create an environment that supports an ongoing process of becoming culturally competent.

ACQUIRING LINGUISTIC COMPETENCE

Health educators need to understand the intricacy of linguistic competence in order to become linguistically competent. The NCCC (2006) defines *linguistic competence* as "the capacity of an organization and its personnel to communicate effectively, and convey information in a manner that is easily understood by diverse audiences including persons of limited English proficiency, those who have low literacy skills or are not literate, and individuals with disabilities" (para. 9).

Linguistic competence includes, but is not limited to, the use of (1) "bilingual/bicultural or multilingual/multicultural staff"; (2) "cross-cultural communication approaches"; (3) "foreign language interpretation services including distance technologies"; (4) "sign language interpretation services"; (5) "multilingual telecommunication systems"; (6) "print materials in easy to read, low literacy, picture and symbol formats"; (7) "materials in alternative formats (e.g., audiotape, Braille, enlarged print)"; (8) "materials developed and tested for specific cultural, ethnic and linguistic groups"; (9) "translation services" (for legally binding documents and educational materials, for example); and (10) "ethnic media in languages other than English" (for example, television, radio, and newspapers) (NCCC, 2006). Linguistic competence requires that the individual and the organization have the capacity to respond effectively to the health literacy needs of the populations served. The organization must have policies, structures, practices, procedures, and dedicated resources that support this capacity.

SUPPORTING CULTURAL AND LINGUISTIC COMPETENCE IN HEALTH EDUCATION

In 1994, the American Association for Health Education (AAHE) became a leader in promoting cultural sensitivity among health educators when it published *Cultural Awareness and Sensitivity: Guidelines for Health Educators.* Although the recommendations released at that time were accurate and still serve as a starting point for working with diverse groups, today's health educators need to be more than just sensitive to cultural groups; they need to be culturally and linguistically competent as well. The approach to the cultural competence process has continued to evolve, and in 2006, AAHE published an official position paper on cultural competency and health education (this document is reproduced at the end of this book, in Appendix A). This position statement acknowledges the fact that due to cultural differences, health promotion interventions found to be effective in one ethnic or racial group cannot be assumed to be equally effective with another group. Prevention strategies must be culturally appropriate and group-specific if they are to effectively serve each of various underserved populations. Finally, AAHE's continuing efforts to address cultural competence and diversity efforts in the field of health education have been a motive force behind this book.

In 2002, the Society for Public Health Education published "SOPHE's Resolution to Eliminate Racial and Ethnic Health Disparities: Process and Recommendations for Accountability," which not only identified the health disparity problem but also explored lessons learned and offered recommendations for decreasing health disparities. In 2005, SOPHE invited some eighty-five researchers and practitioners to its Inaugural Summit to Eliminate Racial and Ethnic Health Disparities, with the purpose of developing a research agenda focused on eliminating health disparities by promoting research dealing with cultural issues (Airhihenbuwa, 2006). Moreover, SOPHE's annual meeting in 2007 focused on the elimination of health disparities through the collaboration of traditional and nontraditional partners. Similarly, the American Public Health Association (APHA) has also played a role in addressing cultural competence and health disparities through a series of sessions at APHA annual meetings, through the publication of books addressing these topics, and through promoting and supporting special interest groups and caucuses.

Although the field of health education has made some progress in addressing cultural and linguistic competence, the fields of medicine, nursing, and social work have taken active steps to address health care disparities and to provide culturally appropriate services (Dana, Dayger Behn, & Gonwa, 1992; Goode, Jones, & Mason, 2002). In addition, several models for addressing cultural competence in the field of health care, as described in previous chapters, have been developed in the last two decades (Purnell & Paulanka, 2003; Campinha-Bacote, 1998). However, the field of health education continues to lag behind in addressing cultural and linguistic competence for its people. To the knowledge of this chapter's authors, only two models have been developed to address the impact of culture in health promotion and disease prevention (Airhihenbuwa, 1995) and to address culture when planning health promotion programs for multicultural groups (Huff & Kline, 1999). In addition, as reflected throughout in the sources used in this book, materials related to cultural and linguistic competence and specifically developed for health educators are limited; most of the materials and textbooks used in health education to address cultural issues were written for other fields.

Moreover, our field's lack of focus on cultural issues is evident in the fact that none of the seminal documents in health education (for example, the report produced by the Role Delineation Project and the research agenda of the Society for Public Health Education) specifically address diversity in health education. The recent National Health Educator Competencies Update Project (CUP) (National Commission for Health Education Credentialing [NCHEC], Society for Public Health Education [SOPHE], and American Association for Health Education [AAHE], 2006) also fails to address cultural and linguistic competence as a core competence for health educators. In fact, the new CUP competency-based hierarchical model only briefly addresses (in four of the sub-competencies for entry-level health educators) diversity, cultural sensitivity, and the use of appropriate language (NCHEC, SOPHE, & AAHE, 2006). Thus the profession of health education would benefit from the development of discipline-specific standards that address culturally and linguistically competent health education programs. The development and implementation of cultural and linguistic competence standards across the health education field would encourage the development and implementation of culturally and linguistically appropriate health education programs (Luquis & Pérez, 2005, 2006; Luquis et al., 2006). Moreover, professional accreditation bodies such as the AAHE-National Council for Accreditation of Teacher Education, the Council on Education for Public Health, the SOPHE-AAHE Baccalaureate Program Approval Committee (SABPAC), and the National Commission for Health Education Credentialing should establish cultural and linguistic competence requirements to ensure standardized objectives and content areas throughout the professional preparation of health educators, health promoters, and public health professionals (Luquis et al., 2006).

STRATEGIES TO INCORPORATE CULTURAL AND LINGUISTIC COMPETENCE INTO HEALTH EDUCATION

In a multicultural and diverse society, health educators and other health professionals alike must strive to achieve cultural and linguistic competence and to incorporate cultural competence training into health education and promotion programs. In order to accomplish this goal, health educators do not need to become experts on every racial, ethnic, cultural, and diverse group residing in the United States, but they do need to be cognizant of differences that may affect their ability to reach target populations, and be proficient in using techniques to bridge cultural divisions (Luquis & Pérez, 2003). Health educators can begin to acquire these abilities by pursuing some of the following strategies.

First, health educators must learn to recognize the importance of culture and respect diversity. Culture influences many aspects of our lives, our families, and our communities, and also how we operate in society. Culture may be characterized by factors such as national origin; customs and traditions; length of residency in the United States; language; age; generation; gender and sexual orientation; religious beliefs; political beliefs; perceptions of family and community; perceptions of health, well-being, and disability; physical ability or limitations; socioeconomic status; educational level; geographical location; and family and household composition (USDHHS, 2003). Thus health educators need to understand all the factors surrounding culture and diversity and how they affect different groups' views of health and health education. For example, the REACH initiative has identified culture and history as one of its key principles in the development of effective community-based strategies and interventions (CDC, 2007).

Second, health educators should maintain a current profile of the cultural composition of their community of interest. One of the most important steps in the development of health education programs is performing the needs assessment. By maintaining a current profile of the population they serve (see the case study in Chapter One, for example), health educators will be prepared to identify the specific, culturally related needs of the community, such as learning style and education, language and interpreter services needed, level of health literacy, housing availability, and other health-related services. Information included in this community profile should be updated frequently, because given ongoing demographic changes, such data can change rapidly (USDHHS, 2003).

Third, health organizations, community-based organizations, schools, worksites, and other health-related agencies should provide ongoing cultural and linguistic competence training to health educators and other health staff. As stated throughout this book, the development of cultural and linguistic competence is an essential element in the professional preparation of health educators. In previous studies the chapter authors found that health educators who had attended cultural diversity training or education programs had achieved a higher level of cultural competence than those who had not attended such programs (Luquis & Pérez, 2005, 2006). This training should include basic cultural competence principles, concepts, terminology, and frameworks and also discussion about cultural values and traditions, family values, linguistics and literacy, help-seeking behavior, and cross-cultural outreach techniques and strategies, among other issues (USDHHS, 2003).

Fourth, health educators must involve *cultural brokers* from the targeted racial and ethnic groups during the development of health education programs. These cultural brokers can include community leaders and organizations representing diverse cultural groups. Collaborating with organizations and leaders who are knowledgeable about the community is the most effective way of gaining information about the community and assists health educators in assessing needs, creating community profiles, gaining trust with community members, and ensuring that strategies are culturally and linguistically appropriate (USDHHS, 2003). In addition, community leaders and key organizations can act as catalysts for change in the community, including forging unique partnerships, which may be essential in the development of effective health education and promotion programs (CDC, 2007).

Fifth, health educators must ensure that health education programs and services are culturally and linguistically appropriate. For example, language can be a major barrier in the provision of health promotion and disease prevention services. Health educators must ensure that written health information is translated into one or more languages, as appropriate for the community to be served, and must consider the literacy level of the target population when developing written materials (USDHHS, 2003). Chapter Eight discussed the importance of culturally and linguistically appropriate health communication and provided suggestions for addressing this issue in health promotion. Chapter Eight also pointed out that effective communication is foundational for the health education profession. Clearly, it is essential for health promotion specialists to learn to communicate across cultures, following the recommendations throughout this book.

Finally, health educators must continuously assess and evaluate the level of cultural and linguistic competence in programs that are under way. Self-assessment and process evaluation are keys to ensuring that health education programs are as effective as possible. Self-assessment will measure how health practitioners and health organizations are serving diverse populations (NCCC, 2006). The NCCC (2006) provides tools and processes for self-assessment that determine the level of cultural and linguistic competence of both the organization and the individuals working within it. Health educators should use these tools to ensure that they and their organizations are effective in serving the diverse population in the United States.

STANDARDS FOR CULTURAL AND LINGUISTIC COMPETENCE IN HEALTH EDUCATION

Cultural and linguistic competence in health education focuses on the key issues of a trained workforce and health education and prevention programs. The following standards are proposed for health educators. They are based on an extensive review of the professional literature, many years of work experience, and the authors' own experiences.

A Workforce Trained for Cultural and Linguistic Competence

■ Professional preparation programs in health education must offer cultural competence courses that transmit and discuss the history, traditions, values, belief systems, acculturation, and language of the major racial and ethnic groups in the United States.

As stated in Chapter Nine, professional preparation programs must include awareness-based, knowledge-based, and skills-based objectives in their required courses to prepare students to become culturally competent professionals.

■ Professional health educators must participate in continuing education designed to enhance their ability to become culturally and linguistically competent and to update the skills they learned in classroom training and in their work experience. In order to promote continued professional development among certified health educator specialists (CHESs), the NCHEC should set a minimum number of continuing education contact hours (CECHs) in the area of cultural and linguistic competence as part of the seventy-five CECHs needed over the five-year certification period.

Health Education Programs Designed for Cultural and Linguistic Competence

■ Health educators must conduct needs assessments that collect racial, ethnic, or cultural group–specific demographic characteristics, including age, gender, social class, education and literacy, religion and spirituality, and language preferences, among others, in order to properly assess the needs for health education programs and then to incorporate the local meaning and understanding of the health-illness continuum as well as the differences of symptom expression in the prevention messages that they deliver.

■ Health educators must use culturally and linguistically appropriate tools to collect data that will help them understand the attitudes and beliefs and also the educational, social, and economic conditions in the community and incorporate this information when developing, implementing, and evaluating health education and prevention programs.

■ Health educators must work with members of their target communities and make them integral members of the program team during the development, implementation, and evaluation of health education and prevention programs.

■ Health educators must use the targeted racial, ethnic, or cultural group's preferred language during the development, implementation, and evaluation of a health education and prevention program. Health educators should not use health education and prevention messages that are simply translated literally from the English language, as they may not convey the intended message in the group's preferred language.

■ Health educators must make it a priority to empower racial, ethnic, and cultural communities to ensure that health education and prevention programs are long-lasting and self-sustaining.

■ Health educators must ensure that health education and prevention programs are accessible, appropriate, and equitable to all racial, ethnic, and cultural groups in the community.

CONCLUSION

The increasing racial and ethnic diversification of the U.S. population is making it very clear that we need to incorporate the concept of cultural and linguistic competence into every aspect of the planning, implementation, and evaluation process of health education and promotion programs. It has also become clear that cultural and linguistic competence constitutes approaches that can help to eliminate health disparities among the diverse segments of the population. Throughout this book, the chapter authors have explored strategies to incorporate cultural and linguistic competence into the development and implementation of materials, programs, and learning opportunities that take into account the specific needs of different racial, ethnic, and cultural groups.

POINTS TO REMEMBER

- Health educators need to understand that cultural and linguistic competence are an integral part of the development, implementation, and evaluation of health education and promotion programs.

- Health educators need to promote cultural and linguistic competence in order to work effectively with the individuals or communities served by their organizations and to address these individuals' or communities' health needs.

- We already know a number of good strategies for incorporating cultural and linguistic competence into health education.

- It is time for our profession to develop standards that address cultural and linguistic competence in health education programs and in the preparation of health education professionals. This chapter offers an initial set of such standards.

KEY TERMS

Cultural competence	Health promotion
Health disparities	Linguistic competence
Health education	

REFERENCES

Airhihenbuwa, C. O. (1995). *Health and culture: Beyond the western paradigm*. Thousand Oaks, CA: Sage.

Airhihenbuwa, C. O. (2006). The inaugural SOPHE summit on eliminating racial and ethnic health disparities. *Health Promotion Practice, 3*, 293–295.

American Association for Health Education. (1994). *Cultural awareness and sensitivity: Guidelines for health educators*. Reston, VA: Author.

Brach, C., & Fraser, I. (2000). Can cultural competency reduce racial disparities? A review and conceptual model. *Medical Care Research and Review, 57*(Suppl. 1), 181–217. Retrieved November 5, 2007, from http://mcr .sagepub.com/cgi/content/abstract/57/suppl_1/181.

Campinha-Bacote, J. (1998). *The process of cultural competence in the delivery of healthcare services: A culturally competent model of care* (3rd ed.). Cincinnati, OH: Transcultural C.A.R.E. Associates.

Centers for Disease Control and Prevention. (2007). *REACHing across the divide: Finding solutions to health disparities*. Atlanta, GA: Author.

Centers for Disease Control and Prevention. (n.d.). *Racial and ethnic approaches to community health: REACH U.S.* Retrieved November 19, 2007, from http://www.cdc.gov/reach/index.htm.

Cohen, E., & Goode, T. D. (1999), revised by Goode, T. D., & Dunne, C. (2003). *Rationale for cultural competence in primary care* (Policy Brief 1). Washington, DC: National Center for Cultural Competence, Georgetown University Center for Child and Human Development.

Cross, T. L., Bazron, B. J., Dennis, K. W., & Isaacs, M. R. (1989). *Toward a culturally competent system of care: A monograph on effective services for minority children who are severely emotionally disturbed*. Washington, DC: Georgetown University Child Development Center, Child and Adolescent Service System Program.

Dana, R. H., Dayger Behn, J., & Gonwa, T. (1992). A checklist for the examination of cultural competence. *Research on Social Work Practice, 2*(2), 220–233.

Denboba, D. L., Bragdon, J. L., Epstein, L. G., Garthright, K., & Goldman, T. M. (1998). Reducing health disparities through cultural competence. *Journal of Health Education, 29*(5), S47–S53.

Diversity Rx. (2003, March 5). *Why is cultural competence important for health professionals?* Retrieved November 9, 2007, from http://www.diversityrx.org/HTML/MOCPT1.htm.

Goode, T., Jones, W., & Mason, J. (2002). *A guide to planning and implementing cultural competence organization self-assessment*. Washington, DC: National Center for Cultural Competence, Georgetown University Child Development Center. Retrieved November 17, 2007, from http://ww11.georgetown.edu/research/guc chd/nccc/documents/ncccorgselfassess.pdf.

Goode, T., & Sockalingam, S. (2000). Cultural competence: Developing policies to address the health care needs of culturally diverse clientele. *Home Health Care Management & Practice, 12*(5), 49–55.

Health Resources and Services Administration, HIV/AIDS Bureau. (2002). *HRSA Care ACTION: Mitigating health disparities through cultural competence*. Retrieved November 19, 2007, from http://hab.hrsa.gov/publications/august2002.htm.

Huff, R. M., & Kline, M. V. (1999). *The cultural assessment framework*. In R. M. Huff & M. V. Kline (Eds.), *Promoting health in multicultural populations: A handbook for practitioners* (pp. 481–499). Thousand Oaks, CA: Sage.

Institute of Medicine. (2004). *In the nation's compelling interest: Ensuring diversity in the health care workforce*. Retrieved October 10, 2007, from http://www.iom.edu/report.asp?id=18287.

King, M., Sims, A., & Osher, D. (n.d.). *How is cultural competence integrated in education?* Retrieved October 31, 2007, from http://cecp.air.org/cultural/Q_integrated.htm.

Luquis, R. R., & Pérez, M. A. (2003). Achieving cultural competence: The challenges for health educators. *Journal of Health Education, 34*(3), 131–138.

Luquis, R. R., & Pérez, M. A. (2005). Health educators and cultural competence: Implications for the profession. *American Journal of Health Studies, 20*(3/4), 156–163.

Luquis, R. R., & Pérez, M. A. (2006). Cultural competency among school health educators. *Journal of Cultural Diversity, 13*(4), 217–222.

Luquis, R. R., Pérez, M. A., & Young, K. (2006). Cultural competence development in health education professional preparation programs. *American Journal of Health Education, 37*(4), 233–241.

Marín, G., & Burhansstipanov, L., Connell, C. M., Gielen, A. C., Helitzer-Allen, D., Lorig, K., et al. (1994). A research agenda for health education among underserved populations. *Health Education & Behavior Quarterly, 22*(3), 346–364.

National Center for Cultural Competence. (2002). Developing cultural competence in health care settings. *Pediatric Nursing, 28*(2), 133–137.

National Center for Cultural Competence. (2006). *Conceptual frameworks/models, guiding values and principles*. Retrieved March 5, 2007, from http://www11.georgetown.edu/research/gucchd/nccc/foundations/frameworks.html.

National Commission for Health Education Credentialing, Society for Public Health Education, & American Association for Health Education. (2006). *A competency-based framework for health educators—2006*. Whitehall, PA: Author.

Office of Minority Health. (2000). *National standards on culturally and linguistically appropriate services (CLAS)*. Retrieved October 20, 2007, from http://www.omhrc.gov/templates/browse.aspx?lvl=2&lvlID=15.

Pérez, M. A., Gonzalez, A., & Pinzon-Pérez, H. (2006). Cultural competence in health care systems: A case study. *California Journal of Health Promotion, 4*(1), 102–108.

Purnell, L. D., & Paulanka, B. J. (2003). *Transcultural diversity and health care*. In L. D. Purnell & B. J. Paulanka (Eds.), *Transcultural health care: A culturally competent approach* (2nd ed., pp. 1–39). Philadelphia: Davis.

U.S. Census Bureau. (2004). *U.S. interim projections by age, sex, race, and Hispanic origin*. Retrieved November 19, 2007, from http://www.census.gov/ipc/www/usinterimproj.

U.S. Department of Health and Human Services. (2000). *Healthy people 2010: Understanding and improving health* (2nd ed.). Washington, DC: Government Printing Office.

U.S. Department of Health and Human Services. (2003). *Developing cultural competence in disaster mental health programs: Guiding principles and recommendations* (DHHS SMA 3828). Rockville, MD: U.S. Department of Health and Human Services, Substance Abuse and Mental Health Services Administration, Center for Mental Health Services.

APPENDIX

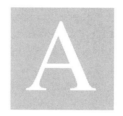

A POSITION STATEMENT OF THE AMERICAN ASSOCIATION FOR HEALTH EDUCATION, APRIL 2006

The American Association for Health Education advances the profession while serving health educators and others who strive to promote the health of all people.

CULTURAL COMPETENCY IN HEALTH EDUCATION

Position

The American Association for Health Education advocates that health educators must strive to achieve cultural competency by understanding the meaning of culture, its complexity within each group, and its effect on health decisions and practices. The preparation of culturally competent health educators needs to begin at all institutions offering undergraduate and graduate degree programs in health education; this preparation should include, but not be limited to, internships with schools and community based organizations working with diverse populations. In addition, health educators need to seek continuing professional development throughout their careers to enhance their understanding about terms such as race, culture, ethnicity, diversity, and the most recent research and practices related to cultural competency. Finally, health educators need to incorporate the concept of cultural competence into every aspect of the planning, implementation, and evaluation of health education and promotion programs.

Rationale

Health educators provide services, in a variety of settings, to a wide variety of individuals from diverse cultural and ethnic backgrounds. As the population becomes more racially, ethnically, and culturally diverse, cultural competency in health education and health promotion becomes fundamental. Given their prominent role in improving the health of the population, it is imperative that health educators possess culturally and linguistically appropriate skills that will enable them to interact effectively with various target populations, thereby increasing health literacy.[1]

The Joint Committee on Health Education and Promotion Terminology[2] defines the term *cultural competence* as: "The ability of an individual to understand and respect values, attitudes, beliefs, and mores that differ across cultures, and to consider and respond appropriately to these differences in planning, implementing, and evaluating health education and promotion programs and interventions." According to the Census Bureau (2000),[3] the U.S. population has reached its most diverse composition. In addition, population projections suggest that the number of White non-Hispanics will continue to decrease in the next few decades. This racial and ethnic diversification of the U.S. population further establishes the need to incorporate the concept of cultural competence into every aspect of health education and promotion programs, as well as into the training of the next generation of health educators. Moreover, culturally competent health interventions have been described as an approach to achieve the goals of Healthy People 2010.[4, 5] Finally, cultural competency is a natural evolution from the cultural awareness and sensitivity advocated by the American Association for Health Education in its book entitled *Cultural Awareness and Sensitivity: Guidelines for Health Educators.*[6]

The American Association for Health Education is an association of the American Alliance for Health, Physical Education, Recreation, and Dance: 1900 Association Drive, Reston, VA 20191; telephone: 703-476-3437; fax: 703-476-6638; e-mail: aahe@aahperd.org.

NOTES

1. Luquis, R., & Pérez, M. Achieving cultural competence: The challenges for health educators. *American Journal of Health Education.* 2003; 34(3): 131–138.

2. Report of the 2000 Joint Committee on Health Education and Promotion Terminology. *American Journal of Health Education.* March/April 2001; 32(2): 11.

3. U.S. Census Bureau. *United States Census 2000.* 2000. Available at: http://www
    .census.gov. Accessed January 24, 2005.

4. Denboba, D. L., Bragdon, J. L., Epstein, L. G., Garthright, K., & McCann Gold-
    man, T. Reducing health disparities through cultural competence. *American
    Journal of Health Education.* 1998; 29(5): S47-S53.

5. Cohen, E., & Goode, T. D; revised by Goode, T. D., & Dunne, C. Policy Brief 1:
    Rationale for Cultural Competence in Primary Care. 2003. Washington, DC:
    National Center for Cultural Competence, Georgetown University Center for
    Child and Human Development.

6. Cultural Awareness and Sensitivity: Guidelines for Health Educators. Association
    for the Advancement of Health Education (AAHE)/AAHPERD, 1994. Reston,
    VA 20191. www.aahperd.org/aahe

APPENDIX

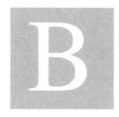

WEB RESOURCES FOR UNDERSTANDING HEALTH DISPARITIES

Agency for Health Care Research and Quality: National Health Disparities Report	http://www.ahrq.gov/qual/Nhdr05/nhdr05
California Department of Health Service: Multicultural Health Disparities	http://www.dhs.ca.gov/hisp/chs/OHIR/ Publications/OtherReports/MHD051703.pdf
Community Health and Elimination of Health Disparities	http://www.calendow.org/Category .aspx?id=308&ItemID=208
Community Health and Health Disparities	http://www.preventioninstitute.org/ healthdis.html
Eliminating Health Disparities	http://www.amsa.org/disparities
Eliminating Racial and Ethnic Health Disparities	http://www.cdc.gov/omhd/Topic/ HealthDisparities.html

Fogarty International Center	http://www.nih.gov/fic
Healthy People 2010	http://www.healthypeople.gov
Institute of Medicine	http://www.iom.edu
Kaiser Family Foundation: A Weekly Look at Health Care Disparities	http://www.kaisernetwork.org/dailyreports/repdisparities.cfm
National Association of School Psychologists	http://nasponline.org/resources/culturalcompetence/index.aspx
National Center for Complementary and Alternative Medicine	http://nccam.nih.gov
National Center for Cultural Competence	http://www11.georgetown.edu/research/gucchd/nccc
National Center for Research Resources	http://www.ncrr.nih.gov
National Institutes of Health Program of Action: Addressing Health Disparities	http://healthdisparities.nih.gov
National Library of Medicine	http://www.nlm.nih.gov
Office of AIDS Research	http://www.nih.gov/od/oar/index.htm
Office of Behavioral and Social Sciences Research	http://www1.od.nih.gov/obssr/obssr.htm
Office of Disease Prevention	http://odp.od.nih.gov
Office of Minority Health	http://www.omhrc.gov
Office of Research on Minority Health	http://www1.od.nih.gov/ORMH/main.html
Public Health Reports	http://www.publichealthreports.org/userfiles/117_5/117426.pdf

Substance Abuse and Mental Health Services Administration	http://samhsa.gov/about
U.S. Department of Health and Human Services, Office of Minority Health: Think Cultural	http://www.thinkculturalhealth.org
Warren Grant Magnuson Clinical Center	http://www.cc.nih.gov

APPENDIX

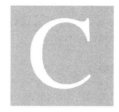

KNOWN HEALTH DISPARITIES AMONG RACIAL AND ETHNIC GROUPS

AFRICAN AMERICAN

Cancer

- In 2003, African American men were 1.4 times as likely to have new cases of lung and prostate cancer as non-Hispanic white men were.

- African American men were twice as likely to have new cases of stomach cancer as non-Hispanic white men were.

- African American men had lower five-year cancer survival rates for lung and pancreatic cancer than non-Hispanic white men did.

- In 2003, African American men were 2.4 times as likely to die from prostate cancer as non-Hispanic white men were.

- In 2003, African American women were 10 percent less likely to have been diagnosed with breast cancer; however, they were 36 percent more likely to die from breast cancer than non-Hispanic white women were.

- In 2003, African American women were 2.3 times as likely to have been diagnosed with stomach cancer, and they were 2.2 times as likely to die from stomach cancer as non-Hispanic white women were.

Diabetes

- African American adults were 2.1 times more likely than non-Hispanic white adults to have been diagnosed with diabetes by a physician.

- In 2002, African American men were 2.1 times as likely to start treatment for end-stage renal disease related to diabetes as non-Hispanic white men were.

- In 2003, African Americans with diabetes were 1.8 times as likely as whites with diabetes to be hospitalized.

- In 2003, African Americans were 2.1 times as likely as non-Hispanic whites to die from diabetes.

Heart Disease

- In 2003, African American men were 30 percent more likely to die from heart disease than non-Hispanic white men were.

- African Americans were 1.5 times as likely as non-Hispanic whites to have high blood pressure.

- African American women were 1.6 times as likely as non-Hispanic white women to be obese.

HIV/AIDS

- Although African Americans make up only 13 percent of the total U.S. population, they accounted for 50 percent of the HIV/AIDS cases in 2004.

- African American males had more than 8 times the AIDS rate of non-Hispanic white males.

- African American females had more than 22 times the AIDS rate of non-Hispanic white females.

- African American men were more than 9 times as likely to die from HIV/AIDS as non-Hispanic white men were.

- African American women were more than 21 times as likely to die from HIV/AIDS as non-Hispanic white women were.

Immunization

- In 2004, African Americans aged 65 and older were 30 percent less likely than non-Hispanic whites of the same age group to have received an influenza (flu) shot in the past 12 months.

- In 2005, African Americans aged 65 and older were 30 percent less likely than non-Hispanic whites of the same age group to have ever received the pneumonia shot.

- Although African American children aged 19 to 35 months had comparable rates of immunization for hepatitis, influenza, MMR (measles-mumps-rubella), and polio, they were slightly less likely to be fully immunized than were non-Hispanic white children.

Infant Mortality

- In 2003, African Americans had 2.4 times the infant mortality rate of non-Hispanic whites.

- African American infants were almost 4 times as likely to die from causes related to low birth weight as non-Hispanic white infants were.

- African Americans had 2.2 times the sudden infant death syndrome (SIDS) mortality rate of non-Hispanic whites.

- African American mothers were 2.6 times as likely as non-Hispanic white mothers to begin prenatal care in the third trimester or to not receive prenatal care at all.

Stroke

- African American adults were 30 percent more likely than their white adult counterparts to have a stroke.

- African American males were 50 percent more likely to die from a stroke than were their white adult counterparts.

- Analysis from a CDC health interview survey reveals that African American stroke survivors were more likely to become disabled and have difficulty with activities of daily living than were their non-Hispanic white counterparts.

AMERICAN INDIAN AND ALASKA NATIVE

Cancer

- In 2002, American Indian and Alaska Native men were 30 percent less likely to have prostate cancer than non-Hispanic white men were.

- In 2002, American Indian and Alaska Native women were 30 percent less likely to have breast cancer than non-Hispanic white women were.

- American Indian and Alaska Native men were twice as likely to be diagnosed with stomach and liver cancers as white men were.

- American Indian women were 20 percent more likely to die from cervical cancer than white women were.

Diabetes

- American Indian and Alaska Native adults were 2.3 times as likely as white adults to be diagnosed with diabetes.

- American Indian and Alaska Natives were twice as likely as non-Hispanic whites to die from diabetes in 2003.

- American Indian and Alaska Native adults were 1.6 times as likely as white adults to be obese.

- American Indian and Alaska Native adults were 1.3 times as likely as white adults to have high blood pressure.

Heart Disease

- American Indian and Alaska Native adults are 1.2 times as likely as white adults to have heart disease.

- American Indian and Alaska Native adults are 1.4 times as likely as white adults to be current cigarette smokers.

- American Indian and Alaska Native adults are 1.6 times as likely as white adults to be obese.

- American Indian and Alaska Native adults are 1.3 times as likely as white adults to have high blood pressure.

HIV/AIDS

- American Indian and Alaska Natives have a 40 percent higher AIDS rates than their non-Hispanic white counterparts do.

- American Indian and Alaska Native men have a 10 percent higher AIDS rate than non-Hispanic white men do.

- American Indian and Alaska Native women have 3 times the AIDS rate of non-Hispanic white women.

Immunization

- In 2004, American Indian and Alaska Native children aged 19 to 35 months received the recommended doses of vaccines for measles, mumps, rubella, Hib

(Haemophilus influenzae type b), polio, and chicken pox at the same rate as non-Hispanic white children.

▪ In 2004, American Indian and Alaska Native adults aged 18 to 64 years were slightly less likely than their non-Hispanic white counterparts to have received the influenza (flu) shot in the past 12 months.

Infant Mortality

▪ American Indians and Alaska Natives have 1.5 times the infant mortality rate of non-Hispanic whites.

▪ American Indian and Alaska Native babies are 2.2 times as likely as non-Hispanic white babies to die from sudden infant death syndrome (SIDS), and they are 1.4 times as likely to die from complications related to low birth weight or congenital malformations.

▪ American Indian and Alaska Native infants are 3.6 times as likely as non-Hispanic white infants to have mothers who began prenatal care in the third trimester or did not receive prenatal care at all.

Stroke

▪ In general, American Indian and Alaska Native adults are 60 percent more likely to have a stroke than their white adult counterparts are.

▪ American Indian and Alaska Native women have twice the rate of stroke that white women do.

▪ American Indian and Alaska Native adults are more likely to be obese than white adults are, and they are more likely to have high blood pressure.

ASIAN AMERICAN AND PACIFIC ISLANDER

Cancer

▪ In 2003, Asian and Pacific Islander men were 40 percent less likely to have prostate cancer than non-Hispanic white men were.

▪ In 2003, Asian and Pacific Islander women were 30 percent less likely to have breast cancer than non-Hispanic white women were.

▪ In 2003, Asian and Pacific Islander women were 1.2 times as likely to have cervical cancer as non-Hispanic white women were.

▪ Asian and Pacific Islander men and women have a higher incidence and mortality rates for stomach and liver cancer than non-Hispanic whites do.

Diabetes

■ In Hawaii, Native Hawaiians have more than twice the rate of diabetes of whites.

■ Asians are 20 percent less likely than non-Hispanic whites to die from diabetes.

■ In Hawaii, Native Hawaiians are more than 5.7 times as likely as whites living in Hawaii to die from diabetes.

■ Filipinos living in Hawaii have more than 3 times the death rate due to diabetes of whites living in Hawaii.

Heart Disease

■ Overall, Asian and Pacific Islander adults are less likely than non-Hispanic white adults to have heart disease, and they are also less likely to die from heart disease.

HIV/AIDS

■ Asians and Pacific Islanders have lower AIDS rates than their non-Hispanic white counterparts, and they are less likely to die of HIV/AIDS.

■ One Asian and Pacific Islander child was diagnosed with AIDS in 2004.

Immunization

■ In 2004, Asian and Pacific Islander adults aged 65 years and older were 40 percent less likely than non-Hispanic white adults of the same age group to have ever received the pneumonia shot.

■ In 2003, Asian and Pacific Islander children aged 19 to 35 months reached the Healthy People goal for immunizations for Hib (Haemophilus influenzae type b), hepatitis B, MMR (measles-mumps-rubella), polio, and chicken pox.

Infant Mortality

■ Among Asians and Pacific Islanders, sudden infant death syndrome (SIDS) is the third leading cause of infant mortality.

■ The infant mortality rate for Asians and Pacific Islanders was 2.8 times greater for mothers under 20 years old than it was for mothers aged 25 to 29.

Stroke

■ In general, Asian and Pacific Islander adults are less likely than non-Hispanic white adults to die from a stroke.

■ In general, Asian and Pacific Islander adults have lower rates of being overweight or obese and lower rates of hypertension than white adults do, and they are also less likely to be current cigarette smokers.

HISPANIC (OR LATINO)

Cancer

- In 2003, Hispanic men were 19 percent less likely to have prostate cancer than non-Hispanic white men were.

- In 2003, Hispanic women were 39 percent less likely to have breast cancer than non-Hispanic white women were.

- Hispanic men and women have higher incidence and mortality rates for stomach and liver cancer than non-Hispanic white men and women do.

- In 2003, Hispanic women were 2.2 times as likely as non-Hispanic white women to be diagnosed with cervical cancer.

Diabetes

- Mexican American adults were 2 times more likely than non-Hispanic white adults to have been diagnosed with diabetes by a physician.

- In 2002, Hispanic men were 1.5 times as likely as non-Hispanic white men to start treatment for end-stage renal disease related to diabetes.

- In 2003, Hispanics were 1.5 times as likely as non-Hispanic whites to die from diabetes.

Heart Disease

- In 2004, Hispanics were 10 percent less likely to have heart disease than non-Hispanic whites were.

- In 2003, Mexican American men were 30 percent less likely to die from heart disease than non-Hispanic white men were.

- Mexican American women were 1.2 times more likely than non-Hispanic white women to be obese.

HIV/AIDS

- Hispanics accounted for 18 percent of HIV/AIDS cases in 2004.

- Hispanic males had over 3 times the AIDS rate of non-Hispanic white males.

- Hispanic females had over 5 times the AIDS rate of non-Hispanic white females.

- Hispanic men were 2.7 times as likely to die from HIV/AIDS as non-Hispanic white men were.

- Hispanic women were 4.5 times as likely to die from HIV/AIDS as non-Hispanic white women were.

Immunization

- In 2004, Hispanic adults aged 65 and older were 20 percent less likely than non-Hispanic whites of the same age group to have received the influenza (flu) shot in the past 12 months.

- In 2004, Hispanic adults aged 65 and older were 40 percent less likely than non-Hispanic whites of the same age group to have ever received the pneumonia shot.

- Although Hispanic children aged 19 to 35 months had comparable rates of immunization for hepatitis, influenza, MMR (measles-mumps-rubella), and polio, they were slightly less likely to be fully immunized than non-Hispanic white children were.

Infant Mortality

- In 2003, infant mortality rates for Hispanic subpopulations ranged from 4.6 per 1,000 live births to 8.2 per 1,000 live births, compared to the non-Hispanic white infant mortality rate of 5.7 per 1,000 live births.

- In 2003, Puerto Ricans had 1.4 times the infant mortality rate of non-Hispanic whites.

- Puerto Rican infants were 2.1 times as likely as non-Hispanic white infants to die from causes related to low birth weight.

- Mexican American mothers were 2.5 times as likely as non-Hispanic white mothers to begin prenatal care in the third trimester or to not receive prenatal care at all.

Stroke

- In 2003, Hispanic men were 20 percent less likely to die from a stroke than non-Hispanic white men were.

- In 2003, Hispanic women were 30 percent less likely to die from a stroke than non-Hispanic white women were.

Source: Adapted from Office of Minority Health (2007). *Minority population profile.* Retrieved September 17, 2007, from http://www.omhrc.gov/templates/browse.aspx ?lvl=1&lvlID=5.

APPENDIX

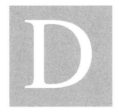

WEB RESOURCES FOR WORKING WITH THE ELDERLY

Administration on Aging (AOA)	http://www.aoa.gov
Agency for Healthcare Research and Quality resource	www.guidelines.gov
American Society on Aging (ASA)	http://www.asaging.org
Center on Aging, Health & Humanities	http://www.gwumc.edu/cahh
Centers for Elders and Youth in the Arts	http://www.ioaging.org/programs/art/ceya.html
Core Curriculum in Ethnogeriatrics Modules (Collaborative on Ethnographic Education)	http://www.stanford.edu/group/ethnoger/ebooks/intro.pdf
Elders Share the Arts (ESTA)	http://www.elderssharethearts.org
Generations United	http://www.gu.org

Gerontological Society of America (GSA)	http://www.geron.org
International Council on Active Aging	http://www.icaa.cc
National Center for Creative Aging	http://www.creativeaging.org
National Center for Health Statistics	http://www.cdc.gov/nchs
National Center for Research Resources	http://www.ncrr.nia.gov
National Council on Aging (NCOA)	http://www.ncoa.org
National Endowment for the Arts (NEA)	http://www.nea.gov
National Institute on Aging	http://www.nia.hih.gov
National Institutes of Health	http://www.nih.gov
Society for Arts in Healthcare	http://www.the.SAH.org

AUTHOR INDEX

SUBJECT INDEX

269

Polk State College
Lakeland Library

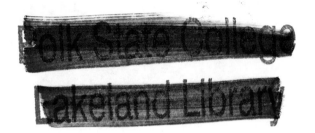

Polk State College
Lakeland Library